MENTAL HEALTH AWARENESS

PRACTICAL SKILLS FOR FIRST RESPONDERS

Marc Laferriere
Stephanie Miloknay

emond ▪ Toronto, Canada ▪ 2018

Emond Montgomery Publications Limited
60 Shaftesbury Avenue
Toronto ON M4T 1A3
http://www.emond.ca/highered

Printed in Canada.
Reprinted November 2020.

We acknowledge the financial support of the Government of Canada. Canadä

Vice president, publishing: Anthony Rezek
Publisher: Lindsay Sutherland
Director, development and production: Kelly Dickson
Developmental editor: Daphne Scriabin
Production supervisor: Laura Bast
Copy editor: Cindy Fujimoto
Typesetter and text designer: Janette Thompson
Permissions editor: Lisa Brant
Proofreader: Gillian Scobie
Indexer: Andrew Little
Cover image: BABAROGA/Shutterstock

Library and Archives Canada Cataloguing in Publication
Laferriere, Marc, author
Mental health awareness : practical skills for first responders / Marc Laferriere, Stephanie Miloknay.

Includes index.
ISBN 978-1-77255-255-3 (softcover)

1. Mental health—Study and teaching. 2. First responders—Training of.
I. Miloknay, Stephanie, author II. Title.

RA790.8.L34 2018 616.890071 C2017-906751-6

For my wife, Bekah, who teaches me daily
that love really does conquer all. Thank you for building
this life together and for all of your love and support.
You're the greatest thing there is.

—Marc Laferriere

I would like to dedicate this work to every mentor,
co-worker, peer, and victim that I have had the privilege of
knowing that helped shape my experiences as a first responder.
Through both the good and the bad, I learned. Thank you to
Emond Publishing for supporting this important topic.

—Stephanie Miloknay

BRIEF TABLE OF CONTENTS

DETAILED TABLE OF CONTENTS

PREFACE

There are hundreds of books about counselling and mental health aimed squarely at psychiatrists, psychologists, and social workers. It is wonderful and they are needed.

This book was created because it is also needed. It is needed to help justice and helping professionals, front-line workers, and the students hoping to join their ranks. These professionals work with individuals living with mental health issues and also have to contend with unique mental health challenges within their industries. Experts, persons with lived experience, and educators in Canada have lamented for quite some time this obvious gap in the teaching literature.

Trainers and educators have taken texts made for other professions and tried to make them fit their needs, but this has never been ideal. We have heard again and again from educators, professionals, and students that they are tired of trying to make material that was not written for them fit in the absence of something better.

Law enforcement officers, firefighters, paramedics, military personnel, correctional officers, search and rescue workers, nurses, residential workers, victim services, dispatchers, and other front-line professionals will benefit from this text, which looks at mental health issues through a lens designed specifically for the valuable work they do.

And it is valuable work being done by these resilient professionals. They deserve a text written specifically for them by authors who have worked on the front lines and gone on to become mental health professionals and educators.

The text is divided into four parts:

PART 1 (Chapters 1–3)

Part 1 of the text is an overview of the history of mental health and how it has intersected with the Canadian justice system. Following **Case Study 1, Chapter 1** delves into a real-world scenario of how stigma experienced by previous generations can affect individuals to this day. **Chapter 2** looks at the modern history of mental health and justice and how individuals move through and between justice and mental health systems. **Chapter 3** has been written to help readers recognize multidisciplinary partnerships that have been created to help police in their role as first responders to incidents involving people with mental health issues.

PART 2 (Chapters 4–7)

Part 2 addresses the most common mental health issues first responders and others will come across in their work as justice and helping professionals. **Case Study 2** asks readers to compare different attributes and supports that may drastically change outcomes for persons living with mental health issues. **Chapter 4** looks at depression and anxiety disorders and helps the reader to move away from common misunderstandings of these mental health diagnoses. **Chapter 5** focuses on a variety of addictions and related mental health issues persons may struggle with. **Chapter 6** examines personality disorders and schizophrenia—less common but very serious mental health conditions—while **Chapter 7** discusses suicide and how to intervene and recognize signs that someone may be contemplating taking their own life.

PART 3 (Chapters 8–10)

Part 3 examines specific techniques for first responders and other related professionals who intervene with a multitude of persons in crisis. **Case Study 3** explores how peculiar behaviour can spiral if left untreated or if it becomes compounded by other factors. **Chapter 8** helps the reader classify various services that are available for persons living with mental illness and what role these services can play in treatment. **Chapter 9** takes the reader through critical analysis of issues such as stigma, barriers to mental health treatment, and the ethics of working with mentally ill individuals despite differences between first responders and other professionals who may be required to work on the same case(s). **Chapter 10** is focused on working with victims and identifying strategies and resources to help meet their unique needs.

PART 4 (Chapters 11–12)

The final portion of the text begins with **Case Study 4**, which investigates how organizations might respond to increasing difficulties in retention in the justice and helping professions due to the personal toll this kind of work can take on individuals. **Chapter 11** reviews a variety of controversial topics related to the vocations this book is meant to serve. **Chapter 12** explores numerous ways Canadian organizations have responded to tragedies that may have been avoided while also exploring gaps in current responses to mental health crises. This chapter also analyses how resiliency in individuals and organizations helps workers deal with stressors and challenges to providing service to their communities.

This book offers a Canadian perspective on the challenges first response workers and related professionals face in identifying and interacting with individuals living with mental health issues. It takes a look at the history of mental health interventions to provide a context for how we got here and addresses the emerging trends in the justice and helping professions related to mental health.

This book also explores controversial issues related to how we address mental health as individual professionals and as organizations. Throughout the text, and specifically in the **"Voices from the Field"** sections, a number of real-life scenarios from a variety of professional perspectives are explored to help readers go beyond the theoretical and become more self-reflective.

We wrote this book because we wished it had been around before and during our time as front-line justice and helping professionals. As educators, we are so glad to have it published and to be able to utilize it to help new generations of front-line workers and those wishing to enter the related professions. You make our communities better and we want to support you in that valuable work.

Acknowledgments

The authors would like to thank Lindsay Sutherland and the entire team at Emond for their enthusiasm and encouragement throughout this process. From our first meeting, we knew we had a great partner to work with. Thanks as well to Daphne Scriabin for keeping our eyes on the prize and our noses to the grindstone with a deft touch that allowed us to learn so much about the process of writing; Cindy Fujimoto for her excellent insights and suggestions, which improved the book in numerous and substantial ways; Gillian Scobie, for her keen eye as a proofreader; Sean Thomson for his help as a research assistant for several of the chapters; our families and friends for their unrelenting support (and coffee!); all our former front-line co-workers for your friendship and solidarity during shifts both difficult and delightful; and to our colleagues and students at Mohawk College—you are amazing partners in teaching and learning.

The authors and Emond would also like to thank: Catherine Marion, Sheridan College; Julie Muravsky, Humber College; Ralph Ashford, Fleming College; and Derek Davies, St Lawrence College for reviewing the manuscript.

ABOUT THE AUTHORS

Marc Laferriere is a professor in the Department of Social Services and Justice Studies and a former coordinator of the Community Justice Services program at Mohawk College.

He is an award-winning educator and has been featured on a variety of television and print publications discussing issues of mental health, systems change, and community development. He is the recipient of the YMCA Peace Medallion for his efforts in social work, child and youth work, and community advocacy.

Marc has worked on the front lines of the mental health field in a variety of capacities with organizations such as Pioneer Youth Services, Avalon Children's Residences, and Moncton Youth Residences. He was also a clinical social worker for Woodview Mental Health and Autism Services and the Grand River Community Health Centre and was the BSW Practicum Coordinator for Wilfrid Laurier University.

Marc holds a Bachelor of Arts from the University of Ottawa, as well as an Honours Bachelor of Social Work and a Masters in Social Work from Lakehead University. Recently he has completed the Leadership, Organizing and Action: Leading Change program at Harvard University's Kennedy School.

Stephanie Miloknay is a professor and the coordinator of the Police Foundations program at Mohawk College. She retired holding the rank of sergeant after serving 24 years with the Halton Regional Police Service. During her career, she obtained extensive experience in the areas of front-line enforcement, crisis intervention, investigations, and policy development.

Stephanie held a secondment at the Ministry of Community Safety and Correctional Service supporting the Policing Standards Section by providing general operational expertise and advice in relation to current policing issues. She has been a member of the Hostage/Crisis Negotiator team, receiving certification through the Canadian Police College; was trained in Critical Incident Stress Management; and was a team leader with the Halton Regional Police Service's Peer Support Team.

She received her Bachelor of Science degree in psychology from the University of Toronto and her Masters degree in social work from McMaster University. Stephanie is also certified in Cognitive Behavioural Therapy and operated a private practice providing therapeutic support to clients with mood disorders such as depression and anxiety.

INTRODUCTION

Who should read this book? This book is for first responders—all law enforcement officers, firefighters, paramedics, correctional staff, search and rescue personnel, dispatchers, nurses, and other front-line and helping professionals. This book will also be beneficial to family members, friends, supervisors, managers, and commanders who seek to gain a better understanding of how they can support those who are exposed to traumatic and cumulative stress. Clergy and other mental health professionals may also find this book helpful as they deliver support to first responders.

PART 1

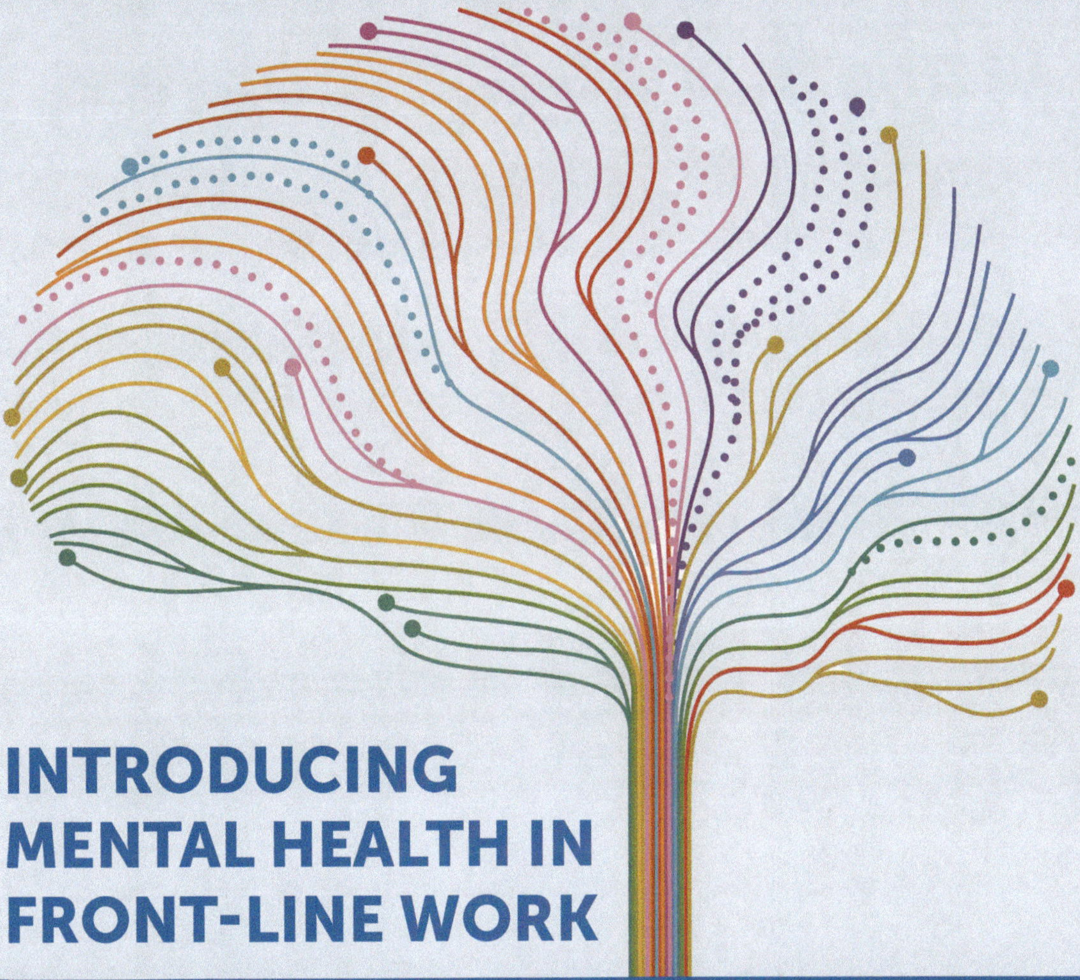

INTRODUCING MENTAL HEALTH IN FRONT-LINE WORK

CASE STUDY 1

Dustin is a 38-year-old male living in Winnipeg, Manitoba. He is a person living with schizophrenia, which was diagnosed when he was 24 years old. He often feels that this part of his life is misunderstood.

First, his diagnosis is not the biggest part of his life—he has only had two **psychotic breaks** since his diagnosis. Second, when people find out that he is a person living with this mental health issue, they tend to believe it is a multiple personality disorder. This is a common misconception popularized by the media and it is difficult to shake.

psychotic break
symptoms can vary from minor delusions to serious depression and violent outbursts in reaction to hallucinations that cause the sufferer to lose a connection with reality; mostly associated with psychosis or drug-induced psychosis

Dustin's mental health is fairly stable because of the medication he takes and he is involved in some regular counselling and self-care. Dustin grew up in a family with a multitude of mental health issues. His fraternal grandmother was institutionalized for mental health issues and he heard horrible stories about that process during his childhood. In fact, because of how he felt about the treatment his grandmother received, he did not seek help for his own growing mental health issues until he was well into his twenties and away from his parents.

The stigma surrounding mental health that Dustin felt from his peers while growing up was enough to make him want to keep his issues to himself. In addition to that, his family held on to the stigma attached to various mental health systems, and his fear of being locked up and abused in the same way his grandmother was kept him from seeking help.

Dustin did not accept help until he had a mental health issue at college that resulted in the police coming to his dorm. He spent two weeks at the St. Boniface Hospital in Winnipeg, and has seen a variety of medical and mental health professionals since then.

After discharge from the hospital, he attended an outpatient program for six weeks, which he went to nearly every day, and then he found a variety of peer support programs and group counselling programs. He saw a counsellor for a while, too.

Dustin's diagnosis does not define him, but despite that, his mental health issue has affected his life. He graduated a year later than the others in his class because of the timing of his hospitalization and after-treatment. Dustin found it difficult to get close to people for a while after he was hospitalized because after he disclosed his illness to two friends and an intimate partner, they did not take that news very well. He also started to feel less close to one of his aunts, who rarely talks to him anymore since his diagnosis.

However, he did become closer with his parents, who drove to Winnipeg from their home in Sudbury to help him after his hospitalization, and he later met and married someone who has been very supportive of his journey in life. When he had another psychotic episode in his late twenties he lost his job and had to downsize to a more affordable apartment, but Dustin and his spouse have rebounded financially since then.

DISCUSSION QUESTIONS

1. What are some of the ways that mental health has affected Dustin's life?
2. Have the historical issues that stigmatize mental health affected Dustin?
3. What are some of the strengths and positive assets Dustin has used to move forward after his diagnosis?

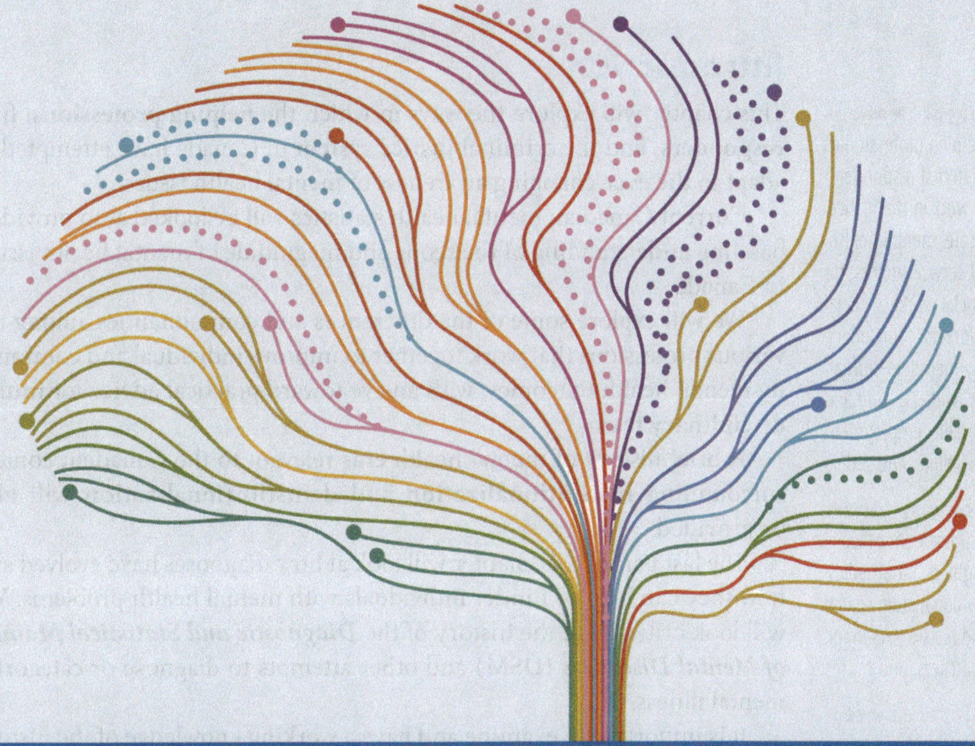

1 JUSTICE AND INJUSTICE
A Brief History of Mental Health and Justice in Canada

LEARNING OUTCOMES

After reading this chapter, you will be able to:

- Understand and use a variety of terms from the various helping professions.
- Discuss how mental health was perceived in Canadian history.
- Recognize distinct eras of mental health response in North America and identify the challenges and improvements made in each era.
- Discuss the process of adaptation that has occurred in response to mental health in the justice system and society.
- Understand the usefulness and controversies surrounding the *Diagnostic and Statistical Manual of Mental Disorders*.
- Critically assess the pros and cons of a mental health diagnosis.
- Critically assess the efficacy of historical anti-stigma efforts.
- Identify improvements and challenges that have occurred in the response of the Canadian justice system to mental health issues.

Introduction

helping professions all helping professionals (other than first responders) who work in the justice, health care, mental health, or social service sectors; for example, social workers, social service workers, counsellors, clergy members, human services workers, child and youth workers, employment counsellors, and others

first responders all law enforcement officers, firefighters, paramedics, correctional staff, search and rescue personnel, dispatchers, and nurses

justice system all professions related to the administration of the law and the criminal justice system, including police, attorneys, paralegals, court workers, probation officers, and so on

multidisciplinary team an approach in which professionals from a variety of professions work together with an individual on a topic or a specific set of problems

institutionalization the practice of confining individuals or groups of people in residential institutions such as asylums, prisons, and mental health hospitals

This chapter will explore the ways in which the **helping professions**, **first responders**, and the criminal **justice system** in Canada have attempted to adapt to the ever-changing awareness of mental health issues.

Current Canadian mental health statistics will be looked at to provide a baseline understanding of the scope and magnitude of mental health issues in Canada.

We will explore some of the differences and commonalities among the various professions that work together to improve individual and community mental health outcomes, with an eye toward practical advice for **multidisciplinary teams**.

A brief history of mental health eras relevant to the Canadian context surrounding **institutionalization** and **deinstitutionalization** will also be provided.

The last part of this chapter will look at how diagnoses have evolved and how they can help or hinder individuals with mental health problems. We will look critically at the history of the ***Diagnostic and Statistical Manual of Mental Disorders*** **(DSM)** and other attempts to diagnose or categorize mental illness.

It is important to examine and have a working knowledge of the history of societal responses to mental health problems in order to develop an understanding of and a context for how to respond to current mental health issues.

The material in Chapter 1 will lead us into the next two chapters, where we will explore more current developments in the helping professions.

Today's Approach

> Canada's inattention to the promotion of mental health and its tendency to devalue and segregate (either physically or socially or both) those who experience mental illness has deep historical roots.
>
> —Archibald Kaiser (2008)

Our approach to mental health today in our social services, courts, and public systems, including first responders and the justice system, is built on a history of prejudice, misunderstanding, and ignorance about mental health and how it affects individuals, families, and communities.

At the same time, these systems have taken steps to evolve and adapt to the challenges of treating those living with mental illness, both fairly under the law and effectively in the health care system. Society's understanding of these issues has grown, and yet many of the positions taken by the justice, health care, and helping professions have, for better or for worse, generated great interest from the general public.

There is a fascination with mental health issues in our policies, in our pop culture, and in our news media. Stories about those who live with mental health issues have permeated our consciousness. We've all seen representations of mental illness as the motivator for the villain in a horror movie or read the extreme stories of violence perpetrated by a few people living with mental health problems.

What we don't see as often—although improvements are being made—are the stories of the vast majority of those living with mental health issues who cope and strive daily to do well.

Taking a look at statistics will help give us a better sense of the scope of mental health issues in Canada than looking at select media reports or pop culture portrayals. According to Statistics Canada, in 2012, 10.1 percent of the population over the age of 15 (2.8 million Canadians) had "symptoms consistent with at least one of the following mental or substance-use disorders: major depressive episode, bipolar disorder, generalized anxiety disorder, and abuse of or dependence on alcohol, cannabis or other drugs" (Pearson, Janz, & Ali, 2013).

The same report looked at lifetime rates for mood disorders or substance-use disorders. It found that 3.5 million Canadians met the criteria for living with a mood disorder in their lifetime, while nearly 6 million Canadians met the criteria for substance-use disorders in their lifetime (Pearson et al., 2013).

deinstitutionalization
societal push to move away from confining people living with mental health issues in institutions and instead offering treatment in community settings

***Diagnostic and Statistical Manual of Mental Disorders* (DSM)**
the standard North American text for classifying and diagnosing mental disorders

DISCUSSION QUESTIONS

1. Can you list three negative portrayals of a person living with mental health issues that you have seen in a book, movie, or television show? Can you list five positive examples?
2. Try to find three positive examples of real-life stories of people living with mental health issues. Can you find three negative or tragic examples?
3. What effects might decades of negative media portrayals of people who live with mental health issues have on our perceptions of mental health?

This means that in 2012 (the most recent census data available on the subject), one in three Canadians (9.1 million people) met the criteria to have one of six mental health or substance-use disorders in their lifetime. See Table 1.1 for a more detailed breakdown of this information (Pearson et al., 2013).

TABLE 1.1 Rates of selected mental or substance use disorders, lifetime and 12-month, Canada, household population 15 years of age and older, 2012

	LIFETIME	12-MONTH
	%	
Mental or substance use disorders[1]	**33.1**	**10.1**
Substance use disorder[2]	21.6	4.4
Alcohol abuse or dependence	18.1	3.2
Cannabis abuse or dependence	6.8	1.3
Other drug abuse or dependence (excluding cannabis)	4.0	0.7
Mood disorder[3]	12.6	5.4
Major depressive episode	11.3	4.7
Bipolar disorder	2.6	1.5
Generalized anxiety disorder	8.7	2.6

NOTES

1. **Mental or substance use disorders** comprise substance use disorders, mood disorders, and generalized anxiety disorder. However, these three disorders cannot be added to create this rate because these three categories are not mutually exclusive, that is, people may have a profile consistent with one or more of these disorders.
2. **Substance use disorder** includes alcohol abuse or dependence, cannabis abuse or dependence, and other drug abuse or dependence.
3. **Mood disorder** includes depression (major depressive episode) and bipolar disorder.

Source: Statistics Canada, 2012.

DISCUSSION QUESTIONS

1. What might the overall rate be if all mental health and substance abuse disorders were accounted for?
2. Would that number be substantial enough to help change the commonly held belief that mental health issues affect only a small number of Canadians?
3. When someone is living with a mental health issue, who else might be affected by it?

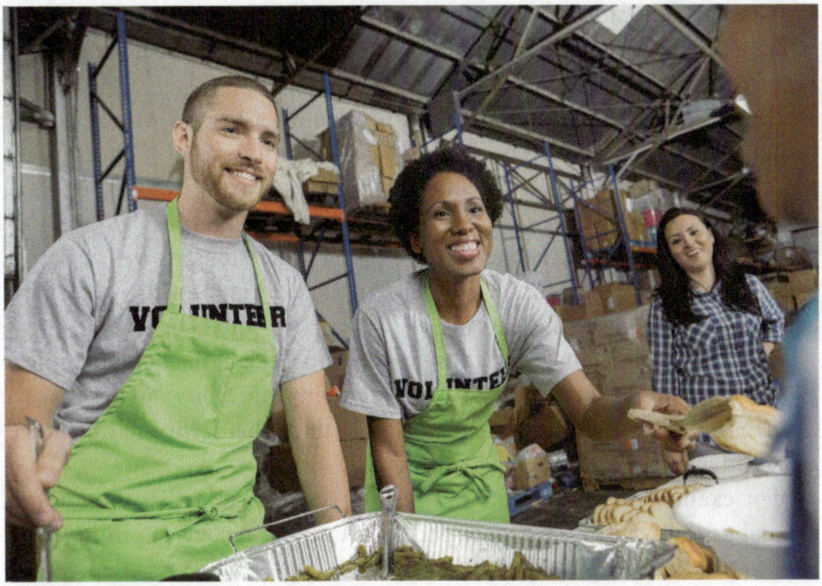

The helping professions include many jobs that assist those in need, including jobs that work directly with issues of poverty and food security.

What's in a Name?

The term "helping professions" is used often in this book. This term is used broadly to include any service provider, other than a first responder, who intervenes to help an individual, family, or community experiencing a mental health issue.

A "helping profession" could be that of child and youth worker, victim services worker, social worker, social service worker, counsellor, parole officer, early childhood educator, court worker, or peer support worker, as well as many other positions in the justice, health care, mental health, and social service sectors. Because these professions involve interacting with people who regularly experience mental health difficulties, this book will be of benefit to all of them.

We see in practice that many helping professionals and first responders work together on multidisciplinary teams for the benefit of individuals and communities when it comes to mental health. It is not unusual for a police officer to work with a mental health professional in the field or for a social worker at a child welfare agency to work hand in hand with an early childhood educator and a counsellor to address different aspects of an individual's mental health issue.

These collaborations across the helping professions can help to address difficult and layered issues in an individual's life and are the reality of work in the helping professions.

There are a variety of terms used to identify a person with a mental health issue. Some helping professions use the term patient. Others might use client, service user, person in recovery, person with lived experience, participant, consumer, or survivor, among many other terms.

Terminology often changes in the helping professions, as well as across other professions. In this book—just like in the working world—you will be exposed to a variety of these terms.

Working professionals and those wishing to work in the helping professions should understand the terms used in their professions and use that set of terms, while at the same time being aware that other terms may be heard and used when collaborating with others.

For example, a police officer may report to the press that there was a "sexual assault victim" at a local park, who is now recovering in hospital. The hospital staff might call that same person a "patient." When that person is discharged and sees a psychotherapist for assessment, the term "client" would likely be used. After an assessment, the person will be referred to a sexual assault centre for trauma counselling, where the term "survivor" is used. This person may attend group therapy, where the term "participant" is used. Years later, if the person joins an advocacy organization that focuses on improving the lives of those who have been sexually assaulted and sits on their board of directors, the term "person with lived experience" is applied; in this context, the person shows those who are helped by, donate to, or volunteer with the organization that someone with a personal history with these issues is helping to make decisions for the organization.

Now that person has had six identifiers applied to him or her. This might be seen as confusing; however, it's not unusual for those who are navigating through the helping professions. There are many debates about identifiers. Is "patient" too passive? Is "consumer" too commercial? Is "victim" disempowering? Is "client" too general?

The reality is that the conversation about this is still evolving and likely will be for some time. Furthermore, multiple professions all bring their own jargon, context, and history to the helping professions, which makes the use of universal identifiers unlikely. If an individual has a particular preference regarding how they identify, it should be used. No matter the phraseology, the importance of working with the individual to better engage with that person is paramount.

How Has Mental Health Been Treated Historically?

While we have certainly come a long way from superstitious beliefs about mental illness, Western culture has had a variety of reactions to mental health issues. Some changes have been positive, resulting in an increase in understanding of, supports for, and dialogue around a variety of disorders.

It could be said that we have come a long way because we started in such a deficit position when it comes to understanding mental health. As recently as the 18th century, a brutal surgical procedure known as trepanning, in which a hole was bored into a patient's head and bone was removed, was used to treat mental health issues such as mania or depression (Gross, 2009, p. 122). It was thought that this procedure could cure madness by letting fumes and vapours out (p. 16).

Within our modern history, Canadians living with mental health issues were often forced into segregation from society and placed in asylums and institutions (Braslow, 1994; Panksepp, 2004). Poor conditions and abuse were common, although the initial intent of the asylum movement was for more progressive, compassionate, and effective treatment of persons living with mental health issues (Sussman, 1998).

Dorothea Dix is credited with popularizing the asylum movement (Gollaher, 1993; Panksepp, 2004). She saw that the mentally ill were wrongly being sent to prisons and almshouses and thought that public care in institutions, hospitals, and asylums would be more effective and more decent than what she observed in workhouses, prisons, almshouses, and even private homes (Gollaher, 1993). Almshouses were homes or communities built by charitable individuals or organizations to house the poor and others who could no longer work.

While addressing the Massachusetts legislature, Dix gave a well-researched and impassioned report on the things she saw happening to people living with mental illness, which included seeing people held "in cages, closets, cellars, stalls, pens! Chained, naked, beaten with rods, and lashed into obedience" (Dix, 2006).

Dix's idea was to treat these sufferers in humane hospitals with more compassionate care as a moral alternative to the horrendous abuses she had witnessed (Ianacone, 1976). She toured North America and Europe speaking to the need to find compassionate alternatives to treating and housing those with mental illnesses, and the idea took root in Western culture (Greenstone, 1979).

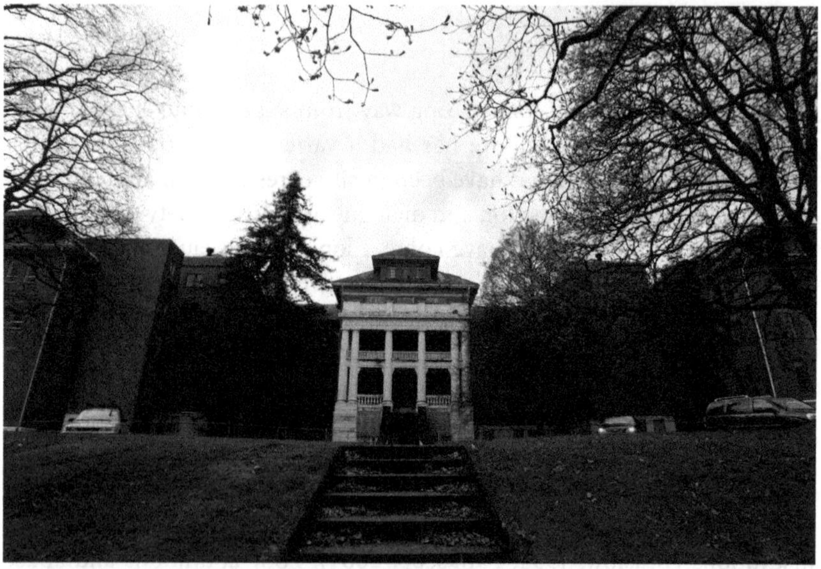

Institutions for mental health were at one time called insane asylums and were viewed by society as places to avoid, which led many people living with mental health problems not to seek help for fear of being institutionalized.

Psychiatric asylums were created as places where those living with mental health "could rest and receive personal care intended to restore their health," and there was hope that this would curb the "demonization and imprisonment" that many who suffered from mental illness had faced (Government of Canada, 2006).

From 1845 to 1914, asylums were opened in Canada, with the first of these institutions opening in Quebec (Sussman, 1998). That first institution was called Beauport, but was also known as the Quebec Lunatic Asylum. In 1855 it was estimated that 2,802 "lunatics" were "present within the borders of Canada" (Insane in Canada, 1855, p. 328). The Toronto Asylum, which was built for 250 patients, was reportedly treating 400 individuals at that time, while Beauport was beyond its 150-patient limit. As an editorialist for *The Medical Chronicle* wrote in 1855, "The country wants these Institutions for the Insane—a common humanity demands them; and the country, for the sake of unfortunate humanity, must have them" (p. 329).

Canadians saw the creation of the asylum system in Canada in the latter part of the 19th century as an approach to serving those with mental health needs that was humanitarian and would help to remove them from poor houses and prisons (Government of Canada, 2006).

While the theoretical reasoning behind this approach appeared sound and supportive, in fact these asylums were too large, lacked individual attention and effectiveness for patients, and ultimately served to "remove those with mental illness from the public sphere" (Government of Canada, 2006). The institutions commonly became overcrowded and treatment standards began to slip (Greenland, Griffin, & Hoffman, 2001). While an exact number of all asylum patients in Canada during the asylum era is difficult to come by because of the lacklustre recordkeeping across many institutions, some statistics exist to help shed light on the impact of asylums. From 1883 to 1937, the Toronto Hospital for the Insane reported 15,365 admissions, with 700 to 1,200 patients in the institution at any given time (Reaume 1997, pp. 67–68).

Generally, people feared medical institutionalization in asylums in Canada "because of their unsanitary conditions and the fact that few people left them healed." These facilities "were seen as places where the most unfortunate went to die and thus were avoided by all except the very poor" (Miron, 2006, p. 23). Asylum physicians (also known as alienists) used drugs as "chemical restraints, not much better and sometimes worse than physical restraints, the straitjackets and muffs that were also regarded as necessary evils" (Braslow, 1999).

In the asylum era, patients were subjected to all sorts of indignities in the name of safety, control, and therapy. Commonplace therapies included being wrapped in warm or cold sheets and tied to a bed, being given continuous baths that could last hours or days, having electroconvulsive treatment (which is still used in a modified form today), sterilization, fever therapy (where patients were injected with a form of benign malaria), and lobotomies (Braslow, 1999). In the 1850s, a variety of scandals plagued the Canadian asylum system, from accusations of staff impregnating patients to reports that the bodies of the dead were being used inappropriately by medical professionals (Miron, 2006, p. 23). Many asylum inmates reported sexual and physical

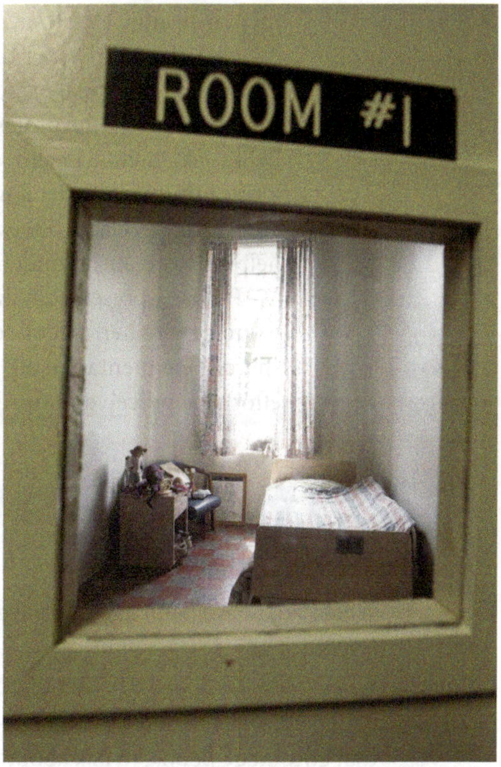

An example of a room in a mental health institution where, for the patient's safety, staff can supervise the patient's actions.

abuse by other inmates and staff. These accusations were often met with "denial or silence" by asylum officials (Reaume, 1997).

Furthermore, asylum tourism was a popular activity in Canada (Miron, 2006, p. 19). This was a practice where members of the public were invited to tour asylums and mental institutions. These tours were not limited to professionals looking to enhance their knowledge of best practices. It is estimated that in Canada alone, tens of thousands of casual observers participated in this type of tourism (p. 19). In 1877, during a fall fair, the London Asylum reported 1,700 tourists on their grounds in only three days (p. 68).

Initially only a small group of professionals and experts associated with asylums in the 19th century wanted to see the practice of casual tourism end. Many experts of the day saw the practice as "progressive, advantageous, beneficial and even necessary" (p. 134).

At the time, those working in asylums argued that giving the public access to the grounds to view the patients helped to raise awareness about mental health. However, it could also be argued that the practice treated patients like oddities for the entertainment of others (pp. 23, 28). It remains a colourful historical example of the extreme choices that those working on the front lines in the profession had to make with regard to people who were living with mental health issues. Should we isolate individuals or is exposure a good thing for societal understanding? What is the right balance between access and privacy? Does access like this remove **social stigma**? Are we helping to create an understanding or are we exploiting the pain of others?

social stigma the association of shame, negativity, public disapproval, disgrace, and/or poor character unfairly associated with people who have a particular characteristic, such as those living with a mental health disorder

Perhaps present-day helping professionals will one day look back and wonder whether recent social media campaigns that encourage others to share their mental health issues were constructive and helpful. Will these efforts be perceived positively or negatively in the future?

DISCUSSION QUESTIONS

1. What might have been some positive outcomes of having casual tourists visit insane asylums?
2. What might have been detrimental about having casual tourists visit insane asylums?
3. What are some of the positive outcomes of mass media and social media campaigns that encourage people to talk about their mental health issues in public forums?
4. What are some of the potential negative consequences of mass media and social media campaigns for those living with mental illness?

The Deinstitutionalization Era

Starting in the mid-1950s, pharmaceutical medications were beginning to be seen as more effective in treating mental illness than they had been in previous generations. In the United States in 1955 over half a million Americans were patients in the public mental health hospitals of the day. This number began to decline shortly thereafter, and most credit this to the introduction of chlorpromazine, also known as Thorazine, and other **antipsychotic**, **antidepressant**, and **antianxiety medications** (Whitaker, 2005, p. 23). Canada saw a similar patient population trend, with total mental hospital patients reaching a high of 59,308 in 1960 but dropping over 40 percent by 1971 to 34,183 (Kedward, Eastwood, Allodi, & Duckworth,1974).

While these pharmacological therapies may have been seen at the time as a suitable replacement for asylum care, they "did not fundamentally replace the need for care and attention" (Dyck, 2011). Other dimensions of care were still required within community settings for those leaving institutions and those expectations were not met. Once again, the societal response to mental illness was well-meaning reform, but once again its execution was not all that was hoped for.

Many scholars and historians agree that the trend toward deinstitutionalization ran parallel to a few other developments in Western society. In 1952, certain medications used to combat mental health issues became more widely available. In the same year, the first mental health classification system was released, and, as mentioned earlier, it is known as the *Diagnostic and Statistical Manual of Mental Disorders*. In 1957, the *Hospital Insurance and Diagnostic Services Act* was passed by the Government of Canada, moving funds to and prioritizing and dedicating smaller clinics and local hospital wings to mental health services instead of large institutions. This ensured that no new large mental asylums or institutions would be built and that, over time, care would be moved to smaller health care centres. The assumption was made that by folding mental health services into the public health care system and community services there would be a decrease in stigma (Dyck, 2011).

It is understandable why this assumption was made. If individuals needing help, and their families, were afraid of being sent to institutions where there were allegations of mistreatment, unsanitary conditions, few positive results reported, and long-term stays forced on patients, it is reasonable to believe that many would hide their mental health concerns. Along with the stigma about mental health issues, there was also a stigma attached to the asylum system. Hospitals and other community settings would have been

antipsychotic medications
used to treat psychotic symptoms such as delusions, hallucinations and mania; can also be used to treat severe depression and bipolar disorders; examples include Risperidal and Seroquel

antidepressant medications
prescription drugs used to treat depression and depressive symptoms by increasing the availability of neurotransmitters in the brain; examples include Cymbalta, Effexor, and Wellbutrin

antianxiety medications
used to treat anxiety disorders such as generalized anxiety disorder, social anxiety disorder, and panic attacks; examples include Ativan, Valium, and Xanax

more attractive or at least more palatable to those living with mental health issues, as well as to the rest of the population.

However, while there were serious problems inherent in long-stay institutional settings, there were notable problems with the new proposition of health-care-system and community-based responses to mental health and mental illness.

Psychiatric issues were now being seen more often in family medicine and emergency rooms by professionals without specific expertise; services were no longer provided by a single service provider but instead by a "complicated matrix of services" and multiple governmental and provincial departments, including the health care system; and housing and other **social services** were increasing the **red tape** involved in getting access to them. Scholars and those in the psychiatric profession suggested that the transition toward "the new face of mental health had been sorely underfunded, under-resourced and overpopulated" (Dyck, 2011). While leaving an institutional setting was a good solution for some people, others found themselves in communities that were under-serviced and without proper opportunities for housing, adequate mental health services, and employment.

social services
public services that provide benefits or assistance to those in need

red tape
excessive and/or complex paperwork, routines, and procedures that delay needed services

Many former asylum patients who had spent a great portion of their lives in institutions had lost the social, community, and/or family supports required for their successful transition back into society. Accessing services became a "revolving door" process for persons with chronic mental illness.

revolving door syndrome
continued pattern of re-admission into programs, services, or care due to relapse into mental illness

The **revolving door syndrome**, or phenomenon, is not something that affected only those leaving institutions. It also affected those who were never let into long-stay institutions. Revolving door syndrome is the process in which a person goes through an ongoing cycle of discharge and readmission into hospitals, other mental health services facilities, or even prison (Voineskos, 1976).

psychotic disorders
mental health disorders that can include hallucinations, deluded thinking, and abnormal perceptions

non-psychotic disorders
mood, anxiety, and other disorders that do not co-occur with psychotic symptoms

Research into hospitalization rates for mental health issues showed that readmission rates had increased substantially in Canada: in Ontario alone, the rate of readmission for patients with **psychotic disorders** increased from 25 percent in 1941 to 70 percent in 1971. For Ontarians with **non-psychotic disorders**, the rate of readmission went from 16 percent to 52 percent in the same 30-year time frame. According to the research, the figures for all of Canada were, on the whole, comparable (Martin, Kedward, & Eastwood, 1976). This meant that many people received acute care when longer-term care was required, which led to the exacerbation of mental health issues and more pressure on the person living with mental health and their loved ones.

Well-regarded mental health historian Gerald Grob has theorized that multiple factors were at play in creating mental health's deinstitutionalization era, including but not limited to:

- Psychiatrists beginning to seek and create opportunities in private practice for themselves, which represented a large reorganization of the profession of psychiatry.
- Shifting views about the treatment and care of those living with mental illness. Increased public awareness about the conditions that mentally ill persons were forced to live in within institutionalized settings created a demand for change. The outcry to ramp up legal and political challenges to the system was gaining momentum.
- The creation and use of new prescription medications to treat mild, moderate, and severe mental health issues. These were starting to be seen as an effective part of treatment in ways they had not been previously.
- Growing government involvement in North American mental health research and the creation of public health programs to deal with mental health and **social welfare**. These were seen as more appropriate uses of taxpayer dollars than funding large institutions that were developing bad reputations (1997).

social welfare
provision of assistance to disadvantaged groups or individuals that is organized through government or private social services

A *Canadian Journal of Psychiatry* report by Sealy and Whitehead in 2004 suggested that deinstitutionalization was perhaps not the best term to describe what was happening to those who were leaving large institutions. Instead, this report used the term **transinstitutionalization** to describe the process by which those living with severe mental health issues were now simply being reinstitutionalized into other, mostly smaller institutions such as private and public group residences, nursing homes, emergency rooms, and various parts of the criminal justice system.

transinstitutionalization
reinstitutionalizing people with mental health issues into prisons, group homes, and other residential programs

The various places where a person living with mental health issues might find himself or herself living after deinstitutionalization/transinstitutionalization are:

- **Group homes:** Smaller residential settings with trained staff who are available 24 hours a day to provide special care to those in difficult social situations or who have mental illness or behavioural disorders. These homes are often located in residential neighbourhoods.

group homes
smaller residential setting for those living with mental health issues; trained staff available 24 hours a day for persons who require special care due to difficult social situations, mental illness, or behavioural disorders; often located in residential neighbourhoods

nursing homes
residential facilities equipped to house and care for the elderly and/or people with chronic illness; trained staff, including medical staff, are available 24 hours a day

hospitals
health care institutions for treatment of acute health issues or injury

penitentiaries/prisons
facilities established for the confinement of persons who have committed crimes or are awaiting trial

shelters for the homeless
service that provides temporary residence for individuals who are living on the streets

- **Nursing homes:** Residential facilities that are equipped to house and care for the elderly and/or people with chronic illnesses. Trained staff include medical staff who are available 24 hours a day.
- **Hospitals:** Health care institutions for the treatment of acute health issues or injuries.
- **Penitentiaries/prisons:** Facilities established for the confinement of those who have committed crimes or are awaiting trial.
- **Shelters for the homeless:** Temporary residences for those who live on the streets. These facilities are usually open for only part of the day.

VOICES FROM THE FIELD

A chapter feature exposing you to the opinions and practices of those working in the helping fields. In these features we are hoping to expose readers to a variety of opinions from a variety of helping professionals. These are intended to be taken as opportunities to engage in discussion. You may or may not agree with the opinions expressed but we hope more than anything for you to engage in the material with an open yet critical eye. Use these as an opportunity to engage in discussion about the topics and opinions presented throughout the book.

VOICES FROM THE FIELD

Was Deinstitutionalization Really Such a Bad Thing?

By Dorothy Cotton, Ph.D., C. Psych., Psychologist

There is a tendency to swear gently under one's breath whenever the word "deinstitutionalization" is mentioned. Deinstitutionalization is widely held to be responsible for many of the evils of the world—homelessness, the increasing incarceration of people with mental illnesses, increased demands on police time, the black plague, holes in the ozone layer, racism, listeria, and so on.

No one, including me, would disagree that there is a very real problem of increasing interactions between police and people with mental illness—but is deinstitutionalization really the culprit?

Deinstitutionalization actually began a very long time ago—back in the 1950s. The initial driving force behind the movement was not so much political, or based on some idealistic philosophy, as it was driven by the fact that new treatments had been developed—pharmacological treatments to be precise. People who were previously untreatable and unstable became treatable and able to function outside of institutions.

However, treatment was not the only factor contributing to deinstitutionalization. Human rights came into play as well. Somewhere along the line, it occurred to policy makers that people with mental illnesses were entitled to the same kinds of rights and liberties that other Canadians enjoyed. The path here was not dissimilar from the path followed by women, various ethnic and minority groups, people with physical disabilities, and/or people of varying sexual orientations. All of these groups at some point in our not-so-distant history were arbitrarily denied their rights because they were different—and as we all know, it is a short leap from "different" to "bad and scary" or even "deficient and lesser."

We seem to have largely gotten over that as far as most of these groups are concerned. But in regard to people with mental illnesses—well, we are not there yet.

Is the reason that police spend so much time with people with mental illnesses an indication that we need more psychiatric hospital beds? I will concede this is an empirical question and it is not outside the realm of possibility that a *few* more beds might make a difference. But I remain unconvinced that it would make a large difference. The vast majority of people who have mental illnesses and interact with police would not ever get admitted to hospital even if there were beds. And if they don't need hospital beds, then what do they need?

- **They need access to services.** But "services" and "hospital beds" are not the same thing. No one would argue that you need to be admitted to hospital for a broken leg or an ear infection. Ditto for the vast majority of mental illnesses.
- **They need tolerance from the public.** How many interactions between police and a person with a mental illness are initiated by some panicked member of the public who has made the very common—and erroneous—link between "mental illness" and "dangerous."
- **They need understanding and realistic assessment from police.** How many interactions between police and people with mental illness go south because the officer has started with the assumption that mental illness equals danger? I often point out that the very same people that police feel threatened by are dealt with on a daily basis by unarmed nurses and

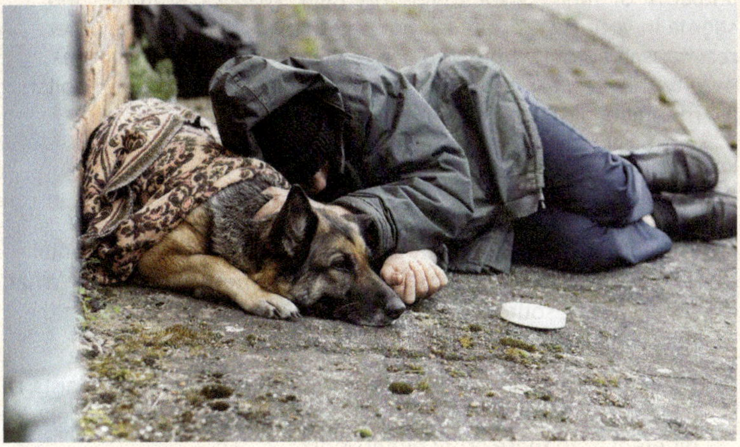

Housing issues are part of a larger set of issues that can have a dire effect on the ability to get the help that is needed to become or stay healthy.

psychologists and other mental health professionals. We deal with it without use of force. It *can* be done.

- **They need housing.** Early data from the Mental Health Commission's *At Home* study, which provides housing to people who were homeless and ineligible for most housing, indicates that when people have housing, their interactions with the police decrease. Hardly a surprising correlation.
- **They need jobs.** You don't have to review a whole lot of research to know that unemployed people get into less trouble than employed people. Sure, it's a bit of a vicious circle—employers are reluctant to hire people with mental illnesses. Research suggests that employers would rather hire someone with a criminal record than with a history of mental illness. Employers have a whole lot more trouble re-integrating people with mental health problems back into the workplace after a period of illness than they do with people with physical illness. Think of your own workplace and how people with mental health problems are treated—both when they are at work and when they are away. It's a common refrain from people with mental health problems that when they are off sick with the flu or heart disease, people are lined up at their door with casseroles and good wishes. When you are off for depression? Not so much.

Are interactions with people with mental illness an increasing burden for police services? Obviously. Should the police be the front line of the mental health system? Probably not.

What can you do? You start from where you have some power and control—and maybe that is internally. Work on attitudes and stigma in your own organization. And then work on all the other *real* causal factors where you can: agitate for housing, for community services, for educating the public, for more research dollars for mental health, for better employment strategies.

Deinstitutionalization? It's not really the main culprit.

Discussion Questions

1. The author states that many calls concerning people with mental illness are initiated by "some panicked member of the public." What other specific sources (people or organizations) might contact the police for assistance?
2. The author compares police officers with nurses and psychologists. Is this a fair comparison? In what ways is the role of law enforcement different from these other professions?
3. What arguments can be made for and against the statement the author makes about police using force? Why is this topic controversial?

The Diagnostic and Statistical Manual of Mental Disorders

In the 20th century, efforts to classify mental disorders became formalized with the creation of the *Diagnostic and Statistical Manual of Mental Disorders*, which is commonly called "the DSM."

In the 19th century, blanket terms such as idiocy or insanity were used to describe mental illness (Torrey & Miller, 2001, p. 336) (see Figure 1.1). Over time efforts were made to further categorize mental illness. In response to variability in diagnosis and confusion by mental health clinicians, a group that would later become known as the American Psychological Association recommended a uniform classification system for mental disorders (Sanders, 2011).

The first manual, published in 1918, was called the *Statistical Manual for the Use of Institutions for the Insane* and it had 22 potential diagnostic categories (Kawa & Giordano, 2012). These 22 original categories included terms such as "senile psychoses," "alcoholic psychoses," "dementia pracox," "paranoia and paranoic conditions," and "involution melancholia" (American Medico-Psychological Association, 1918). These terms are the precursors to terms that became popularized later as senility, alcoholism, dementia, paranoia, and depression.

The first edition of the DSM published in 1952 listed 106 disorders. The latest edition, first published in 2013 (DSM-5, the fifth edition), has 152 disorder classifications listed (McCarron, 2013).

In some ways the updating is fairly straightforward and lacks controversy. For example, sometimes categories were folded into one another as a way of simplifying them or updating language. In the latest edition, the separate diagnoses of **substance abuse** and **substance dependence** were replaced by the common term "substance use disorder."

Other changes are more controversial, such as the removal of the **bereavement** exclusion for diagnosing major depressive disorder. When a person loses a loved one, it can be argued that it is very normal to grieve. The bereavement exclusion meant that clinicians wouldn't treat the normal grieving process as an illness that could lead to more people being medicated for major depressive symptoms when a better fit for treatment might be time, reflection, and/or talk therapy. Another change was a reduction in the criteria required to diagnose attention deficit disorder. Some believe that the number of diagnoses for a variety of mental health issues are already inflated and that a lower number of criteria for diagnosis will cause a rise in misguided pharmaceutical interventions, and pharmaceuticals can have side effects (Wakefield, 2016).

substance abuse
pattern of recurring and harmful substance use (for example, alcohol and/or drugs) that disrupts normal life functions, including the ability to function normally in school, at home, or in the workplace; substance use in situations that present physical hazards, such as driving or operating machinery; and continued use of substances despite social or interpersonal costs

substance dependence
can include an increased tolerance to alcohol and drugs, symptoms of withdrawal when not using, increased consumption, multiple unsuccessful efforts to end use, and so on; occurs when a person adapts or builds a tolerance to repeated exposure to or ingestion of a substance; stopping regular usage causes symptoms of withdrawal

bereavement
normal period of mourning or sadness after the loss of someone or something

FIGURE 1.1 A Little Piece of Mental Health History: Table of Contents from the 1918 *Statistical Manual for the Use of Institutions for the Insane*

CONTENTS

	Page
Foreword	3
Suggestions for the preparation of statistics	7
Statistical cards	8
First admission	8
Readmission	9
Discharge	10
Death	10
Filling in cards	11
Classification of mental diseases	12
Definitions and explanatory notes	14
Traumatic psychoses	14
Senile psychoses	15
Psychoses with cerebral arteriosclerosis	16
General paralysis	16
Psychoses with cerebral syphilis	17
Psychoses with Huntington's chorea	18
Psychoses with brain tumor	18
Psychoses with other brain or nervous diseases	19
Alcoholic psychoses	19
Psychoses due to drugs and other exogenous toxins	20
Psychoses with pellagra	21
Psychoses with other somatic diseases	21
Manic-depressive psychoses	23
Involution melancholia	23
Dementia praecox	24
Paranoia or paranoic conditions	25
Epileptic psychoses	25
Psychoneuroses and neuroses	26
Psychoses with constitutional psychopathic inferiority	27
Psychoses with mental deficiency	28
Undiagnosed psychoses	29
Not insane	29
Statistical tables recommended	30
Directions for the preparation of statistical tables	31
Table 1. General information	
Table 2. Financial statement	
Table 3. Movement of population	
Table 4. Nativity	
Table 5. Citizenship	
Table 6. Psychoses of first admissions	
Table 7. Race	

6

	Page
Table 8. Age of first admissions	36
Table 9. Degree of education	37
Table 10. Environment	37
Table 11. Economic condition	37
Table 12. Use of alcohol	38
Table 13. Marital condition	38
Table 14. Psychoses of readmissions	38
Table 15. Discharges	38
Table 16. Causes of death	39
Table 17. Age at time of death	40
Table 18. Duration of hospital life	40

The 1918 manual was the precursor of the DSM. The DSM has become the standard text in the modern era for diagnosing and classifying mental health. Note the 22 original mental health classifications found in the 1918 manual.

Asperger's syndrome was removed from the latest DSM; it became part of the broader autism spectrum disorder.

The change with regard to Asperger's syndrome is particularly interesting because it speaks to the power and problem of diagnosis. For some people, having a diagnosis can be helpful because it provides some clarity about why individuals and families are experiencing certain issues. Also, a diagnosis can be practical in helping to find the right help and can provide access to appropriate services. In-person and online support communities can also be found for a specific diagnosis and they provide comfort and a place to explore what others have done to help them cope or thrive.

When a diagnosis is changed or taken away, it is possible to lose access to support programs that have been relied on for help. A person may no longer qualify for certain social services, including income, housing, and medical supports. The person may feel as though a part of his or her identity has been taken away.

On the other hand, a diagnosis can be incorrect. It can take an individual down a path of institutionalization or into improper and unhelpful medical or psychiatric treatment, which can result in grave consequences. A diagnosis can also be stigmatizing, making a person feel as though he or she is different from others and defined by a term he or she has only recently become aware of.

Homosexuality was wrongly considered a psychiatric disorder according to the DSM until it was declassified in 1973. At the time, gay, lesbian, and bisexual people who were already dealing with a lot of stigma and societal pressure about their sexuality were also told they had a diagnosable illness that required the intervention of mental health professionals; there were psychological theories that homosexuality was a defect and was caused by "hormonal exposure, excessive mothering, inadequate or hostile fathering, sexual abuse, etc." (Drescher, 2015). Because these theories were codified in the DSM, it led to them being seen as legitimate scientific theories.

Being told you are either ill or immoral when you are neither is problematic and the diagnosis added to societal stigma. Even among mental health professionals who were gay there was a "realistic fear of adverse professional consequences for coming out at the time" (Drescher, 2015). Even though homosexuality was removed from the in DSM-II in 1973, it was replaced by a new diagnosis called Sexual Orientation Disturbance that focused on it being an illness only for those who wanted to change their homosexuality due to feelings of distress. This wasn't removed until the publication of DSM-III in 1987 (Drescher, 2015).

The problem with diagnoses such as these is that they not only add to stigma, but create real-world practical problems and issues for large groups of well people who are wrongly classified as unwell.

Dr. Robert McCarron, who works as an internist-psychiatrist, succinctly describes how difficult it is to diagnose and treat mental illnesses in contrast to physical diseases. He wrote that

> [t]he practice of medicine is an imperfect science, with the constant struggle of diagnostic and therapeutic uncertainty. This applies to the complex and dynamic field of psychiatry. Although recent advances help us to better understand, categorize, and treat psychiatric disorders (such as depression, bipolar disorder, anxiety, and substance misuse), there is more work to be done. It is easier to reliably diagnose and treat disorders when a specific cause is known. For example, most urinary tract infections can be quickly diagnosed and treated. Blood glucose levels can be reliably quantified. Most bone fractures can be accurately diagnosed by observing objective clinical features and radiologic findings. It is much more challenging to diagnose and treat disabling conditions that lack objective data, such as dysfunctional and maladaptive behavioral disorders (2013).

Mental health straddles several professional lines and touches more people than we realize. For example, families, loved ones, colleagues, and many others can be living within the orbit of a person who is living with a mental health issue. In addition to the personal dimension, an affected individual might interact with medical professionals, the justice system, social services, and other front-line workers across the multidisciplinary landscape. These interactions can be positive or negative and can have a great impact either way, and this is why it has never been more important for professionals across the spectrum to incorporate understanding about mental health into their work.

The next chapter will show how mental health and the various helping professions have intersected recently, but we cannot study current trends without understanding the basic historical concepts that were shared in this chapter. Studying the past helps us to avoid repeating mistakes so that we can move forward and help others more effectively. This work will continue to adapt and evolve, just as practitioners in the helping professions will adapt and evolve to better meet the needs of individuals and communities.

POINTS TO REMEMBER

- ✓ Mental health issues are common over the course of life and are emerging as core issues for those in the helping professions whose work is related to justice, health care, and social services. This work takes place across professions in multidisciplinary teams in communities across Canada.
- ✓ Current ways of working with mental health issues are in many ways a vast improvement over the era of institutionalization. While begun with good intentions, the mass institutionalization of those living with mental health issues led to stigmatization, generally poor treatment outcomes, and deterioration of the civil rights of many individuals.
- ✓ While categorizing and diagnosing mental health problems can help those who are afflicted, to researchers and those helping on the front lines, a mental health diagnosis is not all that defines someone. No matter which helping profession we are in, we must continue to strive to treat people as complex individuals who are worthy of dignity and respect while continuing to improve our knowledge of mental health issues and the best practices for treatment within our communities.

KEY TERMS

antianxiety medications, 15
antidepressant medications, 15
antipsychotic medications, 15
bereavement, 21
deinstitutionalization, 7
Diagnostic and Statistical Manual of Mental Disorders (DSM), 7
first responders, 6
group homes, 17
helping professions, 6
hospitals, 18
institutionalization, 6
justice system, 6
multidisciplinary team, 6
non-psychotic disorders, 16
nursing homes, 18
penitentiaries/prisons, 18
psychotic break, 3
psychotic disorders, 16
red tape, 16
revolving door syndrome, 16
shelters for the homeless, 18
social services, 16
social stigma, 14
social welfare, 17
substance abuse, 21
substance dependence, 21
transinstitutionalization, 17

REFERENCES

American Medico-Psychological Association. (1918). *Statistical manual for the use of institutions for the insane*. New York: State Hospital Press.

American Psychiatric Association. (2013). *Diagnostic and statistical manual of mental disorders* (5th ed.). Washington, DC: Author.

Braslow, J. (1999). Insights: Where biopsychiatry came from: A short history of somatic therapies from 1900 to the 1950s. *The Harvard Mental Health Letter/from Harvard Medical School*, *16*(2), 5–7.

Braslow, J.T. (1994). Punishment or therapy: Patients, doctors, and somatic remedies in the early twentieth century. *Psychiatric Clinics of North America*, *17*(3), 493–513.

Cotton, D. (2014). Was deinstitutionalization really such a bad thing? *Canadian Police Chief Magazine*, *Winter*, 11–12.

Dix, D. (2006). "I tell what I have seen": The reports of asylum reformer Dorothea Dix. *American Journal of Public Health*, *96*(4), 622–624.

Drescher, J. (2015). Out of DSM: Depathologizing homosexuality. *Behavioral Sciences*, *5*(4), 565–575.

Dyck, E. (2011). Dismantling the asylum and charting new pathways into the community: Mental health care in twentieth century Canada. *Histoire sociale/Social history*, *44*(2),181–196.

Gollaher, D.L. (1993). Dorothea Dix and the English origins of the American asylum movement. *Canadian Review of American Studies*, *23*(3), 149–176.

Government of Canada. (2006). The human face of mental health and mental illness in Canada, 2006. Minister of Public Works and Government Services Canada. Catalogue No. HP5-19/2006E. Retrieved from http://www.phac-aspc.gc.ca/publicat/human-humain06/pdf/human_face_e.pdf

Greenland, C., Griffin, J.D., & Hoffman, B.F. (2001). Psychiatry in Canada from 1951 to 2001. In Q. Rae-Grant (Ed.), *Psychiatry in Canada: 50 years, 1951–2001* (pp. 1–16).

Greenstone, J.D. (1979). Dorothea Dix and Jane Addams: From transcendentalism to pragmatism in American social reform. *The Social Service Review*, *53*(4), 527–559.

Grob, G.N. (1995). American psychiatry: From hospital to community in modern America. *Caduceus (Springfield, Ill.)*, *12*(3), 49–54.

Grob, G.N. (1997). Deinstitutionalization: The illusion of policy. *Journal of Policy History*, *9*(1), 48–73.

Gross, C.G. (2009). *A hole in the head: More tales in the history of neuroscience*. Cambridge, MA: MIT Press.

Hospital Insurance and Diagnostic Services Act, 1957 [replaced by the *Canada Health Act*, RSC 1985, c C-6].

Ianacone, B.P. (1976). Historical overview: From charity to rights. *Temple Law Quarterly*, *50*, 953.

Insane in Canada. (1855). *The Medical Chronicle*, pp. 326–329.

Kaiser, H.A. (2008). Mental health and Canadian society: Historical perspectives. *Health Law Review*, *16*(3), 79.

Kawa, S., & Giordano, J. (2012). A brief historicity of the *Diagnostic and Statistical Manual of Mental Disorders:* Issues and implications for the future of psychiatric canon and practice. *Philosophy, Ethics, and Humanities in Medicine*, *7*(1), 1.

Kedward, H.B., Eastwood, M.R., Allodi, F., & Duckworth, G.S. (1974). The evaluation of chronic psychiatric care. *Canadian Medical Association Journal*, *110*(5), 519.

Martin, B.A., Kedward, H.B., & Eastwood, M.R. (1976). Hospitalization for mental illness: Evaluation of admission trends from 1941 to 1971. *Canadian Medical Association Journal*, *115*(4), 322.

McCarron, R.M. (2013). The DSM-5 and the art of medicine: Certainly uncertain. *Annals of Internal Medicine*, *159*(5), 360–361.

Mental Health Commission of Canada. (2008). *At home/Chez soi*. Retrieved from https://www.mentalhealthcommission.ca/English/at-home

Miron, J. (2006). "Open to the public": Touring Ontario asylums in the nineteenth century. In J.E. Moran & D. Wright (Eds.), *Mental health and Canadian society: Historical perspectives* (pp. 19–48). Montreal: MQUP.

Miron, J. (2011). *Prisons, asylums, and the public: Institutional visiting in the nineteenth century*. University of Toronto Press.

Panksepp, J. (2004). Biological psychiatry sketched—Past, present, and future. In J. Panksepp (Ed.), *Textbook of biological psychiatry* (pp. 3–32). Hoboken, NJ: Wiley-Liss.

Pearson, C., Janz, T., & Ali, J. (2013). *Mental and substance use disorders in Canada*. Statistics Canada. Retrieved from http://www.statcan.gc.ca/pub/82-624-x/2013001/article/11855-eng.htm

Reaume, G. (1997). Accounts of abuse of patients at the Toronto Hospital for the Insane, 1883–1937. *Canadian Bulletin of Medical History/Bulletin canadien d'histoire de la médecine*, *14*(1), 65–106.

Sanders, J.L. (2011). A distinct language and a historic pendulum: The evolution of the *Diagnostic and Statistical Manual of Mental Disorders*. *Archives of Psychiatric Nursing*, *25*(6), 394–403.

Sealy, P., & Whitehead, P.C. (2004). Forty years of deinstitutionalization of psychiatric services in Canada: An empirical assessment. *Canadian Journal of Psychiatry*, *49*(4), 249–257.

Statistics Canada. (2012). *Canadian community health survey: Mental health*. Catalogue No. 82-624-X. Retrieved from http://www.statcan.gc.ca/pub/82-624-x/2013001/article/tbl/tbl1-eng.htm

Sussman, S. (1998). The first asylums in Canada: A response to neglectful community care and current trends. *The Canadian Journal of Psychiatry*, *43*(3), 260–264.

Torrey, E.F., & Miller, J. (2001). *The invisible plague: The rise of mental illness from 1750 to the present*. New Brunswick, NJ: Rutgers University Press.

Voineskos, G. (1976). Part-time hospitalization programs: The neglected field of community psychiatry. *Canadian Medical Association Journal*, *114*(4), 320.

Wakefield, J.C. (2016). Diagnostic issues and controversies in DSM-5: Return of the false positives problem. *Annual Review of Clinical Psychology*, *12*, 105–132.

Whitaker, R. (2005). Anatomy of an epidemic: Psychiatric drugs and the astonishing rise of mental illness in America. *Ethical Human Sciences and Services*, *7*(1), 23–35.

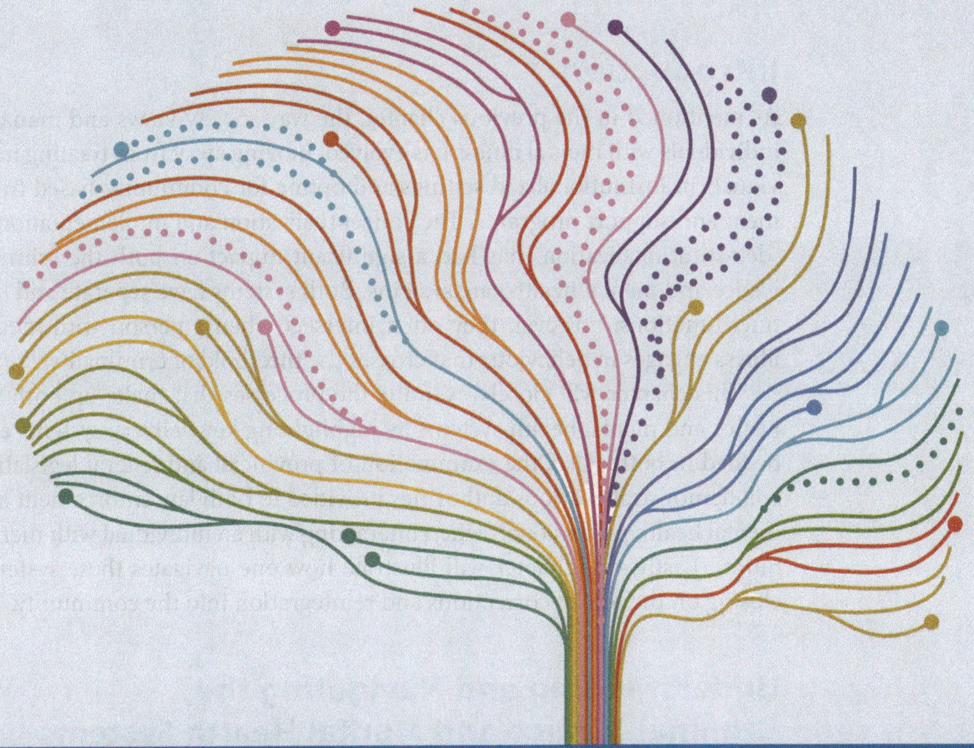

2 CONTEXT IS EVERYTHING

A Look at the Current State of Mental Health in Canada's Criminal Justice System

LEARNING OUTCOMES

After reading this chapter, you will be able to:

- Discuss the legal provisions for the mentally ill under provincial and federal laws (Ontario's *Mental Health Act* and Canada's *Criminal Code*).
- Differentiate between the various criminal court processes.
- Navigate the adult criminal justice and mental health systems.
- Outline the role of corrections and reintegration in Canada.
- Differentiate between the various processes that intersect as an individual moves through the adult criminal justice and mental health systems.

Introduction

As mentioned in the previous chapter, the way society views and manages individuals with mental illness has evolved, moving away from treating individuals in institutionalized settings and opting for community-based treatment and support programs. The conceptualization and implementation of "deinstitutionalization" has had a significant impact on both the criminal justice and mental health care systems. Both systems have separate and distinct functions; however, they often intersect when a person with mental illness engages in behaviour that crosses the threshold of criminality.

This chapter will closely examine the processes that make up both the justice and mental health systems by highlighting key delivery systems embedded in both. Also, the examination of provincial and federal legislation will demonstrate various authorities provided to both law enforcement and mental health professionals when interacting with an individual with mental illness. Lastly, this chapter will illustrate how one navigates these systems, closing on the role of corrections and reintegration into the community.

Understanding and Navigating the Criminal Justice and Mental Health Systems

The criminal justice and mental health systems often intertwine and an individual with mental illness will likely come into contact with one or both during the course of their lifetime. If a person with mental illness is fortunate to have the appropriate family and community supports in place, there is a great chance that he or she will never come into contact with the police. Unfortunately, for some people this is not the case and at some point police intervention may be required.

The Mental Health Act

The police have often been referred to as the "informal first responders" of Canada's mental health system (Adelman, 2003), and this comes as a result of several issues that will be discussed in Chapter 3. However, in short, when an individual is in crisis and there is no immediate support available to him or her, the police are usually dispatched to intervene. The outcome of an interaction between the police and an individual with mental illness relies on three main factors: the behaviour being displayed by the person with mental illness; the knowledge, skills, and abilities of the individual police officer(s); and the parameters of the law.

Section 17 of the ***Mental Health Act*** (MHA) outlines when a police officer can apprehend a person:

***Mental Health Act* (MHA)**
law that regulates the administration of mental health care in Ontario; the main purpose of this law is to regulate the involuntary admission of people into a psychiatric hospital

> 17 Where a police officer has reasonable and probable grounds to believe that a person is acting or has acted in a disorderly manner and has reasonable cause to believe that the person,
>
> (a) has threatened or attempted or is threatening or attempting to cause bodily harm to himself or herself;
>
> (b) has behaved or is behaving violently towards another person or has caused or is causing another person to fear bodily harm from him or her; or
>
> (c) has shown or is showing a lack of competence to care for himself or herself,
>
> and in addition the police officer is of the opinion that the person is apparently suffering from mental disorder of a nature or quality that likely will result in,
>
> (d) serious bodily harm to the person;
>
> (e) serious bodily harm to another person; or
>
> (f) serious physical impairment of the person,
>
> and that it would be dangerous to proceed under section 16 [authorization by a justice of the peace], the police officer may take the person in custody to an appropriate place for examination by a physician.

DISCUSSION QUESTIONS

1. Can you think of an example of when a police officer would have to apprehend someone under the *Mental Health Act*?
2. Do you think the police are given too much authority under this legislation?
3. What issues could arise if the police were not given authority to apprehend someone under the *Mental Health Act*?

Moving Through the Criminal Justice and Mental Health Systems

The following describes the chain of events that could unfold for an individual who is moving through both the criminal justice and mental health systems.[1]

Emergency Department and Community Crisis Support

If an individual has been apprehended by the police under the MHA and *no criminal offence* has been committed, the person will be escorted to the nearest hospital's emergency department to be seen by the attending physician. The attending physician will assess the individual to ascertain whether he or she should be kept (involuntarily) for further assessment by a psychiatrist. If a physician opts to keep the individual in the hospital for assessment, a document called a Form 1 (an application for psychiatric assessment) is signed by the emergency department physician. This document commits the individual to stay at the hospital for up to 72 hours for further assessment. At the end of the 72 hours permitted by a Form 1, the person must either be released, be admitted as a voluntary patient, or continue to be held as an involuntary patient through the use of a Form 3 (a certificate of involuntary admission).

Community Treatment Order (CTO)

Bill 68 (also known as Brian's Law) amended the *Mental Health Act* in 2000 as a result of the tragic death of Brian Smith, an Ottawa television sportscaster. In 1995, he was shot and killed by a man who had been diagnosed with paranoid schizophrenia. Bill 68 fuelled the creation of the **community treatment order (CTO)** (CBC News/The Canadian Press, 2016). These orders allow individuals with a history of in-patient treatment of psychiatric disorders to enjoy the freedom of living within the community and give consent in advance for any treatment or detention that might be required should their condition deteriorate. A CTO is a plan that outlines care that is specific to the individual's needs. It may include medications the person must take and appointments that must be attended in order for the person to be released from a psychiatric facility by a doctor. The concept behind these orders is that the patient will do better in the community than in an institution. These orders are, however, controversial; critics of CTOs believe these orders could be overused and misused.

community treatment order (CTO)
a legal order that sets out the terms under which a person must accept medication and therapy, counselling, management, rehabilitation, and other services while living in the community

[1] Examples are in reference to the province of Ontario, so readers should refer to the specific mental health legislation in the province of their interest.

VOICES FROM THE FIELD

Forced-treatment Orders a Growing Controversy for Mental Health Advocates

By Sue Bailey, The Canadian Press

ST. JOHN'S—They're among the most coercive tools in medicine: community treatment orders [CTOs] can force people with mental illness to accept treatment—or face arrest.

Families and mental health officials say CTOs are a lifeline in desperate situations. But critics say they are dangerously prone to misuse, and jurisdictions across Canada are confronting questions about them.

Newfoundland and Labrador is reviewing how it uses them, while in Alberta they are being studied as part of an overall review of the province's Mental Health Act.

In Ontario, meanwhile, a lawyer says such measures are being over-issued to "the point of abuse." Anita Szigeti, a Toronto-based mental health law specialist, said they have become a convenient tool of control.

"It's supposed to be limited to those who are most chronically unwell with a demonstrated history of revolving-door hospitalization," she said in an interview. "It's being used for many people, if not most people, upon discharge from psychiatric hospital. Routinely."

St. John's lawyer Joan Dawson, who represents a man with schizophrenia, said an order against him last September was imposed without proper notice. Her client at one point went with a police officer under threat of arrest without knowing he was under those provisions, she added.

"A police officer, if they're under order, can enter somebody's house and use physical force to take the person," Dawson said in an interview. "These are law-abiding people.

"The power of the state is huge. It must be balanced with all kinds of safeguards and, in our client's case, it didn't happen. It's appalling."

"The power of the state is huge."

Szigeti said Ontario introduced community treatment orders in 2000 as a less restrictive approach that would typically help about 250 patients in the province avoid involuntary hospital stays. Today, between 5,000 and 6,000 orders are in effect, she said.

Compulsory treatment has strong proponents, especially among psychiatrists and family groups who've watched loved ones refuse help while in the throes of psychosis.

Legislation with community treatment options is in place across most of Canada. It helps ensure patients under such orders, usually renewed every six months and with varying consent requirements, follow medical regimes or be forced back in care. A task force was announced last fall in New Brunswick to craft similar measures in that province.

"Overused to the point of abuse."

But Szigeti said most of her clients resent orders that are difficult to get lifted once issued.

"They are overused to the point of abuse."

Some patients flee the province and cut off all ties with family to escape those controls, she added.

"A lot of the procedural rights and protections that are supposed to be part of the checks and balances to safeguard civil liberties ... are simply not being used."

Forced Treatment in Ontario

A spokesman for Ontario's Ministry of Health said it would take at least two weeks to confirm how many CTOs are in effect. David Jensen also said in an emailed statement that mandatory five-year reviews assess how rights advice is provided.

The most recent review in 2012, by research firm R.A. Malatest & Associates Ltd., noted that orders can be issued for patients who have not been reminded of their legal rights, so long as advisers "make their best effort to contact the consumer."

It also found the number of orders had grown to more than 3,200 by 2010 from an estimated 459 in 2003. It cautioned that with increased comfort with their use "comes the risk of straying from the original purpose of the CTO."

Newfoundland and Labrador's Practice Under Review

Health officials in Newfoundland and Labrador are now reviewing how the orders are used after the Mental Health Care and Treatment Review Board nullified one involving Dawson's client, a 58-year-old man with schizophrenia.

"There appears to have been little to no effort made to ensure compliance with the legislative safeguards, and no mechanism to trigger the automatic review provisions for CTOs," says the ruling, released Feb. 16.

"As stated by the psychiatrist in this matter, there are no CTO protocols or processes in place to ensure compliance with the (Mental Health Care and Treatment) Act."

"There appears to have been little to no effort made to ensure compliance with the legislative safeguards."

Those oversight lapses came eight days after a provincial Supreme Court decision last September in a case involving the same man, Dawson said. Judge William Goodridge ruled a previous CTO was also invalid in part because the psychiatrist did not provide supporting facts that the man met required criteria.

Safeguards to protect vulnerable citizens from "significant state intervention in the context of no criminal activity" must be upheld, Goodridge wrote.

"There is no option for non-compliance or partial compliance with these provisions."

Alberta Liberal Leader David Swann, a former family physician and public health consultant, is part of an ongoing five-year review of that province's Mental Health Act. Concerns about rights protections have come up there too, he said in an interview.

"They're an important contributor to helping patients who are otherwise unmanageable," he said of CTOs used in the province since 2010. "They're also a potential threat to individual rights and freedoms that we have to watch very carefully."

Source: Bailey, 2016.

Discussion Questions

1. What are the benefits of CTOs?
2. What concerns might there be about the use of CTOs?
3. What are the benefits of compulsory (forced) treatment?
4. What steps could be taken to ensure that CTOs are not misused?

The Criminal Code and the Criminal Justice System

Evolution of the Mental Disorder Provisions of the Criminal Code

Accompanying the shift resulting from deinstitutionalization, policies, laws, and the *Criminal Code* have also evolved to reflect the changing societal attitude required to better serve individuals with mental illness.

The provisions of the *Criminal Code* that relate to individuals with mental illness changed significantly in 1992 with the proclamation of Bill C-30. Prior to this time, both policy and law regarding individuals deemed "not criminally responsible" was not codified and detention was determined by the lieutenant governor.

In the mid-1970s the Law Reform Commission of Canada reviewed law and policy in relation to individuals with mental illness and produced 44 recommendations that included appropriate detention and treatment of mentally ill accused that had the rights of the individual and public safety in mind.

In response to the report, in the early 1980s the Department of Justice launched the Mental Disorder Project, which suggested that the provisions of the *Criminal Code* were in conflict with the *Canadian Charter of Rights and Freedoms*.

The Supreme Court of Canada ruling in *R v Swain* declared that the automatic detention of individuals found not guilty by reason of insanity without any hearing to determine the level of danger they pose was in conflict with the Charter.

When Bill C-30 was proclaimed in 1992, the amendment to the law changed the former verdict of "not guilty by reason of insanity" to "not criminally responsible on account of mental disorder" (NCRMD).

In 1999, the Supreme Court of Canada ruled in *Winko v British Columbia (Forensic Psychiatric Institute)* that detention is only warranted if the accused presents a significant threat to society. In cases where there is insufficient evidence to support that the individual is a significant threat, an **absolute discharge** must be issued.

absolute discharge the lowest-level adult sentence that an offender can get; if an offender gets an absolute discharge, a finding of guilt is made but no conviction is registered, and the person is not given any conditions to follow (for example, not even a probation order)

And finally, in 2002, the Standing Committee on Justice and Human Rights conducted a review of the mental health provisions of the *Criminal Code* to address any current issues that had emerged and provided recommendations for a more systematic way to collect data (see Figure 2.1).

Criminal Offence

When police interact with an individual with mental illness, and through investigation it is determined that *a criminal offence has been committed*, the police will make the decision as to whether or not a charge (or charges) will be laid. The police often have the power to use discretion and therefore can make the most appropriate choice for the given situation. The least intrusive action that can be taken is simply the officer providing a "caution,"

FIGURE 2.1 Highlights of Federal Law and Policy Developments Since 1975

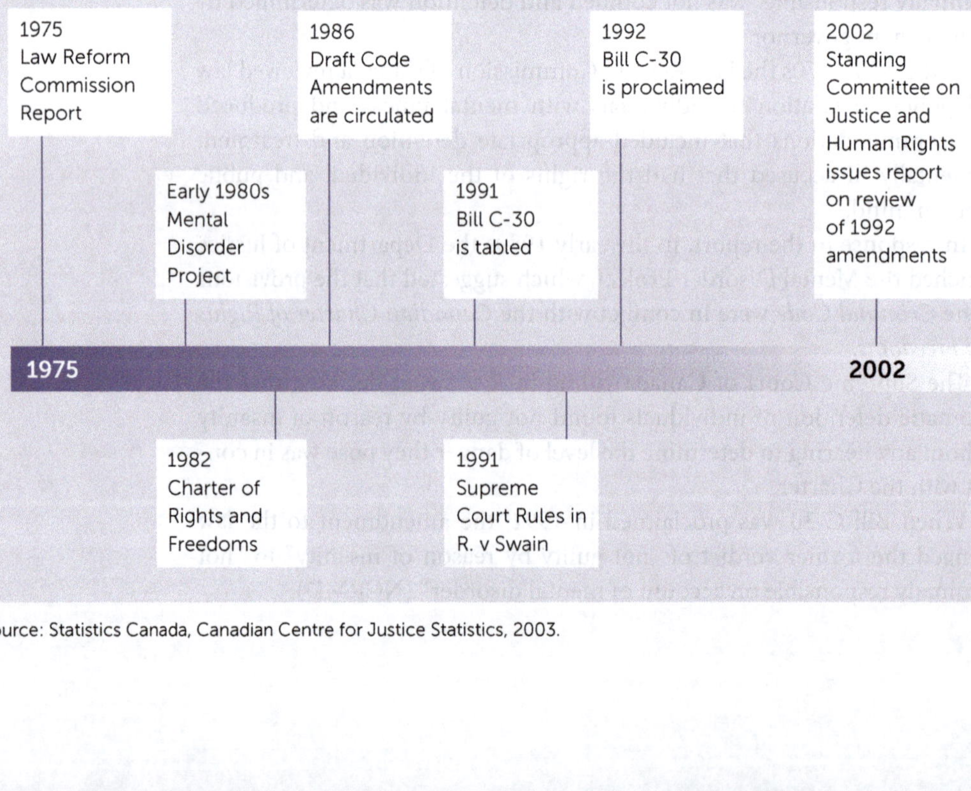

Source: Statistics Canada, Canadian Centre for Justice Statistics, 2003.

or warning, to the individual about the behaviour that warranted police attention. Although a caution can be given, the more common action that would occur is **pre-charge diversion.**

pre-charge diversion
option for police to enter an individual into the mental health system instead of the criminal justice system when certain criteria are met

Pre-charge (Police-Based) Diversion

Pre-charge diversion occurs when a police officer refers an individual to a hospital or other mental health facility instead of involving the person in the criminal justice system. Police officers contemplating diversion will consider several factors to determine whether they should arrest the person or divert them to the mental health system. The primary factors the officer will consider are:

- the seriousness of the offence,
- whether the individual is known to the police (previous contact and nature of that contact), and
- whether there is risk of harm to self or others.

Police may also consider other diversion options such as introducing the individual to a community mental health organization, escorting the person home to his or her family, involving crisis response services to take over custody of the individual, or apprehending the individual under the MHA and delivering him or her to a hospital emergency room.

Some police officers may be hesitant to use diversion options. This may occur because of a lack of services to which individuals can be referred. Other officers may not use this option because of a lack of partnerships or working relationships among the police, hospitals, community crisis centres, and other resource facilities and agencies. Even when diversion options are used, in Ontario any police interaction that involves an apprehension under the MHA will result in the creation of a non-criminal police record.

Arrest to Sentencing: The Criminal Court Process

Arrest and Charges

When the police opt to charge an individual instead of diverting the person through the mental health system, the criminal process commences. If the police are not concerned about public safety, they can process the individual and release him or her from custody on a release form called a "promise to appear" or lay a charge without arrest by issuing a "summons" instead. These notices will inform the individual of the charge and pending court appearance. In the case of a serious offence, or a less serious offence where the officer has concerns about public safety, the police may arrest the individual, charge him or her with a criminal offence, and then hold him or her for a **bail hearing**. The police must bring the individual before a bail court within 24 hours after arrest. It is a fundamental right of all Canadians not to be denied reasonable bail without just cause.

bail hearing
court session in which a judge or justice of the peace decides whether an accused will remain in custody prior to their court date; if the police decide not to release an accused on his or her own, the person must receive a bail hearing with 24 hours of arrest

pre-trial diversion
option for the Crown attorney to enter an individual into the mental health system when certain criteria are met instead of proceeding through the court system

Pre-trial Diversion

After charges have been laid, the Crown attorney has the option not to prosecute and may divert the individual into mental health treatment instead. This is referred to as **pre-trial diversion** or court diversion. For the purposes of diversion away from the criminal justice system, offences are grouped into three categories or levels:

- **Class I:** These are the most minor offences, including shoplifting, causing a disturbance, and possession of a small amount of an illegal substance.
- **Class II:** This includes acts such as uttering threats, public mischief, simple assault, and breaking and entering.
- **Class III:** These are the most severe offences, including assault causing bodily harm, sexual assault, manslaughter, and murder (Makonnen & Alam, 2016).

If the offence is minor and there is no risk to public safety, the Crown may decide that it is in the public's interest to simply withdraw the charge.

In order for the Crown attorney to consider diversion as an option, the following criteria must be considered:

- Is the mental disorder the individual is living with treatable?
- Is there a reasonable prospect of conviction if the case were to go to trial?
- Is the offence alleged eligible for diversion? Only Class I and some Class II offences may be considered for diversion.
- Is there a designated mental health facility or community support agency available to accept the individual as a client for support and treatment?
- Will the individual consent to participating in the diversion program?

Diversion can take place at any stage of the criminal court proceedings, but it is most suitably done before the trial begins. The Crown may suggest diversion; however, in most cases, it is the defence counsel who proposes court diversion and will demonstrate why the accused is suitable for the program. If the accused's case is eligible for diversion, a mental health court support worker will assist with the development of a program that may include community support, supervision, and/or treatment.

If the accused consents to diversion and the program plan, the criminal charges will be **stayed** or dropped. If the charge is stayed, it can be re-instated within the following year in exceptional circumstances if the accused fails to follow the diversion program.

stay (a charge)
stop or suspend court proceedings either indefinitely or until the occurrence of a condition imposed by the court

Bail Hearing

At the bail hearing, it is the Crown attorney who typically will argue why there should be conditions put on an individual's release, or why a person should not be released at all. The justice of the peace who presides over the hearing will opt to deny bail and keep the individual in custody if he or she believes that (1) the individual is a danger to a victim, witness, or the general public, and/or (2) he or she might fail to appear in court.

If released, the individual might have to follow certain conditions, such as

- residing at a specific location;
- staying away from certain people or places;
- limiting travel;
- surrendering his or her passport;
- not possessing weapons or firearms; and/or
- reporting to the police, a probation officer, or bail supervisor.

If bail is granted, the justice may issue a bail order as a precaution to ensure that the individual returns to court.

Types of bail orders include:

- **An undertaking:** A solemn promise, signed by the individual, that he or she will attend court.
- **His or her own recognizance:** A guarantee signed by the individual that he or she will return to court on the set date, or he or she will pay a sum of money. It may be required that the individual deposit this money prior to release.
- **A recognizance with a surety:** Someone (usually a family member or friend) who knows the individual agrees to supervise the individual to ensure court attendance and that imposed conditions are met.

Trial

At the point of trial, the process will vary, depending on what type of offence the individual has been charged with. A "summary conviction" offence is generally less serious that an "indictable" offence. There is also a category of "hybrid" or "dual procedure" offences in which the Crown decides whether to prosecute the case as a summary offence or an indictable offence.

Summary Conviction Offences

Ontario Court of Justice
judges and justices of the peace deliver independent, impartial, and timely justice to thousands of people who come before this court in more than 200 locations across the province; the court deals with approximately 500,000 adult and youth criminal charges, hears millions of provincial offence matters such as traffic tickets, and serves more than 20,000 families

Summary offences are tried in provincial courts, called the **Ontario Court of Justice**, without a jury. The maximum punishment for most summary conviction offences is a fine of $5,000 and/or a jail term of up to six months, although there are some summary conviction offences that are punishable at up to 18 months in jail.

Indictable Offences

Indictable offences are more serious crimes, and include murder. For most indictable offences, the accused has the choice, called an "election," of whether to have his or her trial in the Ontario Court of Justice or in the **Superior Court of Justice**. The most serious indictable offences are always tried at the Superior Court level. Superior Court trials can be held with either a judge and jury or a judge alone. The different court systems for Canada are outlined at the Department of Justice's website: http://www.justice.gc.ca/eng/csj-sjc/just/07.html.

Superior Court of Justice
this court has jurisdiction over criminal, civil, and family cases, and is the largest superior trial court in Canada; the Divisional Court, Small Claims Court, and Family Court are all branches of the Superior Court of Justice

Preliminary Inquiry

Before an indictable offence is tried at the Superior Court, a "preliminary inquiry" is conducted at the provincial level. The purpose of the preliminary inquiry is for the judge or justice of the peace to decide whether there is enough evidence to proceed with the trial. If there is not enough evidence, the case will be dismissed; if there is enough evidence, a full trial will be ordered.

Fitness to Stand Trial

At any time during the criminal process, the Crown or the defence can raise the issue of "fitness to stand trial." However, this is generally done at the bail hearing or the first court appearance. Canadian law presumes that everyone is fit to stand trial unless it is proven otherwise. A person is "unfit to stand trial" if they have a mental illness that prevents them from:

- understanding the nature of the court process.
- understanding the possible consequences of the court process.

- communicating and understanding the instruction of their lawyer.

The court will typically require a psychiatric or fitness assessment to determine whether the accused is fit to stand trial. A typical fitness assessment takes 5 days; however, it can be up to 30 days if the Crown and the defence agree. Under some circumstances, the assessment can be extended up to 60 days.

If, following the assessment, the accused is found fit to stand trial, the criminal process will continue. If, however, the accused is deemed unfit to stand trial, the judge may order the accused to receive treatment for up to 60 days in order to return him or her to a "fit" state. This is sometimes called a "make fit" order. If the accused becomes mentally fit enough to stand trial, the judge can extend the "keep fit" order, which will allow the accused to remain in custody while receiving treatment at a hospital, rather than awaiting trial in a correctional facility.

If the accused is found unfit to stand trial and remains unfit even after treatment, a formal finding of "unfit to stand trial" is made and his or her case is transferred to the Ontario Review Board (ORB). The ORB will make a decision, or disposition, about the case. In some cases, the trial judge may make the initial disposition. The ORB must meet within either 45 days (if the judge did not make a disposition) or 90 days (if the judge did make a disposition) to make a decision. The Board has two choices. It can issue:

- **a detention order:** this means the accused will have to stay in a forensic hospital until the case is reviewed again; or
- **a conditional discharge:** this means that the accused can live in the community under conditions set by the ORB. The ORB will then review the case yearly to decide whether the accused has become fit to stand trial.

The accused will remain under the care of the ORB until:

- he or she becomes fit and is taken back to court to stand trial;
- the Crown cannot prove that it still has a viable case against the accused; or
- the accused is found to be permanently unfit.

If the accused is never likely to become fit and he or she is no longer a danger to the public, the court may decide that it is in the best interests of justice to stay the charges against the individual.

Not Criminally Responsible

not criminally responsible (NCR) when the court finds that a person, because of a mental illness, could not appreciate the nature or consequences of his or her actions, or did not know that the actions were wrong at the time of the act, that person is NCR

Not criminally responsible (NCR) is an important legal defence for individuals who are suffering from a mental illness that made them incapable of understanding their actions at the time they committed a criminal offence. The *Criminal Code* deems everyone to be responsible for his or her own actions unless the contrary is shown. If this comes into question, in most cases the court will order a psychiatric assessment to explore the issue of criminal responsibility. This will be used as medical evidence in a separate hearing to determine whether an accused is, or is not, criminally responsible. Assessment orders for this purpose are usually in force for 30 days, although they can be extended to 60 days if the court deems it necessary. Involuntary treatment during assessment is not allowed. The psychiatric assessment will be presented along with other evidence to determine whether the accused is NCR. If the accused is found NCR, he or she will be placed under the jurisdiction of the ORB. The ORB will make a decision within 45 days about the accused's release based on whether it believes he or she is a danger to the public. In some cases, the trial judge may make the initial disposition. If this occurs, the ORB still makes its own disposition within 90 days. The disposition options of the judge or review board are:

- **Absolute discharge:** If the ORB does not believe that the accused is a significant threat to the public, he or she will be released without conditions. Once an individual receives an absolute discharge, he or she is no longer under the authority of the court or the ORB.
- **Conditional discharge:** The accused will be permitted to live in the community, but with certain conditions. These conditions may include reporting to the hospital or receiving counselling services. If the accused does not follow the conditions set out, he or she can be arrested again. Under a conditional discharge, the accused is still under the authority of the ORB and his or her case is reviewed yearly.
- **Detention order:** A detention order will be given if the ORB believes that the accused will be a significant threat to the public if released. In most cases, the accused would be held in custody in a "forensic hospital." This is a special psychiatric hospital for people who have come into contact with the law. The focus in forensic hospitals is on treatment and rehabilitation, not punishment.

The decision as to which disposition to make is based on whether the accused is believed to be a danger to others, not on the seriousness of the crime that has been committed. This means that if the charge is minor but the accused's mental health state does not improve and he or she is still seen as a potential danger to others, the accused may be under the jurisdiction of the ORB for a longer period than a criminal sentence would have been. However, the ORB is required to order the least restrictive option based on the needs of the accused and the need to protect the public. If the accused is deemed not to require full-time detention, he or she can live in the community, either with the detaining hospital's permission or subject to a conditional discharge.

Sentencing

If the accused is found guilty following a criminal trial, there is a range of sentencing options the judge can choose from. The defence and Crown will be permitted to make suggestions, or submissions, as to the appropriate sentence. In making a decision, the judge will consider the accused's criminal record and personal history, the impact on the victim, and the seriousness of the crime. For some offences there are maximum and minimum sentences that the judge must adhere to. Possible sentences include:

- **Absolute or conditional discharge:** The judge does not always have to convict, even if the accused is found guilty. A discharge can be given for certain offences if it is in the individual's best interest and if it is not contrary to public interest. Under a conditional discharge, the individual must follow certain rules, whereas with an absolute discharge, there are no rules. If an individual is discharged, there will be no criminal record for the offence.
- **Probation:** Probation is a correctional method under which convicted offenders are supervised in the community instead of being imprisoned or after a period of imprisonment has been served. Probation services, which exist in all provinces, are responsible for preparing pre-sentence reports that focus on the accused's background. The reports may suggest that the offender make restitution to the victim, or perform some type of community service as part of his or her punishment. The report may also recommend that the offender be required to take treatment for alcohol or drug problems or accept counselling on mental health concerns or social skills (for example, anger management).

VOICES FROM THE FIELD

Man Who Beheaded Greyhound Bus Passenger Wins Right to Live on His Own—With Daily Monitoring

By Steve Lambert

WINNIPEG—A man who beheaded a fellow passenger on a Greyhound bus in Manitoba has won the right to live on his own eventually.

A Criminal Code Review Board has approved a plan that would allow Vince Li to move out of the group home where he now lives.

Li—who has changed his name to Will Baker—killed Tim McLean during a bus trip along the TransCanada Highway near Portage la Prairie in July 2008.

He was found to be not criminally responsible for the murder because of a mental illness—schizophrenia.

The board reviews Baker's file annually and has ruled he could move out on his own following an updated assessment report that would include conditions for living in the community.

Baker originally was kept in a secure wing at the Selkirk Mental Health Centre, but the board has granted him increasing freedoms almost every year.

The request for more freedom came from Baker's medical team, which said he has been a model patient and understands the need to continue to take anti-psychotic medication.

Even living on his own, he would be subject to several conditions that would include daily monitoring, regular check-ins with mental health professionals and random drug tests.

Baker sat next to the 22-year-old McLean on the bus after the young man smiled at him and asked how he was doing.

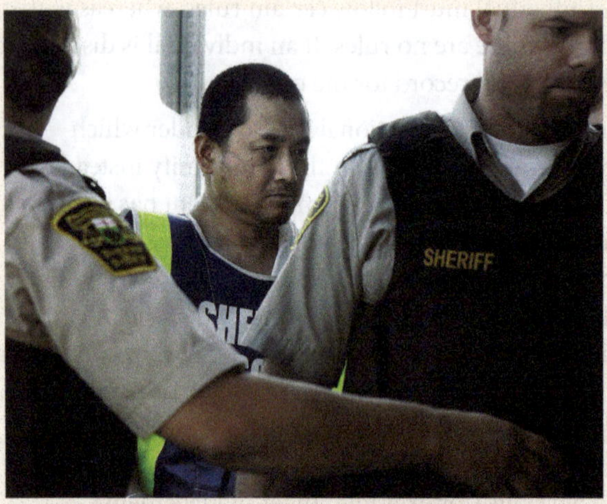

Vince Li was found not criminally responsible.

Baker said he heard the voice of God telling him to kill the young carnival worker or "die immediately." Baker repeatedly stabbed McLean who unsuccessfully fought for his life.

As passengers fled the bus, Baker continued stabbing and mutilating the body before he was arrested.

He won the right to leave the hospital and live in a group home last year.

Supporters say Baker and other people deemed not criminally responsible for their actions deserve the right to rehabilitation and freedom. But opponents, including some politicians and McLean's mother, have opposed the board granting Baker increasing freedom.

Source: Lambert, 2016.

Discussion Questions

1. What are the benefits of Vincent Li being reintegrated into the community?
2. In this case, are individual rights balanced with societal concern for public safety?

- **Conditional sentence:** This involves the individual serving a sentence of less than two years in the community, rather than in jail. The conditions attached to a conditional sentence (for example, house arrest) are generally more restrictive than with a conditional discharge or probation. If the individual breaches the conditions, he or she may have to serve the rest of the sentence in jail. It should be noted that not all offences are eligible for conditional sentences.
- **Fine:** This is a set amount of money that the individual will have to pay to the court as a penalty for the offence that he or she committed. In some cases, this fine is in addition to other penalties, such as probation or jail time.
- **Restitution:** Restitution also involves payment, but, in this case, the money goes to the victim rather than to the court or government. This sum is meant to repay the victim for any injuries or damage to property suffered as a result of the offence.
- **Imprisonment:** Imprisonment is the most serious sentence because it takes away an individual's freedom. If the individual is sentenced to less than two years, he or she will serve time in a provincial correctional institution. A sentence of more than two years is served in a federal penitentiary. In the case of an "intermittent sentence," the individual would go to jail for blocks of time, such as weekends, and be on probation in the community in between these times.

Appeals

The decision made by a judge or jury is not always final. In some cases, a decision made on a criminal case can be reconsidered through an appeal process. A convicted individual can choose to appeal the verdict or just the sentence that was imposed. It is usually the defence that makes the appeal, but the Crown can also appeal if it feels the verdict was wrong or the sentence was inappropriate. Appeals are only made after the trial is over, at which point the case will move to a higher level court. If the case was a summary conviction offence, the appeal will be heard at a Superior Court in the community where the trial was conducted. Appeals for indictable offences are heard at the Ontario Court of Appeal.

At an appeal, a judge will determine whether the trial was conducted properly, whether there were any significant errors made during the trial, whether there was enough evidence to support a conviction, and/or whether the sentence was fair. The appeal court then comes to one of the following decisions:

- **Acquit the accused:** If the evidence does not support the conviction, the appeal court may find the accused not guilty of the offence.
- **Dismiss the appeal:** If the appeal court finds that the trial was properly conducted and the evidence supports the conviction, or there was an error but it was not significant, the court may dismiss the appeal. The appeal court may dismiss an appeal against a sentence if the court is satisfied that the sentence is reflective of the crime.
- **Order a new trial:** The appeal court may set aside the conviction and order a new trial if it finds that the trial was not fairly or properly conducted.
- **Substitute a verdict of guilt:** In a small number of cases, the appeal court may find the offender guilty of an offence and impose a sentence.
- **Vary the sentence:** The appeal court may change the sentence and either increase or lower the sentence, or remove or add penalties (such as a fine or probation).

mental health court specialized court for those who have exhibited criminal behaviour due to mental illness; focuses on treatment and rehabilitation of the individual, rather than punishment

Mental Health Court and Post-Charge Diversion Programs

Mental health courts first appeared in Canada in the late 1990s. Currently, these courts have been launched in Ontario, New Brunswick, Nova Scotia,

Newfoundland, British Columbia, Manitoba, Nunavut, and Yukon. Unlike the adversarial approach taken in the regular criminal court, this court focuses on collaboration and problem solving. Mental health courts attempt to address the underlying issue that caused the individual to come into conflict with the law. There are mental health workers on duty at the court and psychiatrists are available for consultation and assessments. The goal of these courts is to satisfy the criminal law function of protection of the public by addressing individual cases to examine the true causes that lead to conflict with the law. If the participant fails to follow through with their monitored support program, they can be returned to the regular court system. It should be noted that these specialized courts are limited by available resources that vary depending on community size and government funding (Erikson, Campbell, & Lamberti, 2006).

Corrections and Reintegration

For many convicted individuals with mental illness who do not meet the criteria for diversion, perhaps because of the nature of their crime, the consequence of a custodial sentence is a possibility. Provincial jails and federal prisons can be challenging and difficult places for individuals with mental illness. All inmates have a fundamental right to health care, including mental health care. The *Corrections and Conditional Release Act* outlines the obligations of the correctional system to provide this ongoing care.

Correctional Services Canada (CSC) identified 13 percent of male inmates and 29 percent of female inmates in federal prisons as having mental health needs at the time of admission—rates that doubled between 1997 and 2008 (Sapers & Zinger, 2012).

Comprehensive discharge planning is important for all inmates with mental illness to ensure their successful transition back into the community. Failure to be connected to community resources upon discharge is believed to affect recidivism rates, and Brown (2009) confirmed that contact with the criminal justice system following incarceration was significantly higher for inmates with mental illness than for those without (Centre for Addiction and Mental Health, 2013).

FIGURE 2.2 Navigating the Adult Criminal Justice and Mental Health Systems

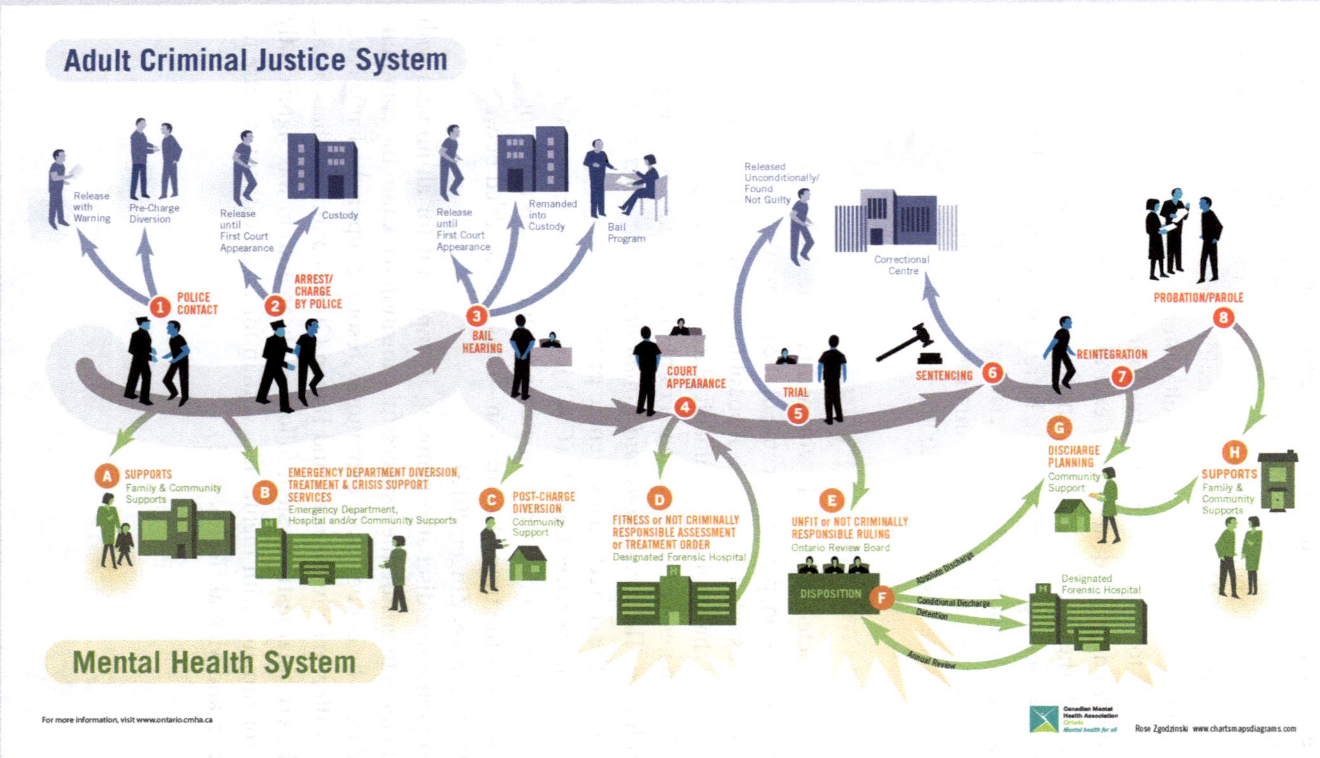

Source: Centre for Addiction and Mental Health, 2015.

POINTS TO REMEMBER

- ✓ This chapter demonstrates that as a result of deinstitutionalization, people with mental illness are at increased risk of coming into contact with the criminal justice system, with police typically being the first point of contact. The justice and helping professions overlap in many areas, and it is important for police to understand that the individuals they deal with may have past history with the mental health system. The many complex and diverse reasons why individuals with mental illness may come into contact with law enforcement must be considered.
- ✓ When changes to the mental health system were being made, the criminal justice system responded by implementing diversion programs and, in some cases, establishing mental health courts. The creation and use of community treatment orders, which continue to be a controversial topic, was discussed. Further, the criminal defence of "not criminally responsible" due to mental illness was discussed to demonstrate the law's view on punishment versus rehabilitation.
- ✓ The criminal justice and mental health system have recognized that a collaborative approach not only serves individuals more effectively and compassionately, but it also serves society at large in keeping low-risk individuals out of the court and correctional systems.

KEY TERMS

absolute discharge, 36
bail hearing, 38
community treatment order (CTO), 32
Mental Health Act (MHA), 31
mental health court, 46
not criminally responsible (NCR), 42
Ontario Court of Justice, 40
pre-charge diversion, 37
pre-trial diversion, 38
stay (a charge), 39
Superior Court of Justice, 40

REFERENCES

Adelman, J. (2003). *Study in blue and grey: Police interventions with people with mental illness: A review of challenges and responses*. Vancouver, BC: Canadian Mental Health Association. Retrieved from http://www.cmha.bc.ca/files/policereport.pdf

Bailey, S. (2016, February 26). *Forced-treatment orders a growing controversy for mental health advocates*. CityNews/The Canadian Press. Retrieved from http://www.citynews.ca/2016/02/26/forced-treatment-orders-a-growing-controversy-for-mental-health-advocates/

Brown, S., St. Amand, M.D., & Zamble, E. (2009, February). The dynamic prediction of criminal recidivism: A three-wave prospective study. *Law and Human Behaviour*, *33*(1), 25–45. Retrieved from https://link.springer.com/article/10.1007/s10979-008-9139-7

Canadian Charter of Rights and Freedoms, Part I of the *Constitution Act, 1982*, being Schedule B to the *Canada Act 1982* (UK), c 11 [Charter].

CBC News/The Canadian Press. (2016, September 24). *Brian's Law constitutional, province's highest court rules*. Retrieved from http://www.cbc.ca/news/canada/ottawa/brians-law-constitutional-court-of-appeal-ontario-1.3762067

Centre for Addiction and Mental Health. (2013, October). *Mental health and criminal justice framework*. Retrieved from https://www.camh.ca/en/hospital/about_camh/influencing_public_policy/Documents/MH_Criminal_Justice_Policy_Framework.pdf

Centre for Addiction and Mental Health. (2015, April 24). *Navigating the adult criminal justice & mental health systems*. Retrieved from http://ontario.cmha.ca/files/2014/06/Adult-Criminal-Justice-Mental-Health-Systems-Map-April-24-2015-FINAL.pdf

Corrections and Conditional Release Act, SC 1992, c 20.

Criminal Code, RSC 1985, c C-46.

Erickson, S.K., Campbell, A., & Lamberti, J.S. (2006). Variations in mental health courts: Challenges, opportunities, and a call for caution. *Community Mental Health Journal*, *42*(4), 335–344.

Greenspan, E.L., Rosenberg, M., & Henein, M. (2017). *Martin's annual Criminal Code*. Toronto: Thomson Reuters.

Lambert, S. (2016, February 25). Man who beheaded Greyhound bus passenger wins right to live on his own—with daily monitoring. *National Post*/The Canadian Press. Retrieved from http://nationalpost.com/news/canada/board-oks-plan-for-man-who-beheaded-bus-passenger-to-eventually-live-on-his-own/

Makonnen, S., & Alam, K. (2016). *Mental health courts in Ontario: A review of the initiation and implementation of the mental health courts across the province*. Provincial Health Services and Justice Coordinating Committee (P-HSJCC). Retrieved from https://www.cmha.ca/wp-content/uploads/2016/11/D2-Mental-Health-Courts-in-Ontario.pdf

Mental Health Act, RSO 1990, c M.7.

R v Swain, [1991] 1 SCR 933.

Sapers, H., & Zinger, I. (2012). Annual report of the Office of the Correctional Investigator 2011–2012. Ottawa, Ontario: The Correctional Investigator of Canada. Retrieved from http://www.oci-bec.gc.ca/cnt/rpt/annrpt/annrpt20112012-eng.aspx

Standing Committee on Justice and Human Rights. (2002). *Review of the mental disorder provisions of the Criminal Code*. Retrieved from http://www.ourcommons.ca/Content/Committee/371/JUST/Reports/RP1032130/justrp14/justrp14-e.pdf

Statistics Canada, Canadian Centre for Justice Statistics. (2003). *Special study on mentally disordered accused and the criminal justice system*. Catalogue No. 85-559-XIE. Retrieved from http://publications.gc.ca/Collection/Statcan/85-559-X/85-559-XIE2002001.pdf

Winko v British Columbia (Forensic Psychiatric Institute), [1999] 2 SCR 625.

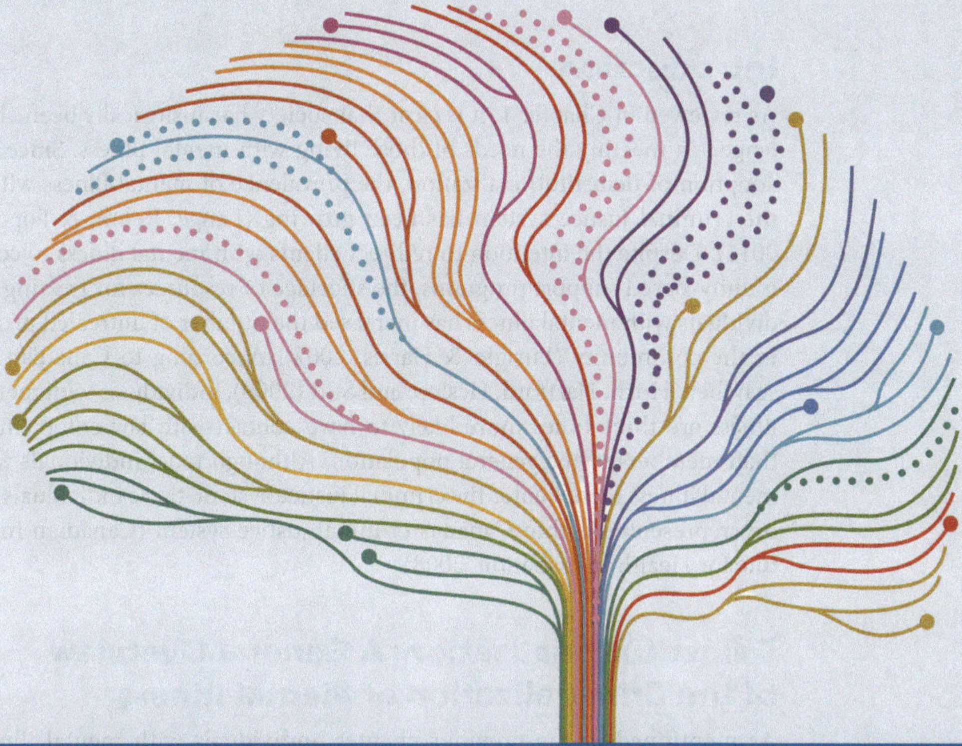

3 DEINSTITUTIONALIZATION
Implications for Law Enforcement

LEARNING OUTCOMES

After reading this chapter, you will be able to:

- Explain the impact of deinstitutionalization on the criminal justice system.
- Recognize the role of police as the "informal first responders" of the mental health system.
- Understand joint law enforcement and community initiatives such as COAST and other mobile crisis-intervention programs.
- Understand the phenomenon known as "suicide by cop."
- Identify improvements in police training and mental health awareness.
- Describe the role of a crisis negotiator.

Introduction

As reviewed in Chapter 1, it is clear that society has historically been challenged in meeting the needs of those living with mental illness. Since the adoption of deinstitutionalization, the prevalence of mental illness within the criminal justice system has been growing (Lange, Rehm, & Popova, 2011). Despite the intention to redirect clients with mental illness to community-based support programs, the shortage of resources for treating individuals with mental illness has increased the number of untreated people in the community (Lurigio & Harris, 2007). According to Canadian researchers Hoch, Hartford, Heslop, and Stitt (2009), individuals with mental illness are three times more likely to have contact with law enforcement than members of the general population. Although most individuals with mental illness do not enter the criminal justice system, these individuals are overrepresented within Canada's criminal justice system (Canadian Institute for Health Information, 2008).

Deinstitutionalization: A General Overview of the Criminalization of Mental Illness

As mentioned in the previous chapter, individuals with mental illness may enter the criminal justice system for a variety of reasons. Societal factors such as substance abuse, poverty, homelessness, and past trauma can increase the risk. Additionally, some individuals with mental illness sometimes behave in ways that warrant police intervention. Regardless of the factors that trigger a criminal justice system response, the overrepresentation of people moving through this system is often referred to as the "criminalization" of mental illness (Centre for Addiction and Mental Health, 2013).

The criminalization of mental illness is linked to numerous factors, the most notable being the lack of available treatments and community supports. Without this access, some individuals with mental illness may engage in behaviour and activities that draw the attention of law enforcement. How police officers choose to handle these interactions determines the fate of an individual's involvement with the criminal justice system and/or mental health system.

The Impact on Law Enforcement

Police officers have been described as the "informal first responders of our mental health system" because of the frequency with which they are in contact with individuals with mental illness (Adelman, 2003). Research suggests that of all the calls police officers respond to, 5 percent of them involve individuals living with mental illness. Of these calls, 60 percent involve some type of alleged criminal behaviour (20 percent of which is deemed violent crime), while the remaining 40 percent of these encounters are a result of a mental health crisis, unusual or bizarre behaviour, and victimization. Further, 40 percent of individuals with a mental illness have been arrested on at least one occasion during their lifetime (Brink et al., 2011). Reviewing statistics gathered in 2007 from police services in Ontario, over 40,000 calls involved individuals with mental illness and 16,000 calls involved the police apprehending the individual under the ***Mental Health Act*** **(MHA)** (Durbin, Lin, & Zaslavska, 2010).

***Mental Health Act* (MHA)**
law that regulates the administration of mental health care in Ontario; the main purpose of this law is to regulate the involuntary admission of people into a psychiatric hospital

Ontario's MHA legislation grants police officers and physicians specific powers to send an individual for a psychiatric assessment. It also grants the court power to have an individual sent to a hospital or psychiatric facility for examination. The MHA permits police officers to apprehend individuals if the officer has reasonable grounds to believe that a person is acting in a disorderly manner and is a threat or at risk of causing harm to themselves or others. Once the apprehension is made, the officer escorts the individual to a health care facility—typically a hospital emergency department, for an examination by a physician.

Apprehension of the individual is not the only option available to the police. In many jurisdictions across the country, police mobile mental health crisis teams exist to assist individuals in crisis. One such program with

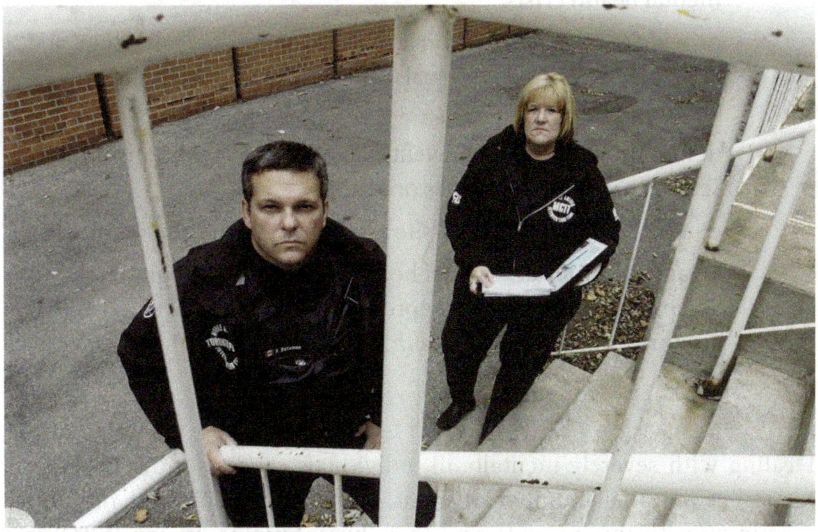

The Toronto Police Service's Mobile Crisis Intervention Team.

Crisis Outreach and Support Team (COAST) one of several mobile crisis teams made up of mental health workers and police officers that assist in mental health-related crisis situations

teams in Ontario is the **Crisis Outreach and Support Team (COAST)**. COAST teams comprise plain-clothes police officers and a mental health worker (for example, a nurse or social worker) who go to the scene to provide support to the individual in crisis. There are similar programs that operate under different titles, such as the Toronto Police Service's "Mobile Crisis Intervention Teams" (MCIT) and the Royal Canadian Mounted Police's "Car 67" program (RCMP, 2015). Regardless of name, all programs attend and respond to calls involving mental health crises, including individuals experiencing suicidal thoughts or self-harm, distorted or psychotic thinking, anxiety, overwhelming depression, or anyone suffering from a temporary breakdown of coping skills.

Crisis Outreach and Support Team (COAST)

The COAST program is a collaborative partnership between participating hospitals and police services in a given jurisdiction. The program partners a mental health nurse or social worker with specially trained plain-clothes police officers to respond to 911 emergency and police-dispatched calls involving individuals experiencing mental health crises. The team responds and will assess and connect a person in crisis with appropriate services. This program alleviates the need for front-line uniform patrol officers, who do not always have the same level of training as COAST officers, to respond.

The mandate of COAST is to:

- enhance the quality of service delivered to people experiencing a mental health crisis.
- provide a secondary response to calls for service, follow-up, and referrals involving individuals with mental illness in their own environment.
- defuse the situation to prevent the individual from causing serious harm to themselves or others.
- conduct an immediate on-site assessment of the person in crisis.
- arrange appropriate mental health treatment through referral to an appropriate agency or apprehend the individual under the authority of the *Mental Health Act*.

suicide by cop (SBC) suicide method in which an individual deliberately behaves in a threatening manner with intent to provoke a lethal response from a law enforcement officer

Suicide by Cop

Dealing with severely mentally ill individuals causes serious challenges for police. A small number of mentally ill people confront the police seemingly with the desire to end their lives. **Suicide by cop (SBC)** is a

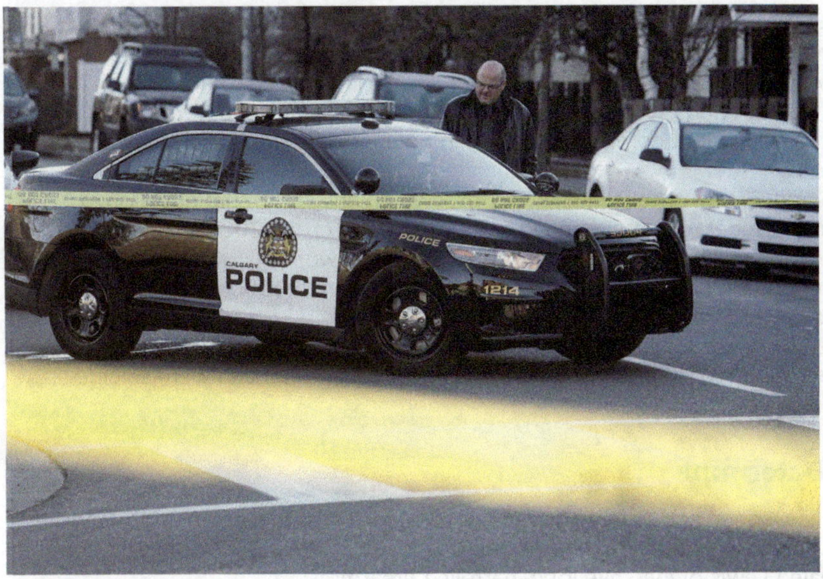

Suicide by cop.

method of suicide that occurs when an individual engages in threatening behaviour in an attempt to be killed by law enforcement. As a phenomenon, SBC falls within the arena of "victim precipitated homicide" (Mohandie, Meloy, & Collins, 2009). To understand the frequency of SBC, research involving a large North American sample found that 36 percent of all officer-involved shootings could be classified as SBC (Mohandie, Meloy, & Collins, 2009).

BOX 3.1 SUICIDE BY COP: A GROWING PHENOMENON

On the evening of July 17, 2010, the RCMP in Okotoks, Alta., received a report of a domestic assault, and about six hours after the initial call, with the emergency response team deployed around his house, 39-year-old Corey Lewis stepped out the door.

"He took up a kneeling stance and raised an object to his shoulder and pointed it at the loudspeaker. The object he was holding appeared to have a silver tip and was dark in colour," according to Cliff Purvis, the executive director of the Alberta Serious Incident Response Team.

Const. Jason Krivoshein had an M-16 assault rifle with a flashlight attached, which he shone on Lewis, 39. Lewis, in a shooting stance, quickly turned toward the light.

"I took my gun off safe and I fired," Krivoshein told an inquiry later. Three of his six shots hit Lewis, who died about an hour later.

The object he was carrying—it was duct-taped to his hands—was an umbrella.

Was this the kind of incident commonly known in police circles and TV dramas as "suicide by cop"?

An inquest now underway in Yellowknife may provide an answer to that question in another case. Karen Lander, 42, was carrying a firearm on March 14, 2012 when she was shot by RCMP, who were responding to a report of a suicidal woman.

It is a phenomenon that has been around since at least the mid-1980s, criminologists and other experts say.

And it may even be growing, according to a 2009 study, which found that 36 percent of officer-involved shootings in a large sample from the U.S. and Canada were suicide by cop.

Not Easy to Determine

In the Okotoks case, police had entered Lewis's home earlier in the evening and one officer said that he saw Lewis holding a rifle, so the police retreated. A check of the long-gun registry revealed Lewis owned five long-barrelled firearms.

Another officer told the inquiry that Lewis' wife Naydene, an Okotoks town councillor, had been concerned her husband had not been taking his antidepressants.

The day after his death, Purvis told a media conference that they had discovered a note on the stairs inside the front door. Then he said, "ASIRT is investigating the possibility that the deceased intended suicide when he engaged the police."

Earlier that year, on Jan. 9, John Wilcox was stopped by an RCMP officer in North Vancouver after he had collided with a parked car and then the officer's police car.

Both men got out of their vehicles, and the officer told an inquest that he ordered Wilcox, 39, to get down on the ground.

He did but then got up, advanced toward the officer while reaching into his pocket. He pulled out a black object and the officer fired, striking Wilcox.

The officer knew Wilcox from a previous domestic disturbance, when Wilcox threatened to shoot the police who had shown up at the scene, the officer told the inquest.

Wilcox, a talented animator, suffered from bipolar disorder. The object he took from his pocket was a cellphone.

After he was shot, Wilcox said, "Why don't you kill me? Just kill me now. Why don't you kill me?" witness Claire McGivern told CBC News.

Wilcox would later die in hospital.

Was this a suicide by cop? The inquest ruled it was homicide, with mental illness a significant condition contributing to death, and no charges were laid.

Simulated Weapon Possession

Determining motives and who is at fault in cases like these poses a challenge for investigators, particularly as, "in the early to mid-1980s, a phenomenon began to emerge in the United States" that people were using a law enforcement response to try and end their own lives, as John Violanti and James Drylie write in their 2008 book, *Copicide: Concepts, Cases, and Controversies of Suicide by Cop*.

The phenomenon has been called suicide by cop since that time, and it has appeared in news headlines since at least 1987. It has also been the subject of a number of books and many professional journal articles.

Incidents seem to be more common. A 1998 study of police shooting cases in Los Angeles County from 1987 to 1997 found that 11 percent of those cases can be classified as suicide by cop.

In the 2009 study mentioned earlier, which was co-authored by Peter Collins of Toronto's Centre for Addiction and Mental Health, 36 percent of officer-involved shootings were classified as suicide by cop.

The study sample included 707 cases from the U.S. and Canada between 1998–2006. It also found that in 19 percent of the cases, the person "simulated weapon possession to accomplish their suicidal intent."

Some other findings from the study, which the authors say is "the largest known sample" of officer-involved shootings [, are that]:

- 95 percent of the suicide-by-cop subjects were male;
- 62 percent of the subjects "had a confirmed or probable mental health history;"
- 48 percent of the confirmed mental health subjects suffered from depression or some form of mood disorder;
- 87 percent of the cases had "suicidal communications by the subject at any point prior to or during the incident;"
- 14 percent of the suicide-by-cop subjects left a suicide note;
- 61 percent of the subjects talked about suicide during the incident and
- 79 percent of those subjects referred specifically to suicide by cop.

Another American study published in 2000 observed that "suicide by cop situations are unpredictably dangerous and require at least the same level of caution as any other type of police intervention with potentially violent persons."

Rebecca Stincelli, a former law enforcement instructor in California and the author of a book titled *Suicide by Cop*, has interviewed survivors of such attempts and says on her website that these people indicated they wanted to be killed by police "because they could not pull the trigger themselves and they knew, when forced with the circumstances, the police officer would respond with deadly force.

Source: CBC News, 2013.

Discussion Questions

1. Why do you believe most suicidal individuals who confront police are male?
2. What additional training might officers receive to better handle these high-risk calls?

Police Training

The Mental Health Commission of Canada (MHCC) was established in 2007, bringing together multidisciplinary experts and professionals from across the helping professions with the mission to improve the mental health system and to address changing attitudes about mental health in Canada. The MHCC launched a study to review situations involving interactions between police and people with mental illness. While police encounters with these individuals vary in nature, it is typically only the high-profile cases that are covered by the media, and these rare incidents are those in which a person with mental illness dies during the interaction with police. The success stories involving the police are seldom highlighted. An incident that results in the death of an individual typically leads to a coroner's inquest, and several inquests have taken place over the past decades. Most of these inquests made recommendations for more and/or improved police training. This has resulted in substantially improved training for police over the past 10 to 15 years (Coleman & Cotton, 2014).

There continues to be a focus on providing adequate interdisciplinary education for police, not only so they better recognize and understand behaviours related to mental illness, but also so they can respond in a more empathetic way, employ de-escalation techniques as needed (to avoid the use of force), and help connect affected individuals with the appropriate community supports and mental health services.

In Canada, basic police training takes place at police colleges such as the Ontario Police College (OPC), Atlantic Police Academy, L'Ecole nationale de police du Quebec (ENPQ), Saskatchewan Police College, and the Justice Institute of British Columbia. Some city police services educate their own officers; for example, Calgary, Edmonton, Lethbridge, Brandon, Halifax, and Winnipeg. RCMP training takes place at the Depot Division in Regina. A few police services provide additional "in-house" training to newly hired officers in addition to the provincial training. Some of these services are Toronto Police, Peel Regional Police, Halton Regional Police, London Police and the Ontario Provincial Police (OPP). In British Columbia, the RCMP and other municipal services are required to participate in mandatory crisis intervention and de-escalation training every three years (RCMP, 2014). In a country the size of Canada, it can be argued that police training generally has been inconsistent, and as such, monitoring and accountability mechanisms are required to ensure police training in mental health is consistent provincially, if not nationally.

It must be made clear that the causes and outcomes of interactions between individuals with mental illness and law enforcement are complex and often fall outside the control of the police. Training for police officers can help to improve interactions with individuals with mental illness to avoid injury and death and to, when possible, avoid the involvement of the criminal justice system. Police education is essential in order to facilitate change, but it is not the only component. Insufficient mental health research and situational factors such as lack of resources, bias, and stigma in the community also affect the overall situation.

VOICES FROM THE FIELD

De-escalation Training for Police

By Yasmeen Krameddine and Peter Silverstone, University of Alberta, and David DeMarco and Robert Hassel, Edmonton Police Service

Police officers are now frequently the first-line responders for those suffering a mental health or addiction problem, but training in handling these cases isn't keeping up with the need.

To counter this, the Edmonton Police Service (EPS) teamed up with the University of Alberta to investigate a new way to improve outcomes. This research was led by Dr. Peter Silverstone and PhD candidate Yasmeen Krameddine, and the results to date are very positive.

The training focuses on improving interactions between police officers and individuals exhibiting various forms of mental illness. What makes it novel is that it uses actors to portray real-life scenarios, developed in close collaboration between police and the University of Alberta.

Police officers then interact with the actors in these scenarios. The goal is to increase skills in active verbal/non-verbal communication, de-escalation techniques, empathetic understanding, and mental health knowledge.

This program is run as a one-day intensive training program with six scenarios: depression, addiction, schizophrenia, alcohol withdrawal, mania, and a suicidal individual.

It allows officers to improve their interactions in real-life situations. One important part of the training is the use of professional actors, who give feedback to the officers after each scenario. This is in addition to feedback from more senior training officers.

The actors are trained to acknowledge both the positive and negative behaviours of each officer during the scenario, giving officers in-depth feedback on how the officer made the actor feel during the interaction. Feedback is crucial for officers to understand how their actions affect the emotions and behaviour of individuals they come in contact with. The actors were trained extensively on verbal and non-verbal communication techniques, and varied their interactions depending on what the officer said or did.

For example, if the officer rolled his or her eyes, didn't listen to what was being said, or tried to rush the actor, the actor would in turn behave more belligerently and less helpfully.

In contrast, if the officer looked engaged, gave the actor his or her attention, and held eye contact, the actor would be more relaxed, helpful, and supply all the information asked for.

Emphasis during the feedback for each scenario was on increasing the expression of empathic feelings and body language expressed to the actors in the scenarios.

After the scenario was complete, the feedback continued to highlight why the actor behaved in certain ways. This allowed police to have an outside perspective of their actions and body language, giving them a better view of how their actions or what they said impacted the way they are viewed.

An example of feedback from an actor would be "when you asked me my name, I felt like you actually cared about me, as a person, so I was comfortable in answering your questions" or "when you told me to calm down it made me angry because your tone suggested you didn't care why I was so angry."

To date, more than 650 police officers have completed this training. Results have been very positive.

Over a six-month period, EPS members demonstrated significant improvements in their communication, empathy, and de-escalation skills, as observed by their supervising officers.

Additionally, there was an improvement in an officer's ability to confidently recognize, respond, and empathetically communicate with individuals in distress.

This supported a 41 percent increase in the actual number and classification of mental health calls, with 19 percent less time being spent on each call, thus an increase in efficiency. Over a six-month period, this led to cost savings of $83,828.

Additionally, police reported feeling significantly more confident in their training and ability to interact with a mentally ill individual. There was also a large decrease (more than 40 percent) in the use of any kind of force when interacting with mentally ill individuals, although there were other internal police initiatives that may have helped this latter figure.

These results show promise, and continue to emphasize the positive effects of this innovative mental health training initiative. What's interesting about the research that was done, and the tips provided, is that little things can make a big difference.

Active listening and expressing empathy in both verbal and non-verbal communication improves outcomes for police officers, particularly when interacting with those who have mental illness and/or addiction problems.

This study also shows that these skills can be taught and improved, and that this leads to true-to-life training and real-life application. Feedback from officers taking part repeatedly said how realistic the scenarios were and that they were able to subsequently incorporate these skills into their daily tasks.

Dos and don'ts for working with people with psychiatric problems

Try to **do** the following:

- **Ask individuals their name in a conversational manner, and offer yours.** This small act of bonding can go a long way in developing an understanding and empathetic relationship.

- **Active listening.** This is done by keeping attention and maintaining eye contact [with] the individual. You can also summarize what they say by repeating it back to them. Nod your head up and down to demonstrate strong non-verbal understanding. If you show you are actively listening, you will increase empathy with the subject, helping you gain any information and insights you need.
- **Use "open" body language.** Body language is an unconscious form of communication that can escalate or de-escalate situations depending how it's used. Keep a calm and relaxed posture, try not to cross your arms, smile and show you're concerned. These behaviours allow the subject to feel safe and trusted.
- **Mirroring.** Copy individuals' body language if you can. It's a powerful way of empathizing using non-verbal communication.
- **Label and confirm their feelings.** Since feelings and emotions are frequently a major cause of problems, labelling their feelings shows you are listening, for example, "It sounds like you're feeling very underappreciated." Confirming also helps them see that their feelings are normal, such as "anyone would feel sad after losing their job."
- **Focus on family.** By asking the person about their family or friends, you can decrease their isolation and remind them that they have people in their life. Examples may be "do you have any children?" and "what would your children do if they no longer had you in their life?"
- **Tell them what you are doing and why.** Research shows that if you explain to the individual what you have to do and why, there will be less chance of aggression and escalation. For example "I am going to have to arrest you because it looks like there are five warrants out for your arrest."

Try **not** to do the following:

- **Telling them to "calm down" or "relax."** These words may make them angry because they feel they're being talked down to and told what to do. This does the opposite of making someone feel calm.
- **Using dominating body language.** Standing over an individual with your feet planted, hands on your waist or on your gun, can indicate control and power. This may make the person feel defensive, powerless, and unimportant. They are less likely to be co-operative. If they're sitting, try instead to crouch down to their level, so you're able to talk to them as equals.
- **Improper mirroring.** Copying isn't always appropriate. If they're shouting, don't shout back, no matter the provocation. Try talking in a softer voice so they have to stop to listen to what you are saying. Also, if the person is scared or anxious, mirroring their body language can exaggerate anxiety and fear, which may escalate the situation. Keep a calm demeanour, even if they are not. Eventually and without realizing it, many subjects will copy your body language.

- **Telling them they shouldn't feel a certain way.** All feelings are real, no matter how outrageous they sound. Do not belittle what the subject is experiencing. For example, if a subject is hearing voices, don't say "no, you don't hear that." Instead, ask more about the situation: "How long have you been hearing them?" or "How do they make you feel?"

Source: Royal Canadian Mounted Police, 2014.

Discussion Questions

1. In what ways could de-escalation training be improved?
2. Should this training be offered to all levels of officers, from new recruits to senior management? If so, why?
3. Can this training assist in reducing the stigma that is associated with mental illness? How?
4. Which other disciplines related to mental health should justice professionals, such as police officers and correctional officers, look to partner with for training?

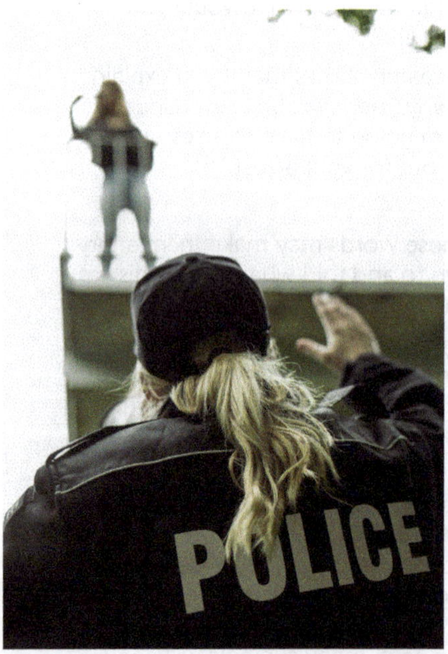

A crisis negotiator at work.

Crisis Negotiators

Crisis negotiators are specially trained police officers who respond to incidents involving hostage and/or barricaded individuals. In some situations, these individuals are suffering from a mental illness and are in an extreme state of crisis. Crisis negotiators assess the psychological profile of a subject in an attempt to determine the most effective strategy for communication and to identify risk factors associated with the subject. Negotiators often work in tandem with a psychiatrist who is available for consultation during a crisis call. Negotiators also assist with the development of surrender plans and work closely with emergency response teams that specialize in tactical rescues.

POINTS TO REMEMBER

- ✓ Deinstitutionalization has had a significant impact on the criminal justice system. The most noticeable impact has been on the police: new demands on officers have made it necessary for them to take on the role of "informal first responders" for the mental health system. In response to this, police services have had to adopt and develop innovative ways to manage the influx of individuals with mental illness who are coming into contact with the criminal justice system.
- ✓ Community initiatives such as COAST and other mobile crisis-intervention programs began to emerge to help manage the increase in calls for service involving individuals in crisis. These programs tend to partner police formally with mental health and other first responders. Also, the profession of law enforcement has seen an increase in officer-involved shootings as a result of the phenomenon known as "suicide by cop."
- ✓ Increases and improvements in police training in relation to mental health awareness and de-escalation techniques have become imperative in addition to the roles that crisis negotiators and emergency response teams play in intervention.

KEY TERMS

REFERENCES

Adelman, J. (2003). *Study in blue and grey: Police interventions with people with mental illness: A review of challenges and responses*. Vancouver, BC: Canadian Mental Health Association. Retrieved from http://www.cmha.bc.ca/wp-content/uploads/2016/07/policereport.pdf

Brink, J., Livingston, J., Desmarais, S., Greaves, C., Maxwell, V., Michalak, E., Parent, R., Verdun-Jones, S., & Weaver, C. (2011). *A study of how people with mental illness perceive and interact with the police*. Calgary: Mental Health Commission of Canada.. Retrieved from http://www.mentalhealthcommission.ca/English/document/437/study-how-people-mental-illness-perceive-and-interact-police

Canadian Institute for Health Information (2008). *Improving the health of Canadians: Mental health, delinquency and criminal activity*. Ottawa: Author. Retrieved from https://secure.cihi.ca/free_products/mh_crime_full_report_apr11_08_e.pdf

CBC News. (2013, February 27). *Suicide by cop, a growing phenomenon*. Retrieved from http://www.cbc.ca/news/canada/suicide-by-cop-a-growing-phenomenon-1.1374212

Centre for Addiction and Mental Health. (2013, October). *Mental health and criminal justice policy framework*. Toronto: Author. Retrieved from https://www.camh.ca/en/hospital/about_camh/influencing_public_policy/Documents/MH_Criminal_Justice_Policy_Framework.pdf

Coleman,T., & Cotton, D. (2014). *TEMPO: Police Interactions: A report towards improving interactions between police and people living with mental health problems*. Mental Health Commission of Canada. Retrieved from https://www.mentalhealthcommission.ca/English/document/36596/tempo-police-interactions-report-towards-improving-interactions-between-police-and-pe

Durbin, J., Lin, E., & Zaslavska, N. (2010). *Impact study, final report: A study of hospital emergency service use, crisis service delivery and police response after mental health system enhancements*. Toronto: Centre for Addiction and Mental Health.

Hoch, J.S., Hartford, K., Heslop, L., & Stitt, L. (2009). Mental illness and police interactions in a mid-sized Canadian city: What the data do and do not say. *Canadian Journal of Community Mental Health 28*(1), 49–66. Retrieved from http://dx.doi.org/10.7870/cjcmh-2009-0005

Lange, S., Rehm, J., & Popova, S. (2011). The effectiveness of criminal justice diversion initiatives in North America: A systematic literature review. *International Journal of Forensic Mental Health*, *10*(3), 200–214. Retrieved from http://dx.doi.org/10.1080/14999013.2011.598218

Lurigio, A.J., & Harris, A. (2007). The mentally ill in the justice system: An overview of historical causes and suggested remedies. *Professional Issues in Criminal Justice*, *2*, 145–169.

Mental Health Act, RSO 1990, c M.7.

Mohandie, K., Meloy, J., & Collins, P. (2009, March). Suicide by cop among officer-involved shooting cases. *Journal of Forensic Science*, *54*, (2).

Royal Canadian Mounted Police [RCMP]. (2014, April 3). De-escalation training for police. *Gazette* magazine, *76*(1). Retrieved from http://www.rcmp-grc.gc.ca/en/gazette/de-escalation-training-police

Royal Canadian Mounted Police. (2015). Enhancing police response to mental health situations. *In Focus*. Retrieved from http://bc.rcmp-grc.gc.ca/ViewPage.action?siteNodeId=2096&languageId=1&contentId=41702

PART 2

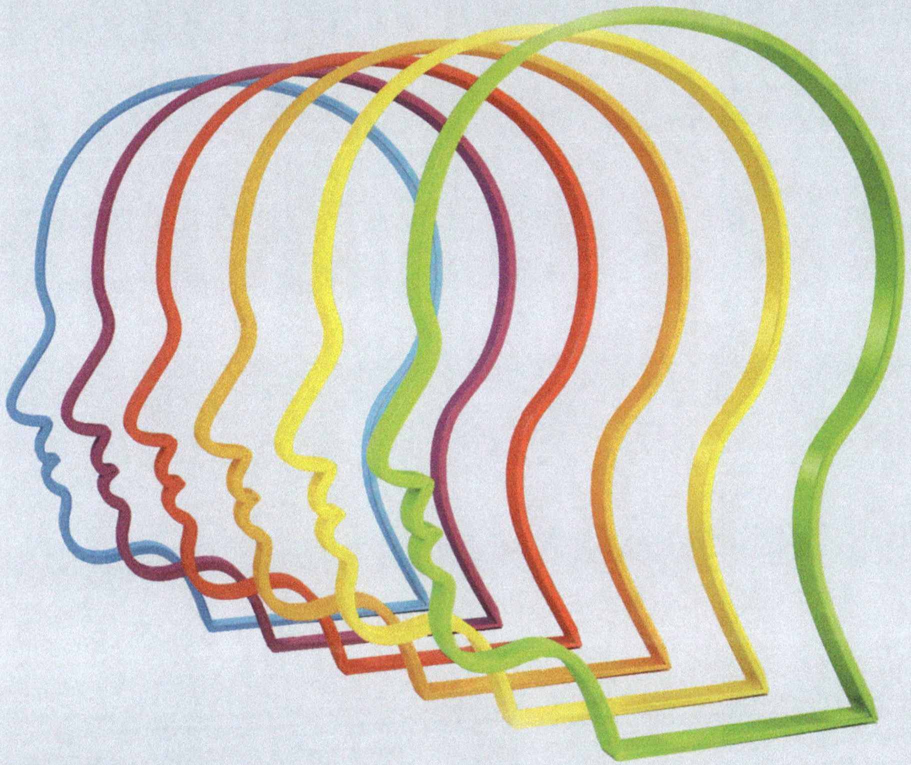

COMMON MENTAL HEALTH ISSUES

CASE STUDY 2

SCENARIO 1

Hank is a 35-year-old middle-class man living in Windsor, Ontario. In general, Hank drinks quite a bit (three or four nights a week) and this sometimes causes problems for him. Hank has a good job in sales, however, and he believes that drinking to the level that he does gives him many opportunities to schmooze with his clients. Great stories of drunken nights are what he is known for.

His wife says that he definitely causes her to worry, and she has seen him very hungover on mornings after his late-night social calls. She also isn't as impressed as his clients seem to be with some of the stories he tells her. She thinks it's not stuff to brag about and worries about how impulsively he acts when he is out on the town "having a good time."

Tonight, Hank is celebrating a night out with some old friends he has not seen since his days in college. His friends are in town for a sales conference and the timing worked out for everyone. Hank and his friends meet at a restaurant. They are dressed in business casual clothing: nice pants or designer dress jeans and collared shirts. Two of them are wearing sports jackets and one is wearing a well-made company windbreaker.

Hank and his wife got into a bit of an argument this evening before he went out, and, to Hank's credit, he does feel bad about some of the things he said. It has been a few hours since the argument took place though, and Hank is feeling great; he makes a mental note to text his wife later. He has had seven drinks so far … or is it eight? He doesn't quite remember.

Hank tells his friends about a pub that shows soccer games from all over the world, and since they used to play a lot of soccer in college, it seems like the right place for them to end their night.

Because they are so drunk, they decide to walk to the pub, not realizing how long it will take. Hank soon realizes that he should have used the washroom prior to leaving for the pub. He tells his buddies to wait for a second and goes into an alley to relieve himself. While in the alley, he remembers that he had wanted to text his wife.

When he takes out his phone, the light from it is noticed by the owner of the building Hank is relieving himself on and the owner comes out and starts to yell at Hank. Hank is embarrassed and flustered, and apologizes as he finishes urinating. He tries to explain what he's doing and when the building owner threatens to call the police, Hank offers him the 30 dollars he has left in his wallet.

Hank's friends come over to apologize for Hank, and the owner, seeing that Hank and his buddies are quite drunk and a little intimidating but friendly, just tells them to get off his property and leave the area. The building owner goes inside and Hank and his friends get to the pub and have a bit of a laugh about Hank always getting into these situations when he is drinking.

SCENARIO 2

Sendhil is a 48-year-old male who also lives in Windsor, Ontario. He served in the military for eight years and has been living with post-traumatic stress disorder (PTSD) after acquiring two injuries in combat that forced him out of service. Originally from North Bay, Sendhil moved to Windsor for a security job in the hospitality industry.

Sendhil feels quite isolated living in Windsor. The loneliness and all the transitions in his life led to a great deal of stress, depression, and anxiety for him. His work started to suffer and he was let go soon after suffering a panic attack at work. Sendhil has a hard time buying into mental health programs—his personal beliefs and a very poor experience with a psychologist as he was leaving the armed forces have cemented that view. He thought about seeking some sort of help when he began to feel things in his life slip while he was working, but did not know where to turn because he wasn't connected with any mental health or helping professionals in Windsor.

Things got worse as Sendhil's money ran out. There was trouble when he acted out aggressively during a meeting with Ontario Works. He regretted his verbal outburst, but was overcome with frustration at the red tape and hoops he had to jump through to get help with his search for employment. Soon after this, he was evicted from his apartment for nonpayment of rent. He lived in a motel for a while, but has now been living on the streets for four years, staying some nights at a local shelter.

These days, Sendhil spends most of his time downtown because of the access to meal programs and shelters. Being downtown provides good opportunities for him to panhandle. One Saturday night when he had to relieve himself he was going to try to use a washroom inside a pub where he has had some success in the past, but decided against it because it the entranceway was unusually busy. Instead, he headed for the alley behind the pub.

A cook on his way out to take a break came out the back entrance while Sendhil was urinating in the alley. The cook started making loud, rude comments to Sendhil, who began to swear at the cook. Police who were on patrol came onto the scene after hearing the shouting.

Sendhil started to experience the feelings of panic he gets during times of stress, and when an officer got close to Sendhil, the officer saw how agitated he was. The cook was fairly calm but was smirking at Sendhil, which infuriated the already exasperated man. The police officer closest to Sendhil noticed that one of his hands was balled into a fist. The officer asked Sendhil to desist and walk out of the alley with him.

Sendhil started shaking and breathing heavily while muttering under his breath. Some swearing was heard through the muttering, and the situation escalated, resulting in Sendhil being arrested for uttering threats. He was taken away in the back of a cruiser as the cook gave his statement about what had happened to an officer who remained behind.

QUESTIONS

1. What are some of the warning signs that Hank displays that he may be living with some mental health issues?
2. What were some of the key factors that led Hank and Sendhil to have different experiences (Hank with a member of the public and Sendhil with members of the justice system) and outcomes despite both of them committing the same initial offence?
3. Where do you see Hank's story going over time? And what about Sendhil's story; how do you think he will end up?

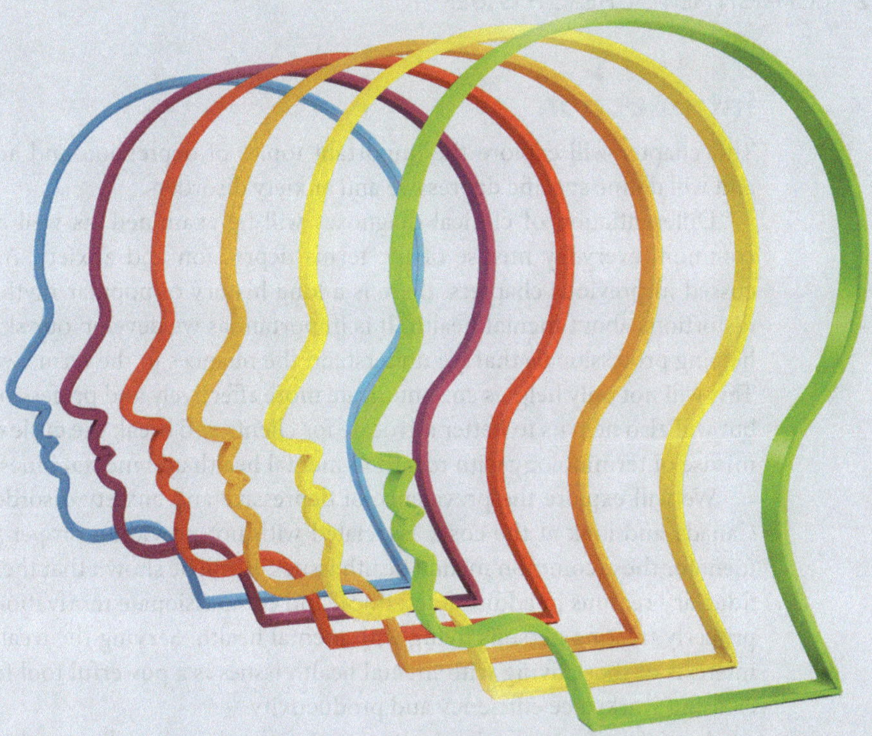

4 DEPRESSION AND ANXIETY

LEARNING OUTCOMES

After reading this chapter, you will be able to:

- Define depression and anxiety and describe their symptoms.
- Categorize a variety of types of depressive disorders and anxiety disorders.
- Identify common misconceptions about depression and anxiety.
- Use effective terminology to describe mental health.
- Define and understand the concepts of absenteeism and presenteeism.
- Differentiate between current best practices with regard to depression and anxiety.
- Select practical options for successful work with individuals who are living with depression and/or anxiety.

Introduction

This chapter will explore the important topics of depression and anxiety and will define specific depressive and anxiety disorders.

Differentiation of clinical diagnoses will be examined, as well as the common, everyday misuse of the terms depression and anxiety. As discussed in previous chapters, there is a long history of popular myths and distortions about mental health. It is important as we develop our skills as helping professionals that we understand the nuances in the terms we use. This will not only help us communicate more effectively and professionally, but will also help us to better advocate for clients and break the cycle of the misuse of terminology with regard to mental health and mental illness.

We will explore the prevalence of depressive and anxiety disorders in Canada and look at the costs associated with not providing proper treatment for these common mental health issues. It will be shown that there are fiduciary reasons in addition to ethical and compassionate motivations for properly treating persons living with mental health. Serving the treatment interests of those living with mental health issues is a powerful tool for increasing workplace efficiency and productivity.

A brief look at effective treatments for the disorders discussed in the chapter will be given, as well as a focus on practical help that front-line professionals can provide to aid persons who are living with these disorders.

You will learn through this chapter that, because they are relatively common, depression and anxiety are difficult, taxing, and expensive issues for Canadian society as a whole. Keep in mind as you read this chapter that there are effective treatments for persons living with these disorders. It is regrettable that so many individuals have to live with these specific mental health issues. However, in Canada, resources for help are widely available, including person-to-person medical and counselling services, therapeutic groups, and even online and telephone assistance. Studying this chapter will grow your skills for helping others who may find themselves living with depression and/or anxiety.

Understanding Depression

> That's the thing about depression: a human being can survive almost anything, as long as she sees the end in sight. But depression is so insidious, and it compounds daily, that it's impossible to ever see the end. The fog is like a cage without a key.
>
> —Elizabeth Wurtzel, *Prozac Nation* (1995)

You might say something like, "I'm so depressed because my favourite restaurant moved across town."

But you're not depressed, you're inconvenienced. You might be frustrated and you could even be sad, but chances are you are not feeling depression in this instance. Many of us often misuse the words "depressed" and "depression." Over time, the use of a technical term can become popularized and the correct meaning will be lost.

This often happens with language. For example, a brand name like Kleenex or Band-Aid will be used to refer to tissues or bandages. People don't mean to downplay or water down terms that are meant to describe serious or specific mental health issues, but the words become part of everyday language. Those who work in the helping professions must become aware of this misuse of language.

depression or depressive disorder feelings of sadness, hopelessness, low self-worth, and/or reduced ability to enjoy previously enjoyable daily activities that persists for a period of longer than two weeks

mood disorder psychological disorder that is marked by an elevation and/or lowering of a person's mood that interferes with daily functioning

Depression or depressive disorder is the most common **mood disorder** in Canada and is sometimes also called clinical depression, major depression, or major depressive disorder (Public Health Agency of Canada, 2016) (see Figure 4.1). In 2012, according to Statistics Canada, 11.3 percent of Canadians identified symptoms that met the criteria for depression within their lifetime (Pearson, Janz, & Ali, 2013). The World Health Organization recently reported that major depressive disorder is the fourth largest contributor to the global burden of disease, and it believes depression will become the second largest burden by 2030 (Mathers & Loncar, 2006). Studies show that depression increases the likelihood of individuals reporting that they have "limitations in self-support care, more disability days, more productivity loss-related costs, poorer physical and emotional health, and an increased use of health services" (Gili et al., 2013).

When individuals live with untreated or ill-treated depression it results in massive costs for workplaces and the economy. In 2016, the Conference Board of Canada studied this issue in great depth and recommended that improved treatment of depression and anxiety disorders would boost the Canadian economy by nearly $50 billion (Sutherland & Stonebridge, 2016).

The understanding of the extent of mental health costs to society continues to grow. Failure to meet the

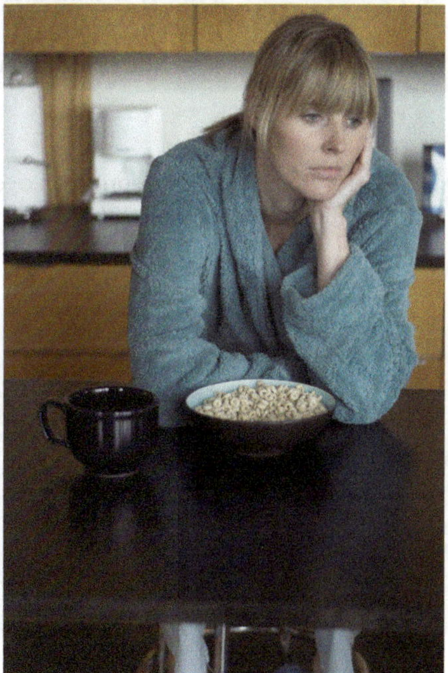

Over 10 percent of Canadians have symptoms of depression, including having a depressed mood for over two weeks that interferes with quality of life.

absenteeism missing work, school, or other responsibilities

presenteeism attending work, school, or other responsibilities but with reduced productivity because of mental or physical illness

mental health needs of organizations and employees can seriously affect productivity due to **absenteeism** and **presenteeism**. While these terms can be used in relation to individuals living with a variety of mental health issues, absenteeism and presenteeism will be used in this chapter as they relate to depression and anxiety because these disorders are prevalent in Canada.

The term absenteeism may be heard often because it is used in both schools and workplaces. When someone misses school, a class, a work shift, or an official function he or she was supposed to attend, he or she may be marked or labelled as "absent," and when this occurs with any regularity it is an obvious cause for concern. A fairly new concept that is being applied by human resource departments and mental health experts across the country is the idea of "presenteeism."

Presenteeism occurs when someone attends his or her work, school, or other function when he or she is ill, but does so with a reduced level of productivity. A person who come to work with the flu will likely be indisposed and unproductive for large portions of his or her workday. The same thing can occur with mental health concerns. Further, because of perceived stigma, a person might be less willing to admit that he or she is struggling with a mental health issue, and this can affect recovery.

FIGURE 4.1 Rates of Depression over 12 Months,[1] by Age and Sex, Canada, Household Population 15 and Older, 2012

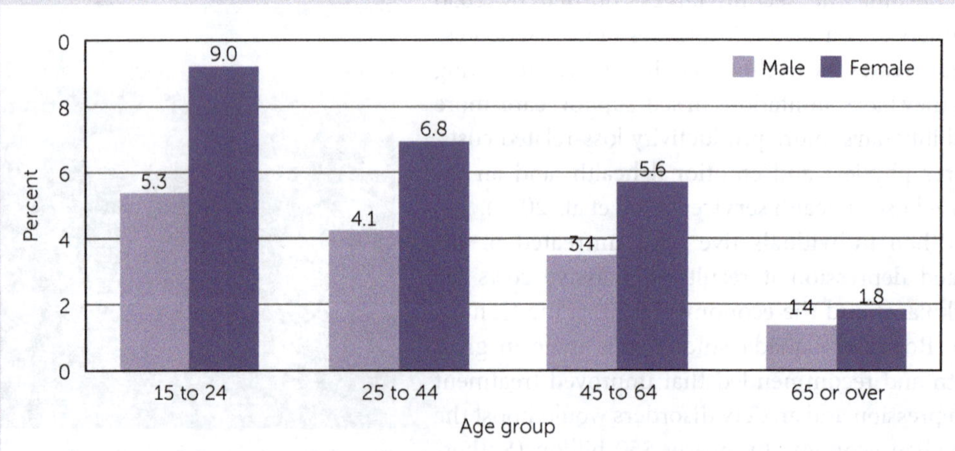

1. Respondents were classified with depression if they met the criteria for this condition in the 12 months prior to the survey.

Source: Pearson, Janz, & Ali, 2013.

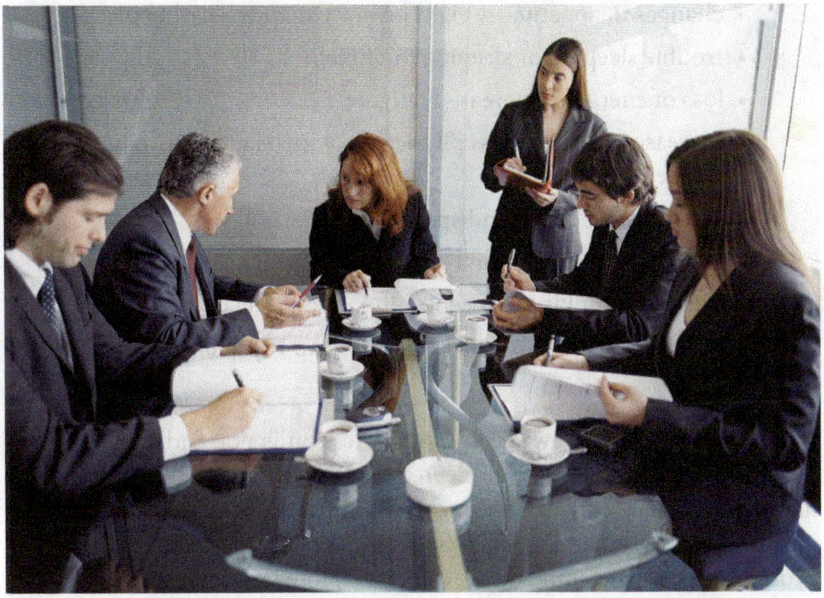

Depression, anxiety, and other mental health disorders cost Canada billions of dollars a year in lost productivity from absenteeism and presenteeism.

Imagine coming to work every day while living with a moderate or severe mental issue and attempting to hide it. In a study looked at by the Conference Board of Canada in its recent report it was estimated that presenteeism due to major depressive disorder alone could cut worker productivity by one-quarter in a given year. That is equal to 60 working days missed in a year because of presenteeism, in addition to days actually missed through absenteeism (Sutherland & Stonebridge, 2016).

The Conference Board of Canada made four strong recommendations to improve mental health outcomes for working Canadians in order to stem the longer-term costs of mental illness: improved treatments, improved workplace programs, initiatives to better integrate those unable to work, and improved integration of services and care (Sutherland & Stonebridge, 2016).

According to the American Psychiatric Association's latest edition of the *Diagnostic and Statistical Manual of Mental Disorders* (the "DSM-5"), the criteria for depression can include a variety of the following symptoms if they occur for two weeks or more:

- feeling sad or having a depressed mood;
- loss of interest or pleasure in activities once enjoyed;

- changes in appetite—weight loss or gain unrelated to dieting;
- trouble sleeping or sleeping too much;
- loss of energy or increased fatigue;
- increase in purposeless physical activity (e.g., hand-wringing or pacing);
- slowed movements and speech;
- feeling worthless or guilty;
- difficulty thinking, concentrating, or making decisions; and
- thoughts of death or suicide (American Psychiatric Association, 2013).

We also need to be aware of what depression is not. Sadness, grief, and feelings of bereavement are not depression. If you were to lose a loved one, have a relationship end, or get downsized from your workplace it would be a normal response to feel grief or sadness. While sadness or the **grieving process** might share some of the same symptoms as depression and while grief can become particularly intense, it is important to note the differences.

grieving process normal process through which an individual deals with the loss of something or someone from their life

Again, the American Psychiatric Association's DSM-5 can be consulted, this time for a succinct description of the differences between depression and grief:

- In grief, painful feelings come in waves, often intermixed with positive memories of the deceased. In major depression, mood and/or interest (pleasure) are decreased for most of a period of two weeks.
- In grief, self-esteem is usually maintained. In major depression, feelings of worthlessness and self-loathing are common.
- For some people, the death of a loved one can bring on major depression. Losing a job or being a victim of a physical assault or a major disaster can lead to depression for some people. When grief and depression co-exist, the grief is more severe and lasts longer than grief without depression. Despite some overlap between grief and depression, they are different. Distinguishing between them can help people get the help, support, and treatment they need (American Psychiatric Association, 2013).

Whether the person you are speaking or working with has depression or grief, many of the tactics explored later in this chapter will be helpful. See Scenario 4.1 to find out why it is important to discern which issue the person may be suffering from.

SCENARIO 4.1

A Lesson in Describing to Other Professionals What We Have Observed

Imagine that you are a child and youth worker who has had to call the police to deal with a young girl (Evie) in your care who has become increasingly hostile and violent, and has begun to describe things that are not happening around her as though they are real.

You call the police because there has been a great deal of property damage, threats of violence, and other inappropriate behaviour. Over the course of this incident, it becomes clear that you and the officer will be travelling with Evie to a nearby hospital to assess her mental health.

At the hospital, Evie has begun to calm down while waiting in a small room in which a mental health nurse is assessing her, with the police nearby to protect Evie and the other people involved in this situation. The nurse asks you some questions privately about her background. You explain that Evie experienced a bad home-visit earlier that week and has been quite sad since then.

You tell the nurse that Evie has depression. Not having other records available, the nurse believes that you mean clinical depression (two weeks of depressed mood or more, not related to a normal grieving process). Evie chooses to not respond when the nurse tries to interview her. Intake into the hospital occurs with very little input from Evie.

Discussion Questions

1. What is the problem in this scenario?
2. How has the child and youth worker misrepresented Evie?
3. Is it possible that decisions will be made at the hospital that might not be the right fit because Evie's symptoms were initially misunderstood? If so, what might those decisions be?

While depression can affect anyone, there are some risk factors that may help you in the assessment process and in a fuller understanding of the disorder. These may work in correlation with each other or one factor may be particularly strong for a person living with depression. Knowing these factors can also help to reduce the stigma associated with depression.

Factors that play a role in the disorder include human biochemistry (chemicals in the brain), genetics (family history of depression), personality (stress tolerance, self-esteem, and pessimism), and environmental factors (poverty, abuse, neglect, and exposure to violence). Be they external or internal factors, we can see how each of these can help to explain why some people are more vulnerable to depression than others (American Psychiatric Association, 2013). In the same way, we can also look at these factors

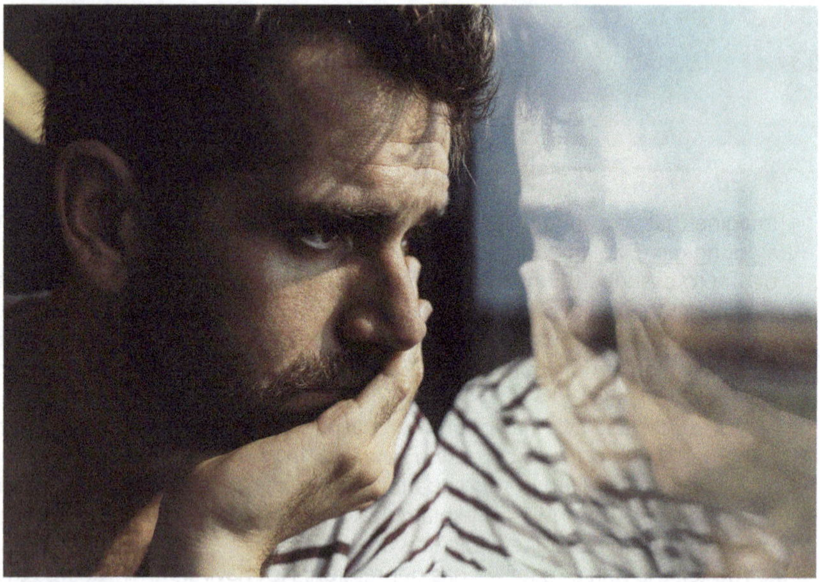

Many factors play a role in depression, including biochemistry, genetics, personality, and environmental issues such as poverty and exposure to violence.

and flip them to see potential assets for the client. One example could be that of a person who has depression but also has strong and positive personality traits. While they might still be vulnerable to the disorder, they might also be able to use these assets to help cope with depression, to seek out counselling, or to communicate their needs effectively.

Depressive Disorders

Now that you know the differences between grief, sadness, and depression, let's take a look at a variety of depressive disorders and what they might help you communicate to other professionals and the affected individuals that you'll be working with.

- **Persistent depressive disorder** is also sometimes called dysthymia and occurs when mood is depressed for two years or more. This may look like major depression for periods of time, followed by symptoms that are more manageable and less severe but that still interrupt the patterns of daily life such as sleep, work, and other regular functioning.

- **Psychotic depression** adds symptoms of psychosis that co-occur with severe depressive mood. For example, a person may find themselves having delusional thoughts or even hallucinating while being depressed. In this state, the delusions and hallucinations tend to be marked by depressive themes that include hopelessness and guilt. The person may at first find him- or herself to be severely depressed and over the course of that depression they will hear voices telling them they are worthless, or have delusions that they are an oppressed historical figure.
- **Seasonal affective disorder (SAD)** sees depressed mood generally occurring in the winter when there are fewer natural opportunities to be exposed to sunlight. With SAD, people become depressed and withdraw from their normal social activities, oversleep, and gain weight during the winter months in a way that doesn't usually happen to them in summer. Sometimes SAD is treated using **light therapy**: the person is instructed to spend time in front of electric lights that are designed to approximate the mood enhancing properties of natural sunlight.
- **Bipolar disorder** is a mood disorder that causes persons living with it to have very low moods that meet the criteria for major depression, but they also experience euphoric highs that are referred to as **mania**. In the manic state, a person living with this disorder may feel invincible, act recklessly, or report very high levels of productivity that would not be achievable within their normal or baseline mood. A person on a manic high might also, conversely, find him- or herself being irritable and have rushing thoughts.
- **Disruptive mood dysregulation disorder** is diagnosed in children who exhibit frequent and intense outbursts of temper, anger, and irritability nearly every day for at least 12 months. This behaviour goes well above moodiness or tantrums, which are a normal part of childhood, and instead requires a clinical response because it tends to impair functioning in more than one place the child frequents. For example, this disorder may cause a child to have poor relationships and poor function at both school and at home.
- **Premenstrual dysphoric disorder (PMDD)** is a severe form of premenstrual syndrome that follows similar patterns of timing, starting 7 to 10 days before a monthly period. While most women

light therapy
method of treating seasonal affective disorder (SAD) that uses exposure to artificial light that approximates sunlight; sometimes referred to as phototherapy

mania
symptom of bipolar disorder that is characterized as a state of persistent and abnormally elevated arousal or mood that can have characteristics of both euphoria and irritability

report some degree of emotional disruption during this time, approximately 5 percent of women experience severe emotional symptomology that can manifest as severe depression, irritability, anxiety, insomnia, and other issues that interfere with the normal activities of daily life. Approximately 15 percent of women who live with PMDD attempt suicide (Harvard Mental Health Letter, 2017).

BOX 4.1 PREGNANCY AND DEPRESSION

Perinatal depression was recently also known as postpartum depression and is sometimes confused with "baby blues," but is far more serious. While baby blues tends to clear within a week or two after giving birth, women who experience perinatal depression have a severe depression during or after delivery. Extreme sadness, exhaustion, and anxiety can overwhelm a mother and undermine her ability to take care of her newborn child and herself. Additionally, severe agitation, suicidal thoughts, and fear of hurting the child or lack of interest in the newborn child may appear alongside obsessive thoughts (Meltzer-Brody, 2011).

In its 2009 report, *What Mothers Say: The Canadian Maternity Experiences Survey*, the Public Health Agency of Canada note that baby blues occurs in up to 80 percent of women, while more severe depression occurs in 10 to 20 percent of women and begins in the first year after giving birth to a child, and can last for months and sometimes years. Psychosis after delivery is rare, but does occur in 0.2 percent of women who give birth in Canada (Bartholomew et al., 2009, p. 206).

Predictors can include depression and anxiety while pregnant, stressful life events beyond the pregnancy, lack of access to social supports, a history of depression, hormonal changes, a negative birth experience, lack of experience with babies, stress in relationships, number of children, and age (Bartholomew, 2009).

Treatment for this depressive disorder can be difficult because prescribing medication during pregnancy can result in complications with and potential risks for the pregnancy. Even after delivery there are potential risks to the child because of exposure to antidepressants in breast milk. However, providing no treatment may also result in risks to the mother and child (Meltzer-Brody, 2011).

Discussion Questions

1. How might someone living with a mental health disorder feel if, because of a pregnancy, he or she had to suspend use of medication that had been working?
2. What might be some of the complications that could occur due to this scenario?
3. What would you find helpful to hear if you were in that situation?

A Primer on Anxiety

Panic is, usually, a sudden going over to the enemy of our imagination.

—Christian Nestell Bovee (1862)

Anxiety and depression are often linked in public health announcements, pamphlets, and books because of their commonality. While it was estimated that in 2012 nearly 3.5 million Canadians over the age of 15 had symptoms consistent with a mood disorder such as depression, 2.4 million Canadians were estimated to have symptomology consistent with generalized anxiety disorder (six months or more of excessive anxiety and worry, with symptoms such as fatigue and concentration issues) within their lifetime (Pearson, Janz, & Ali, 2013).

In 2014, the federal government undertook the Survey on Living with Chronic Diseases in Canada. This was the first time a national survey was created to collect information "on the experiences of Canadians with professionally diagnosed mood and/or anxiety disorders" (Toews, McRae, & O'Donnell, 2016). While physical health diseases such as cancer and diabetes have received numerous federal studies, there have been many fewer

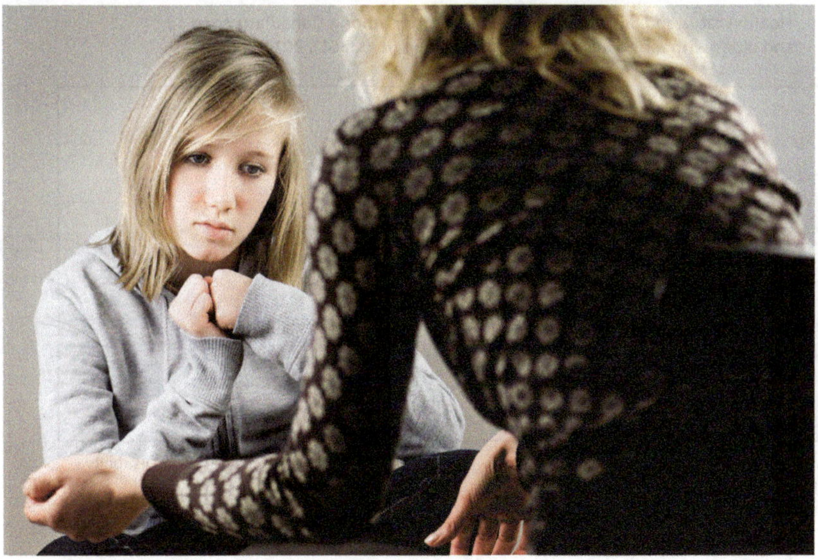

Anxiety is a serious and common mental health issue that presents in a variety of ways and can be misunderstood as shyness.

perinatal depression
severe depression during or after giving birth that involves extreme sadness, exhaustion, and anxiety; also known as postpartum depression

predictor
piece of data that is used to foretell some aspect of future well-being; for example, if individuals with more education tended to have greater economic opportunities, education would be said to be a good predictor of economic opportunity—this does not mean everyone with an education is well off or that everyone without one is poor, but that trends exist that show one is a good predictor of the other

anxiety
disorder characterized by excessive, intrusive, and persistent fear, uneasiness, and apprehension; may also include elements of obsessive and/or compulsive behaviours and panic

studies of mental health diseases with the result that up-to-date information about the prevalence of anxiety and mood disorders in Canada is not easily available.

We do know that addiction (to be covered in Chapter 5), mood disorders, and anxiety disorders affect most Canadians. This may be why mood disorders and anxiety disorders are often found mentioned together in promotional material and literature.

Another reason they are often found mentioned together is the high co-occurrence of mood and anxiety disorders. In the 2014 Survey on Living with Chronic Diseases in Canada study, 31.5 percent of respondents self-reported having both a mood and an anxiety disorder. Furthermore, those who reported having both mood and anxiety disorders were also more likely to report worse general and mental health, more limitations on their activities, more restrictions or modifications required at work, and were more likely to report severe disability (Loukine, O'Donnell, Goldner, McRae, & Allen, 2016) (see Figures 4.2 and 4.3).

FIGURE 4.2 Health Status and Disability

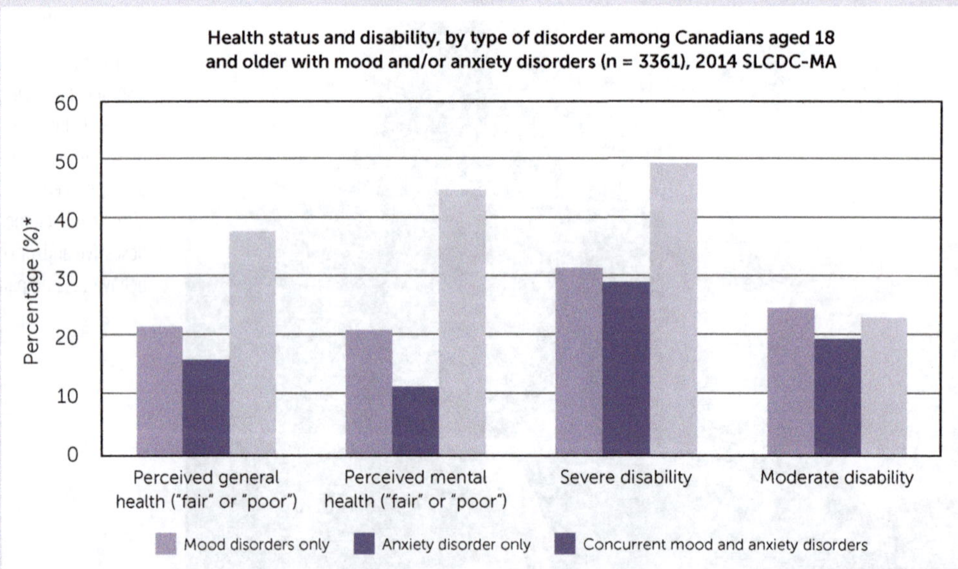

Abbreviation: SLCDC-MA, Survey on Living with Chronic Diseases in Canada—Mood and Anxiety Disorders Component.

* Percentages are based on weighted numbers to reflect the Canadian population aged 18 years and older with mood and/or anxiety disorders living in the 10 provinces.

Source: O'Donnell, Cheung, Bennett, & Lagacé, 2016.

Depression and anxiety are often misunderstood, as shown in the example in Evie's story in Scenario 4.1, above. It is not unusual to overhear people who have some manageable stress, nervousness, or fear throw around phrases like "my anxiety is so bad today" or "I'm very anxious about my exams." This is not done to purposely diminish the impact of clinical anxiety, but is more often done out of a lack of understanding about this mental health issue.

Because these phrases are used so often it can be argued that the power of these words has been diminished. It can also be argued that words like depression and anxiety have become less taboo and more available to those running awareness campaigns. Because most of us have experienced stress, fear, and nervousness, we feel as though we can understand something like anxiety far more readily than some other mental health issues.

FIGURE 4.3 Activity Limitations

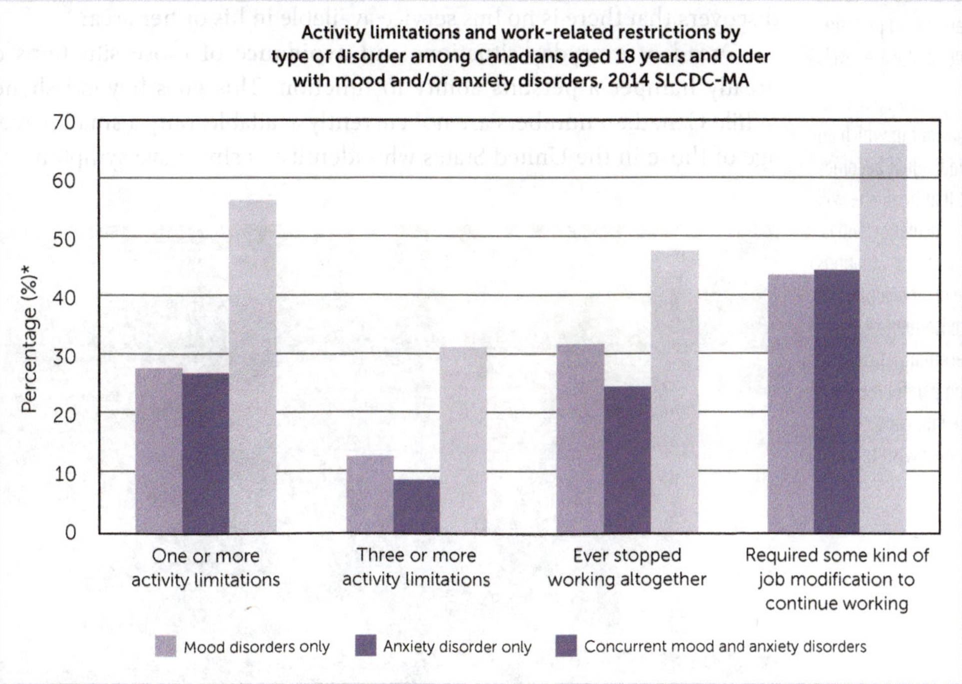

Abbreviation: SLCDC-MA, Survey on Living with Chronic Diseases in Canada—Mood and Anxiety Disorders Component.

* Percentages are based on weighted numbers to reflect the Canadian population aged 18 years and older with mood and/or anxiety disorders living in the 10 provinces.

Source: O'Donnell et al., 2016.

To someone who has had a panic attack or lives with a diagnosable anxiety disorder, the common use of the term "anxiety" does not capture adequately what they may be feeling and living with day to day. The remainder of this chapter is meant to help illuminate these issues and provide a better understanding of what anxiety and anxiety disorders are like to live with, and how to cope and help others cope with this disease.

Normal amounts of anxiety can be useful. Being reasonably worried about an exam might lead someone to study without distractions and take the process more seriously. A normal fear response in a threatening situation can help save a person's life. An example of this would be the **fight-or-flight response** protecting a person's body from danger in a hostile situation.

fight-or-flight response
acute response to stress during which a physiological reaction occurs in response to an event that is perceived as harmful or threatening; may include increased cortisol in the body and increased heart rate, blood pressure, and blood glucose levels

What happens when anxiety spikes without an obvious reason? What if someone becomes extremely anxious and fearful during a needed and routine activity, such as a medical procedure (for example, the person reacts violently toward a nurse who is trying to administer a flu shot)? What happens to a person with anxiety who works out of town and has a serious car accident that results in strong anxiety toward driving when that person discovers that there is no bus service available in his or her area?

Dread of everyday situations and **avoidance** of those situations can greatly hamper a person's ability to function. This goes beyond shyness. While Canadian numbers are not currently available, only a small percentage of those in the United States who identify as shy "have symptoms that

avoidance
behaviour in which an individual becomes insistent that he or she will avoid particular activities, environments, or situations because of a perception of negative consequences (such as becoming anxious or experiencing painful feelings) if they come into contact with the things they wish to avoid

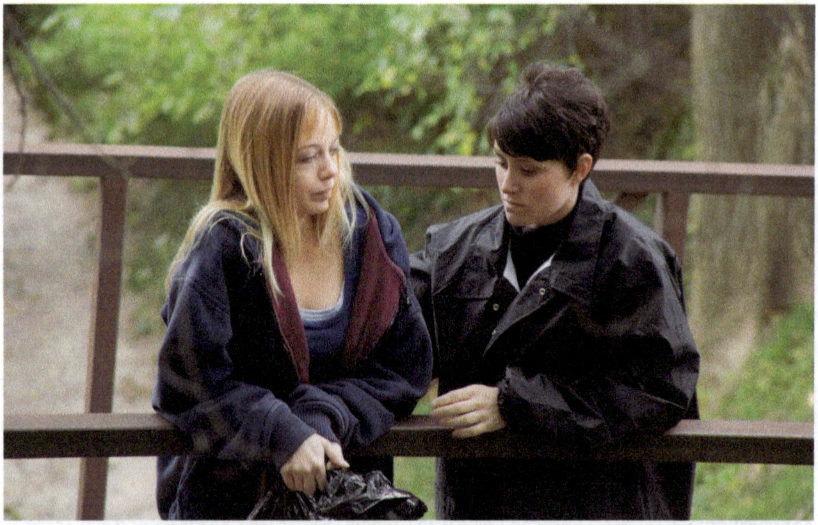

A helping professional can make a huge difference in the life of someone who is struggling. Non-judgmental listening is a valuable skill in helping those in need.

meet the diagnostic criteria for social anxiety disorder" (American Psychiatric Association, 2013). While some levels of anxiety are normal and even helpful, people who live with anxiety disorders tend to have intrusive thoughts and concerns that reoccur and are unhelpful in social situations and in carrying out activities in daily life.

Anxiety Disorders

There are numerous types of anxiety disorders. As with depressive disorders, identifying the specific types of anxiety a person is feeling can lead to insights for treatment and can also serve to educate the general public on the facts of those disorders rather than perpetuating the spread of the myths that exist about them. It is important to note that all these disorders share traits of disproportionate and intense fear and insistent, prolonged worry for those living with them. They are also only considered to be disorders when they create significant distress for the person living with the mental health issue and impair daily living.

The five anxiety disorders listed below have been defined by the Public Health Agency of Canada and will be seen when working in the helping professions:

- **Generalized anxiety disorder:** Excessive anxiety and worry about a number of events or activities that occurs on more days than it does not during a period of at least six months, with associated symptoms such as fatigue and poor concentration.
- **Social anxiety disorder**: Exposure to social or performance situations that almost invariably provokes an immediate anxiety response that may include palpitations, tremors, sweating, gastrointestinal discomfort, diarrhoea, muscle tension, blushing, or confusion, and which may meet the criteria for a panic attack in severe cases.
- **Post-traumatic stress disorder:** Flashbacks, persistent frightening thoughts and memories, anger or irritability in response to a terrifying experience in which physical harm occurred or was threatened (such as rape, child abuse, war, or natural disaster).
- **Panic disorder:** The presence of recurrent, unexpected panic attacks, followed by at least one month of persistent concern about having additional attacks, worry about the implications of an attack or its consequences, or a significant change in behaviour related to attacks. There are three clusters of symptoms: re-experiencing, avoidance and numbing, and arousal.

Panic disorders are sometimes associated with agoraphobia, which is anxiety about, or the avoidance of, places or situations from which escape might be difficult or embarrassing, or in which help may not be available in the event of a panic attack or panic-like symptoms.

The essential feature of a panic attack is a discrete period of intense fear or discomfort that is accompanied by at least four of the following 13 physical symptoms:

- palpitations, increased heart rate, or pounding heart;
- sweating;
- trembling or shaking;
- sensation of shortness of breath or smothering;
- feeling of choking;
- chest pain or discomfort;
- nausea or abdominal distress;
- dizziness, unsteadiness, light-headedness, or fainting;
- de-realization or de-personalization;
- fear of losing control or going crazy;
- fear of dying;
- paresthesia (numbness or tingling sensation);
- chills or hot flashes.

- **Obsessive-compulsive disorder:**
  - **Obsessions:** Persistent thoughts, ideas, impulses, or images that are intrusive and inappropriate and that cause marked anxiety or distress. Individuals with obsessions usually attempt to ignore or suppress such thoughts or impulses or to counteract them with other thoughts or actions (compulsions).
  - **Compulsions:** Repetitive behaviours (such as handwashing, ordering, or checking) or mental acts (such as praying, counting, or repeating words) that occur in response to an obsession or are carried out in a ritualistic way.
  - **Specific phobia:** Marked and persistent fear of clearly discernible objects or situations (such as flying, heights, and animals) (Public Health Agency of Canada, 2002).

Some additional forms of anxiety disorder you may come across while working in the helping professions include:

- **Agoraphobia:** Similar to but different from social anxiety disorder. While social anxiety disorder is focused on scrutiny from others, those living with agoraphobia will avoid social situations because they fear they will develop incapacitating panic-like symptoms and will find it very difficult to escape (American Psychiatric Association, 2013).

- **Separation anxiety:** This disorder will manifest itself as avoidance of social settings because of worries around separation from attachment figures. For example, a child might refuse to go to school if he or she suffers from this disorder. Persons with separation anxiety disorder are often comfortable socially if the person their attachment is fixated on is present (American Psychiatric Association, 2013).

Tips and Treatments for Working with People Who Are Living with Depression and/or Anxiety

Depression and anxiety can be very difficult for those living with either or both disorders. They can also provide challenges for those in the helping professions. While registered social workers, psychotherapists, and psychiatric professionals will use a variety of treatments there is still a great deal that other helping professionals can do to be of service in these situations.

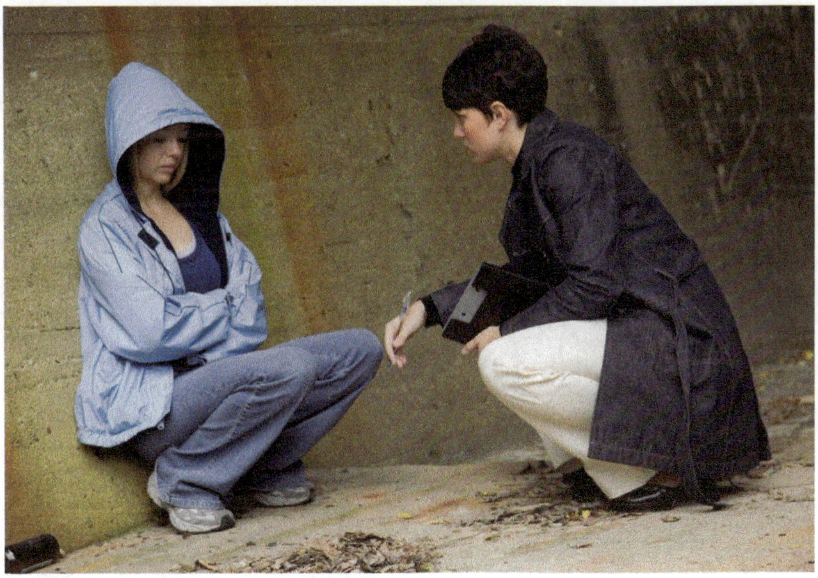

Those in the helping professions sometimes meet people where they are, emotionally, and sometimes geographically.

For example, anyone can offer emotional support to someone struggling with these issues. By truly and actively listening in a non-judgmental manner you can help someone feel heard and start the person moving forward toward more appropriate mental health supports.

active listening form of communication that is helpful in a variety of therapeutic situations; it involves listening to another individual with full concentration and encouraging that person with verbal and non-verbal cues to demonstrate that the listener is paying close attention to what is being said; also sometimes called intentional listening

minimal encouragers subtle verbal ("uh huh") and non-verbal actions (nods, open and attentive posture) that make speakers feel comfortable and listened to

open-ended questions questions that cannot be answered with a yes or no response; fuller and more meaningful answers are encouraged: "how did that make you feel?" is an example

closed questions questions that can usually be answered very briefly or by a yes or no response; for example "when is your birthday?" and "did you bring your lunch to school?" are closed questions

Active listening is a skill that all helping professionals would do well to learn and use in a variety of places in their work, including when working with people living with a mental health issue. Some have described active listening as a "dynamic and interactive process" that goes beyond listening with your ears to using your entire focus as well as showing the other person that you are approaching them with "attention, understanding, [and] empathy" while assessing and using verbal and non-verbal communication (Fradelos & Staikos, 2013).

People show that they are actively listening when they use an appropriate amount of eye contact; are in a listening posture (facing the other person and attentive); and use **minimal encouragers** such as nodding or saying things such as "uh huh," "wow," or "tell me more." Active listeners also allow silence in the conversations they hold so that both sides can take the time to reflect on what is being said, and they make skillful use of **open-ended** and **closed questions**, are adept at **paraphrase**, and can **summarize** a conversation well.

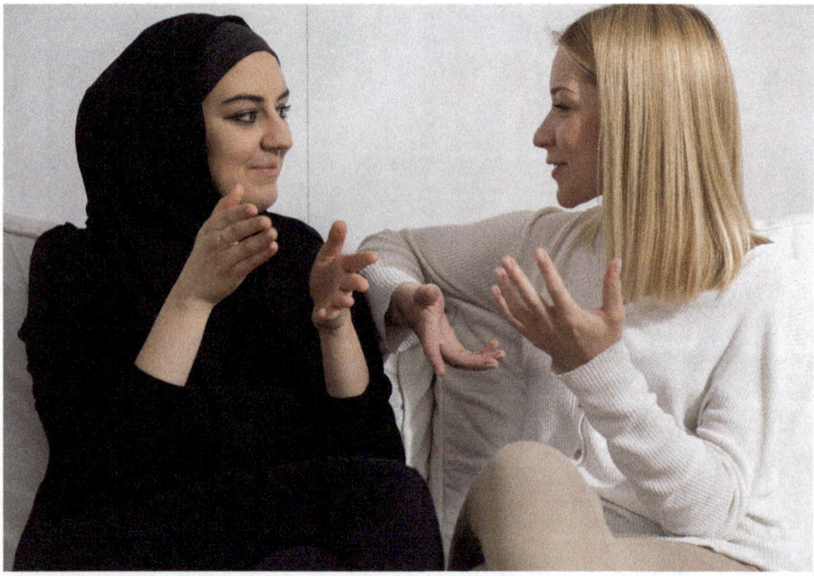

Depression and anxiety are common mental health issues in North America that can affect anyone. Active listening, which takes practice, is a valued skill in the helping professions.

Active listening has been shown time and time again to be a very helpful factor in client satisfaction for many helping professionals across the mental health field, including nurses and other hospital staff, counsellors at telephone crisis centres, those who work with adolescents, and the police (Best, 2008; Coderoni, 2002; Fradelos & Staikos, 2013; Wong et al., 2007; Young, 1989).

paraphrasing restating an individual's words in a new way to demonstrate that he or she has been understood

summarization condensing and clarifying an individual's statements; this is helpful in expressing what has been said as a theme or in helping to draw a conversation or session to a close

No doubt you have spoken with someone who seems really and truly interested in you and what you have to say. Similarly, you've likely experienced the opposite treatment as well. People tend to feel better when they sense they have been heard as opposed to sitting across from someone who is looking at their watch or their interview questions. Imagine how important it would be to you that you were listened to if you were describing a difficult personal situation or your own mental health—especially if it was something you had not ever, or rarely, discussed.

It is important to listen non-judgmentally. People living with anxiety or depression may have made choices in life that you do not personally agree with. Judging individuals' actions as they share with you is not a positive action and does not help you to learn more about their situation or how they can be helped in that moment. While it can be difficult to put aside your personal feelings at times, exercising a non-judgmental attitude when speaking with vulnerable individuals is necessary in a helping relationship.

Even if you are not counselling someone (and only legally registered and qualified persons should be counselling people), you can still use the tenets of the best practices for creating a **therapeutic relationship** when working with people who are living with mental health disorders such as the depressive and anxiety disorders we've explored in this chapter.

therapeutic relationship relationship between an individual and a helping professional that aims to create beneficial changes in the life of the client; also sometimes called a therapeutic alliance or a helping alliance

Some of the best practices for a therapeutic relationship that may be helpful to adopt in the helping professions include having a positive regard for the individual (seeing him or her as worthy of caring about); taking a strengths-based approach (seeking and pointing out the individual's strengths); being genuine and honest; being aware of your own feelings while working with someone; and building rapport through trust, empathy, and hopefulness.

One of the ways to put a practical form of hopefulness to work is through helping the person find a pathway to an appropriate mental health resource in the long term. Letting someone who is living with a mental health issue know that he or she is part of a large group of people who have the same sorts of issues, and that treatment is available and has been known to work, shows a hopeful approach while also helping to provide a practical next step for the person.

medication/pharmacological treatments treatment using legal drugs recommended or prescribed by a medical professional

antidepressants prescription drugs used to treat depression

psychotherapy talk-therapy method used to treat mental disorders

cognitive behavioural therapy (CBT) structured form of talk therapy with a limited number of sessions that helps individuals build an awareness of distorted, negative, or inaccurate thought patterns; the focus of this style of therapy is to change behaviours and thinking to help solve problems

electroconvulsive therapy medical treatment that has been shown to be effective for treating clients with severe depressive disorders: brief electrical stimulation is focused on the brain while the person is under anaesthesia

self-help a variety of processes that are self-directed to improve health or well-being; methods may include using books, online resources, and peer-run support groups with some basis in psychology

Here are some resources, places, and people who can help guide the individuals you are working with:

- Individuals in crisis can talk to someone at a local crisis line or information line such as 211, the Kid's Help Phone, Tele-Health, or a crisis number in your community.
- If your community has drop-in counselling, you can suggest they go there and, if your agency allows for it, offer them transportation.
- Ask whether they would be willing to talk to their doctor, if they have one, and if not, a doctor at a local walk-in clinic.
- Ask whether they have or are currently seeing a social worker, therapist, or psychologist and whether they are willing to talk to that person about their current issues.
- Speak with members of your professional team to see whether there are other options available.
- If a crisis threatens the life or well-being of an individual, 911 or the police should be called.

It will be helpful to let the individuals you are working with know that there are many treatments and therapies that have been shown to work for the majority of those recovering from a depressive disorder; in fact, "between 80 and 90% of people with depression eventually respond well to treatment" and "almost all patients gain some relief from their symptoms" (American Psychiatric Association, 2017).

Some effective treatments for depression include **medication/pharmacological treatments** such as **antidepressants, psychotherapy** (talk therapy), **cognitive behavioural therapy (CBT)**, **electroconvulsive therapy**, **self-help**, and **coping** (American Psychiatric Association, 2017).

Treatment also plays an exceedingly important role in helping persons living with an anxiety disorder improve their quality of life. Meta-analyses of **individual therapy** and **group therapy** treatments for anxiety disorders have shown they can be effective for individuals who present symptoms. Encouraging clients to face their fears through **exposure therapy**, **mindfulness-based cognitive therapy (MBCT)** (which includes meditation, relaxation, and breathing control), and CBT has been shown to be effective. Self-help books and computer-based programs have also shown some effectiveness, as have some forms of pharmacological treatments (Katzman et al., 2014).

When working with individuals in longer-term settings (for example, in a residential-care environment), you should read the recommendations of their medical and mental health professionals and help the individuals abide by the plans set out for them.

coping
use of skills to help tolerate stresses and conflicts and make it easier to live with them

individual therapy
psychotherapy practised in a one-on-one process between a trained therapist and an individual

group therapy
psychotherapy practised in a group setting with a trained therapist guiding the sessions

exposure therapy
used in the treatment of anxiety disorders: an individual is gradually exposed to a feared object or situation while in a safe environment; exposure is increased in the hope of normalizing the object or situation to the individual, thereby, in time, extinguishing the phobia or anxiety

mindfulness-based cognitive therapy (MBCT)
form of psychotherapy that combines principles of CBT with education about a major depressive disorder as well as mindfulness training and meditation techniques

POINTS TO REMEMBER

- ✓ Depression and anxiety are not uncommon in Canada but can be commonly misunderstood because these terms, in an unfortunate but pronounced trend, are being inaccurately used. It is important to note that not all sadness is necessarily depression and not all anxiety is bad. Sometimes these feelings are normal and even helpful.
- ✓ However, there are specific depressive and anxiety disorders. People are complex, and it is possible for an individual to live with depressive and anxiety disorders concurrently.
- ✓ A variety of treatments have been shown to be fairly effective, over time, in treating mental health issues and improving the quality of life for those living with depression and/or anxiety, and in reducing absenteeism and presenteeism in individuals' daily lives.
- ✓ Developing active listening as a skill is something that all front-line helping professionals should do in order to build rapport with the individuals they are trying to help. Active listening has been shown to improve the outcome for individuals suffering from mental illnesses, so be sure to use the active listening skill development tips provided in this chapter.

KEY TERMS

absenteeism, 78
active listening, 92
antidepressants, 94
anxiety, 85
avoidance, 88
closed questions, 92
cognitive behavioural therapy (CBT), 94
coping, 95
depression or depressive disorder, 77
electroconvulsive therapy, 94
exposure therapy, 95
fight-or-flight response, 88
grieving process, 80
group therapy, 95
individual therapy, 95
light therapy, 83
mania, 83
medication/pharmacological treatments, 94
mindfulness-based cognitive therapy (MBCT), 95
minimal encouragers, 92
mood disorder, 77
open-ended questions, 92
paraphrasing, 93
perinatal depression, 85
predictor, 85
presenteeism, 78
psychotherapy, 94
self-help, 94
summarization, 93
therapeutic relationship, 93

REFERENCES

American Psychiatric Association. (2013). *Diagnostic and statistical manual of mental disorders* (5th ed.). Washington, DC: Author.

American Psychiatric Association. (2017). What is depression? *Patients & Families: Depression*. Retrieved from https://www.psychiatry.org/patients-families/depression/what-is-depression

Bartholomew, S., Boscoe, M., Chalmers, B., Dzakpasu, S., Fell, D., Heaman, M., … Young, D. (2009). *What mothers say: The Canadian maternity experiences survey*. Ottawa: Public Health Agency of Canada. Retrieved from http://www.phac-aspc.gc.ca/rhs-ssg/pdf/survey-eng.pdf

Best, A. (2008). Adolescent mental health. *Nursing Standard*, *22*(33), 59.

Bovee, C.N. (1862). *Intuitions and summaries of thought* (Vol. 2). Cambridge: Riverside Press.

Coderoni, G.R. (2002). The relationship between multicultural training for police and effective law enforcement. *FBI Law Enforcement Bulletin*, *71*(11), 16–18.

Fradelos, E., & Staikos, C. (2013). The contribution of active listening to the development of therapeutic relationship in mental health nursing. *Scientific Chronicles/Epistimonika Chronika*, *18*(4), 213–219.

Gili, M., Toro, M.G., Armengol, S., García-Campayo, J., Castro, A., & Roca, M. (2013). Functional impairment in patients with major depressive disorder and comorbid anxiety disorder. *The Canadian Journal of Psychiatry*, *58*(12), 679–686.

Harvard Mental Health Letter. (2009, October). *Treating premenstrual dysphoric disorder*. Retrieved from http://www.health.harvard.edu/womens-health/treating-premenstrual-dysphoric-disorder

Katzman, M.A., Bleau, P., Blier, P., Chokka, P., Kjernisted, K., Van Ameringen, M., & the Canadian Anxiety Guidelines Initiative Group on behalf of the Anxiety Disorders Association of Canada/Association Canadienne des troubles anxieux and McGill University. (2014). Canadian clinical practice guidelines for the management of anxiety, posttraumatic stress and obsessive-compulsive disorders. *BMC Psychiatry*, *14*(Suppl. 1), S1. http://doi.org/10.1186/1471-244X-14-S1-S1

Loukine, L., O'Donnell, S., Goldner, E.M., McRae, L., & Allen, H. (2016). Health status, activity limitations, work-related restrictions and level of disability among Canadians with mood and/or anxiety disorders. *Health Promotion and Chronic Disease Prevention in Canada: Research, Policy and Practice*, *36*(12), 289.

Mathers, C.D., & Loncar, D. (2006). Projections of global mortality and burden of disease from 2002 to 2030. *PLOS Medicine*, *3*(11), e442.

Meltzer-Brody, S. (2011). New insights into perinatal depression: Pathogenesis and treatment during pregnancy and postpartum. *Dialogues in Clinical Neuroscience*, *13*(1), 89–100.

O'Donnell, S., Cheung, R., Bennett, K., & Lagacé, C. (2016). The 2014 survey on living with chronic diseases in Canada on mood and anxiety disorders: A methodological review. Health Promotion and Chronic Disease Prevention in Canada. Retrieved from: https://www.ncbi.nlm.nih.gov/pmc/articles/PMC5387795/

Pearson, C., Janz, T., & Ali, J. (2013). *Mental and substance use disorders in Canada*. Statistics Canada. Catalogue No. 82-624-X. Retrieved from http://www.statcan.gc.ca/pub/82-624-x/2013001/article/11855-eng.htm

Public Health Agency of Canada. (2002). Chapter 4: Anxiety disorders. *A report on mental illnesses in Canada*. Retrieved from http://www.phac-aspc.gc.ca/publicat/miic-mmac/chap_4-eng.php

Public Health Agency of Canada. (2016). What is depression? Retrieved from: http://www.phac-aspc.gc.ca/cd-mc/mi-mm/depression-eng.php

Sutherland, G., & Stonebridge, C. (2016). Healthy brains at work: Estimating the impact of workplace mental health benefits and programs. Ottawa: Conference Board of Canada.

Toews, J., McRae, L., & O'Donnell, S. (2016). 2014 survey on living with chronic diseases in Canada: Mood and anxiety disorders component. *Health Promotion and Chronic Disease Prevention in Canada: Research, Policy and Practice*, *36*(12), Introduction.

Wong, S.Y.S., Cheung, A.Y., Lee, A., Cheung, N., Leung, A., Wong, W., & Chan, K. (2007). Improving general practitioners' interviewing skills in managing patients with depression and anxiety: A randomized controlled clinical trial. *Medical Teacher*, *29*(6), 175. doi:10.1080/01421590601050585

Wurtzel, E. (1995). *Prozac nation: Young and depressed in America.* New York, N.Y.: Riverhead Books.

Young, R. (1989). Helpful behaviors in the crisis center call. *Journal of Community Psychology*, *17*(1), 70–77.

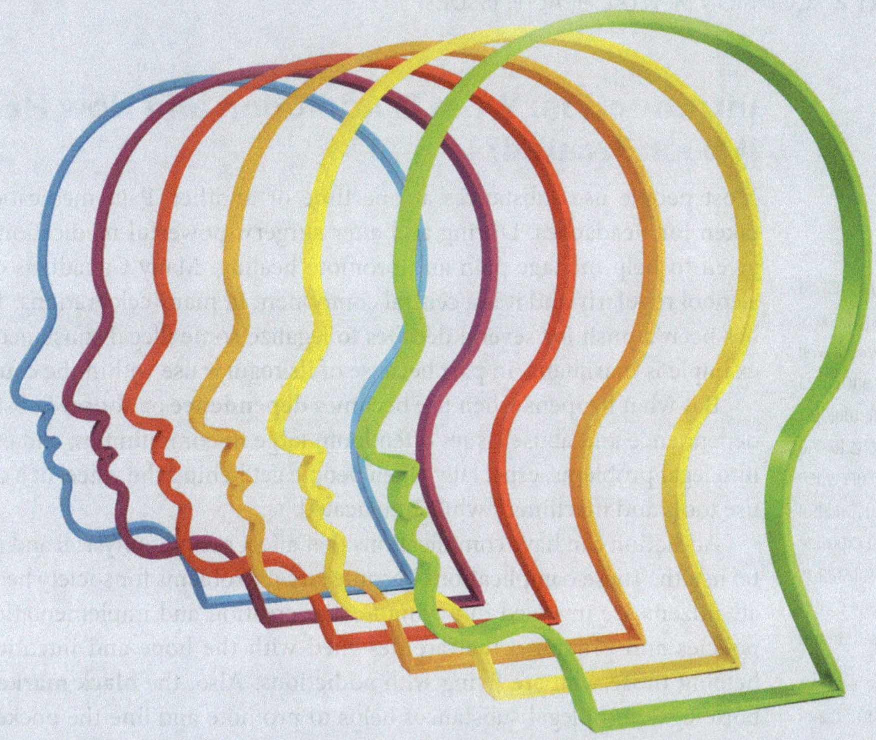

5 CONCURRENT DISORDERS AND ADDICTIONS

LEARNING OUTCOMES

After reading this chapter, you will be able to:

- Give a brief synopsis of Canada's phases of addiction treatment.
- Recognize the signs of addiction, types of addiction, and prevalence of addiction in Canada.
- Use the correct definition of the term "concurrent disorders" and discuss how this category fits into the Canadian mental health system with regard to addiction.
- Assess contentious issues that are related to the justice system's response to drugs, addiction, and substance abuse.
- Examine best practices for intervening and working in environments where addictions and concurrent disorders are prevalent.

Introduction: What Is Addiction and How Has It Been Treated?

substance dependence can include an increased tolerance to alcohol and drugs, symptoms of withdrawal when not using, increased consumption, multiple unsuccessful efforts to end use, and so on; occurs when a person adapts or builds a tolerance to repeated exposure to or ingestion of a substance; stopping regular usage causes symptoms of withdrawal

substance abuse pattern of recurring and harmful substance use (for example, alcohol and/or drugs) that disrupts normal life functions, including the ability to function normally in school, at home, or in the workplace; substance use in situations that present physical hazards, such as driving or operating machinery; and continued use of substances despite social or interpersonal costs

black market trafficking and trade of legal or illegal goods and services in a way that is against the law in order to avoid inspection, quality standards, and/or taxes

substance-use disorder pattern of substance or alcohol use that is problematic, impairs daily living, and causes distress

Most people use substances at one time or another. Pain medication is taken for headaches. During and after surgery, powerful medications are given to help manage pain and promote healing. Many Canadians drink alcohol regularly and it is a central component in many celebrations. There has been a push for several decades to legalize some illegal substances; an example is marijuana, in part because of its regular use within the country.

But what happens when use becomes **dependence** or **abuse**? Substance dependence and abuse issues often loom large in communities, and evolve into legal problems, especially when people get behind the wheel of a car or use tools and machinery while intoxicated.

Addiction can have complications that affect people's physical and mental health. These complications become larger problems for society because all citizens are involved in paying for the creation and implementation of policies and programs that are designed with the hope and intention of helping those who are living with addictions. Also, the **black market** for both legal and illegal substances helps to promote and line the pockets of organized crime, street gangs, and other groups that are often in conflict with the law.

In the fifth and most recent edition of the *Diagnostic and Statistical Manual of Mental Disorders* (the DSM), addiction is classified a few different ways. One of these is **substance use disorders**, which are separated into 10 classes. The 10 classes are listed below, with a few examples for each:

- **Alcohol:** Beer, wine, cider, hard liquor
- **Caffeine:** Coffee, tea, energy drinks, sodas
- **Cannabis:** Marijuana, liquid cannabis, ingestible oils, edibles
- **Hallucinogens:** LSD, PCP, peyote, mescaline, ketamine
- **Inhalants:** Paint thinners, gasoline, glue, nitrous oxide, chloroform, amyl nitrite
- **Opioids:** Codeine, fentanyl, methadone, morphine, oxycodone.
- **Sedatives:** Ambien, clonazepam, diazepam, Valium
- **Hypnotics and anxiolytics:** Clonidine, melatonin, phenobarbital, risperidone
- **Stimulants:** Cocaine, diet pills, Ritalin
- **Tobacco:** Chewing tobacco, cigars, cigarettes

In addition to the classes listed above, there is a temporary category called "other substances" for unknown and newly discovered addictive substances that is used before they are properly identified. With the proliferation of designer drugs and the creative use of everyday materials that can be engineered to become addictive substances, this is an important category to have when something that police and other first responders have yet to learn about hits the market and emergency rooms. Examples of some substances that were in this other category include anabolic steroids and the betel nut that is chewed in some countries to produce a euphoric sensation (American Psychiatric Association, 2013). Drugs such as "bath salts" (popular name for a synthetic stimulant that has been widely reported on in recent years) would also have been in this category when they first appeared on the market before much was known about their origin and effects.

The common trait among all of these classes of drugs and all the types used as examples is that each of them causes

> [d]irect activation of the **brain reward system**, which is involved in the reinforcement of behaviours and the production of memories. They produce such an intense activation of the reward system that normal activities may be neglected. Instead of achieving reward system activation through **adaptive behaviours**, drugs of abuse directly activate the reward pathways. The pharmacological mechanisms by which each class of drugs produces reward are different, but the drugs typically activate the system and produce feelings of pleasure, often referred to as "**a high**" (American Psychiatric Association, 2013).

It is also vital to understand that in addition to substance use disorders there are a suite of conditions that lie under the term **substance-induced disorders**. These include **intoxication**, **withdrawal**, and other mental disorders that can be brought on by the use of substances and medications and they include the following:

- psychotic disorders,
- bipolar and related disorders,
- depressive disorders,
- anxiety disorders,
- obsessive-compulsive and related disorders,
- sleep disorders,
- sexual dysfunctions,

brain reward system
several parts of the brain that are activated by pleasurable stimuli such as food, sex, water, drugs, and alcohol

adaptive behaviours
positive skills that people learn in order to adapt to and function in the activities of daily life

a high
feelings of elation, excitement, and euphoria brought on by intoxication

substance-induced disorders
medical or mental health disorders that are caused directly by the use of substances; an example is substance-induced psychosis

intoxication
state wherein mental and physical control is diminished by the use of alcohol or drugs

withdrawal
often painful set of symptoms that occur when a person stops using a substance that he or she has been using on a regular basis

- delirium, and
- neurocognitive disorders (American Psychiatric Association, 2013).

addiction
habitual or compulsive use of a mood-altering substance or engagement in activities such as gambling

12-step recovery program
group programs whose goal is to help others in recovery avoid negative lifestyle choices related to addiction

Alcoholics Anonymous (AA)
12-step program the primary purpose of which is to help alcoholics achieve a state of sobriety; Narcotics Anonymous provides a similar service for those trying to recover from drugs

For several decades, **addiction** has been treated as a disease with roots related to genetic, biological, social, economic, cultural, and environmental factors, but this was not always the case. In their 2004 report to the Senate of Canada, Kirby and Keon describe addiction treatment in Canada as a process that has had five distinct phases.

Phase One: A lack of attention to treatment was fuelled by moralistic ideals about addiction being caused by issues with will power or personality. Access to treatment was lacklustre and mostly confined to asylums and prison systems. Kirby and Keon theorize that this phase ended in the late 1940s.

Phase Two: This phase began in the late 1940s and continued through to the mid-1960s. It saw attitudes toward addictions begin to change as **12-step recovery programs** like **Alcoholics Anonymous (AA)** were created and saw some success. Government began to support and sponsor these programs and other educational programs that view alcoholism as treatable and preventable.

Phase Three: This phase ran from the middle of the 1960s into the 1980s. During this period, drug use surged in Canada and addiction services expanded to try to meet the need for treatment. From 1970 to 1976, spending on treatment went from $14 million to $70 million in Canada. More individuals were found to be using both drugs and alcohol simultaneously.

Phase Four: This phase began in the 1980s and continued into the early 1990s. Social workers, social services workers, and other non-specialized health and welfare workers became better appreciated as persons who can identify and support substance-abuse treatment. Women, teens, and Indigenous persons began to be treated in large enough numbers to see specific programs developed to serve them. Medical models were still used, but diverse cognitive, behavioural, and social programs were also implemented as part of Canada's Drug Strategy.

Phase Five: This phase began in the early 1990s and continued into the 2000s with an increased awareness of addiction. During this time, these services were integrated into community health and social services structures occurred. Illegal drugs became more potent and the risk of early addiction increased. Opportunities to gamble in person or online in Canada increased and became an emerging concern in the addiction field (Kirby & Keon, 2004).

Since the time of Kirby and Keon's report, an increase in understanding about the impact and treatment of **soft addictions** has occurred, as well as a growing appreciation for **concurrent disorders** within the justice and helping professions. In the present and near future we are likely to see more anti-stigma work occurring on various platforms, from academia to social media.

soft/behavioural/process addictions compulsive behaviours not related to substance use but that are similar in many respects, including dependency and tolerance; for example, gambling

concurrent disorders a state wherein a client lives with co-occurring mental health and addiction issues that affect and interact with one another

It is worth noting that the legalization of marijuana will likely be taking its first tentative steps Canada-wide as this book runs through its first edition. This is the first time in many generations that we will be experiencing a major illegal drug becoming legalized in Canada. The effects this will have on anti-stigmatization efforts, the legal system, and the helping professions, both positive and negative, are unknown but will be of great interest to those in the field.

DISCUSSION QUESTIONS

1. In small groups, pick a phase as described by Kirby and Keon (2004) and discuss what factors might have prevented a person from seeking help for addictions during that time period.
2. When looking at the factors that lead to addiction—genetic, biological, social, economic, cultural, and environmental—which two factors do you think are most important for a justice or helping professional to be aware of?
3. For the current generation of young people, which type of addiction do you think is most prevalent and most damaging overall: alcohol, drugs, gambling, or some other addiction?
4. How can justice and helping professionals help fight stigma about addictions and treatment for addiction?

Prevalence of Addiction and Concurrent Disorders for Adults and Youth in Canada

In 2002, the Canadian Centre on Substance Abuse partnered with federal and provincial levels of government to create a cost-analysis of substance abuse in Canada. The data released in 2006 found the total societal cost of substance abuse to be $39.8 billion. This worked out to $1,267 per Canadian.

Legal substances such as tobacco (42.7 percent) and alcohol (36.6 percent) were a much larger percentage of the estimated cost than illegal drugs (20.7 percent). These figures included the cost of health care services, law enforcement, and productivity losses due to consumption of these substances (Rehm et al., 2006, pp. 1–14).

In 2002, 35.8 percent of criminal court cases in Canada were attributed to alcohol. This worked out to over 130,000 cases in that year alone, with a cost to the public of more than half a billion dollars. In the same year, nearly 25 percent of all adult sentences and 29 percent of all youth sentences could be attributed to alcohol. The costs that year attributed to correctional stays, probation, and parole services for adults and youth involved with alcohol topped $660 million. For that year alone, enforcement for alcohol-related offences, including policing, courts and corrections, were $3.1 billion (Statistics Canada, 2014). With these staggeringly high numbers for just a single addictive substance, it is no wonder that justice and helping professionals need to have an understanding of how addiction works.

The Government of Canada collects substance-use data regularly through the Canadian Tobacco, Alcohol and Drugs Survey (CTADS). This process explores drug use by Canadians 15 years of age and older and is done every two years.

While tobacco smoking is at its lowest rate ever recorded (13 percent or 3.9 million smokers), the prevalence of illicit drug use (including cannabis, cocaine, crack, ecstasy, speed or methamphetamines, hallucinogens, and heroin) increased from 11 percent in 2013 to 13 percent in 2015 (or 3.7 million users) (Statistics Canada, 2017).

Since 1991, the police-reported crime rate has decreased by 50 percent, while the police-reported drug offence rate has increased 52 percent over the same time. (Cotter, Greenland, & Karam, 2015).

The general rate of crime is down, but the rate of drug-related offences is rising rapidly and becoming more of a concern for first responders and helping professionals. In 2013, 67 percent of those offences involved cannabis (Cotter, Greenland, & Karam, 2015). With the legalization of cannabis having been a major issue in the 2015 federal election and the work now being done to legalize some forms of cannabis across the country, this statistic should see a radical change in the near future.

Other drugs commonly found or involved when police intervene include cocaine (16 percent), methamphetamines such as crystal meth (4 percent), heroin (1 percent), and ecstasy (less than 1 percent), while other substances such as barbiturates, LSD, or "date rape" drugs comprise 11 percent of police-reported drug offences combined (Cotter, Greenland, & Karam, 2015) (see Figure 5.2).

FIGURE 5.1 Police-Reported Drug Offences and Police-Reported Crime Rate, Canada, 1977 to 2013

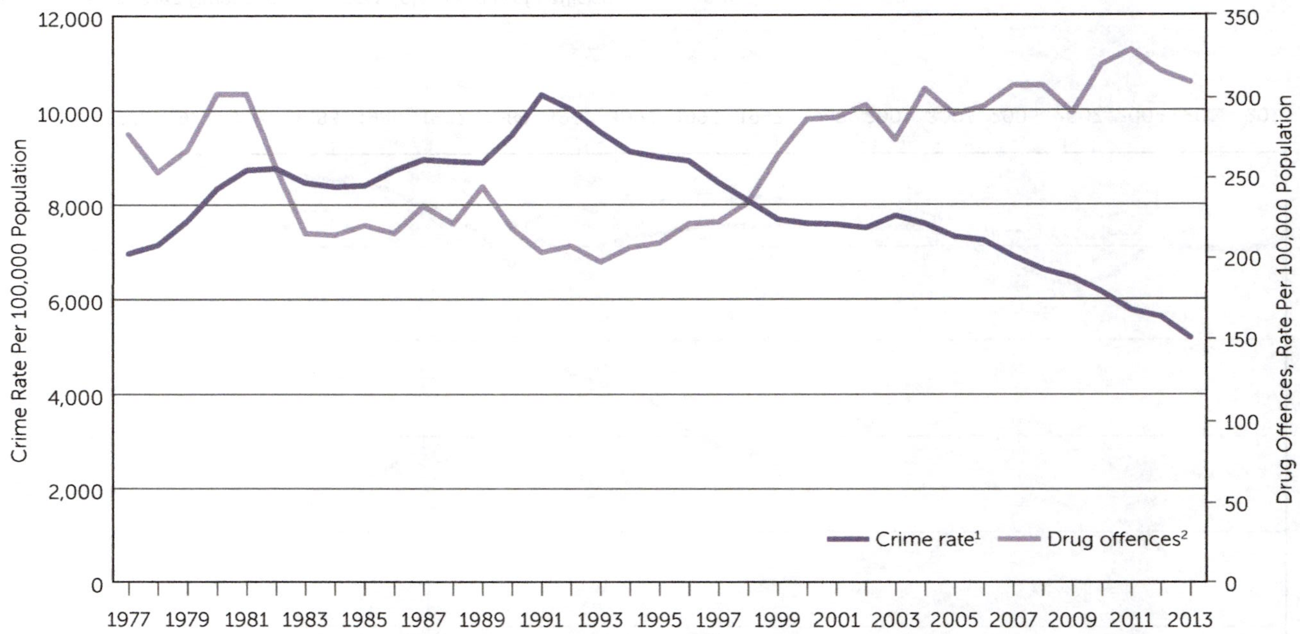

1 Includes all police-reported *Criminal Code* (excluding traffic) violations.

2 Includes possession, trafficking, import/export, and production of cannabis, cocaine, heroin, methamphetamines, ecstasy, precursors and equipment, and other controlled drugs and substances.

See: http://www.statcan.gc.ca/pub/85-002-x/2015001/article/14201-eng.htm

and: http://www.statcan.gc.ca/pub/85-002-x/2015001/article/14201/c-g/desc/desc01-eng.htm

FIGURE 5.2 Police-Reported Drug Offences, by Type of Substance, Canada, 1977 to 2013

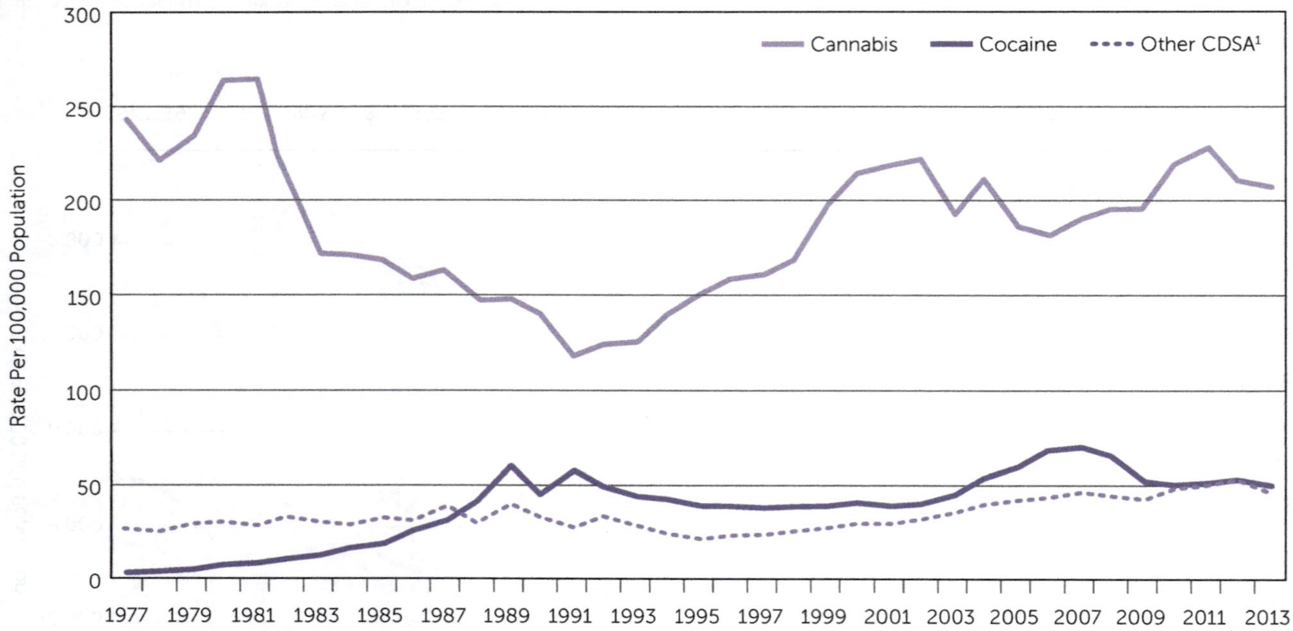

1 Includes the *Controlled Drugs and Substances Act* violations of trafficking, import, export, and production.

Source: Cotter, Greeland, & Karam, 2015.

See: http://www.statcan.gc.ca/pub/85-002-x/2015001/article/14201-eng.htm
and: http://www.statcan.gc.ca/pub/85-002-x/2015001/article/14201/c-g/desc/desc03a-eng.htm

Fentanyl is receiving a lot of attention from police services, the helping professions, and researchers because of its deadly properties and growing reach across the country. In the first 10 months of 2016, British Columbia saw 332 deaths linked to fentanyl, while there were 193 deaths in Alberta. It is estimated that at least 162 opioid deaths were related to fentanyl in Ontario in 2015 (Canadian Press, 2016).

fentanyl
a synthetic opiate originally used as a prescription medication for cancer patients dealing with intense pain; 2 mg of fentanyl (about the same size as 2 grains of salt) can be deadly

All of this has prompted numerous responses from police services in conjunction with community partners across the country. One example of a response to the opioid issue, spearheaded by the Brantford Police Service in Southwestern Ontario, involved the creation of a community roundtable, website, apparel, community forums, and a full public relations campaign to help get the word out about the dangers of fentanyl.

One of the seven action items implemented by the group included providing partnerships to get **naloxone** into the hands of potential users and front-line responders as part of a **harm-reduction strategy** (Allen, 2017). See Box 5.1 for more information.

naloxone
a medication that can reverse the effects of opioid overdose

harm-reduction strategy
strategy meant to reduce the negative consequences of substance use for an individual who is unwilling or unable to completely end his or her use of drugs or alcohol; for example, a counsellor may work with a person who drinks 30 beers a week to try to get them to drink only 15 beers a week

In addition to the costs reported above, the human cost of drug and substance abuse and its intersection with crime is well known. Street prices for a daily **fix** of a substance abuser's drug of choice can be catastrophically high, leading the drug user into all manner of illicit or illegal activities (see nearby Figure 5.3).

Sex work, fraud, break and enters, shoplifting, and car and other types of theft frequently occur because drug users need to quickly obtain the necessary cash required to feed their addiction.

Substance abuse also intersects with the criminal justice system in that the costs to feed an addiction put pressure on the user. This may lead to property crimes, theft, violence, and other unsavoury actions in order to get a fix.

a fix
common slang term that describes an addict getting and using his or her drug or substance of choice

In 2016, VICE Canada spoke to addicts and persons in recovery and asked them about current street prices of substances. While these will vary in different markets across the country and can change due to market forces, this list provides an interesting and somewhat recent snapshot of input from across the country:

- **cocaine:** \$80 a gram
- **prescription opioids:** \$4 a pill
- **heroin:** \$300 a gram
- **crack:** \$80 a gram (Krishnan, 2016)

Some of these costs seem lower than they were in 2014. And there is some data to suggest that as illegal drugs become less costly to purchase, access

BOX 5.1 FENTANYL CAN KILL

by Sean Allen

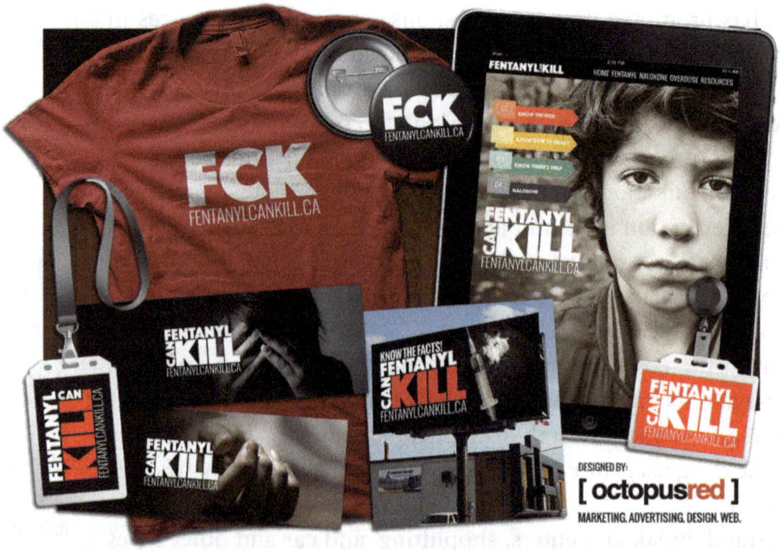

Marketing materials prepared by local firm Octopus Red use a bold, clever acronym from the campaign's website—FentanylCanKill.ca—to spread the message about the dangers of fentanyl and other opioids.—Image by Octopus Red.

March 22, 2017, *Brant News*—Brantford Police Service Chief Geoff Nelson was quick to deflect praise for a community roundtable's response to the rising prevalence of opioid abuse in our community.

"Look at what you've done here," one of the community agency members of the roundtable said to Nelson.

"No. Look at what the community has done here," Nelson replied.

Both were right.

Tuesday was my first time at the table, but this was the fourth meeting of the community roundtable convened by the chief last summer in response to a particularly deadly weekend of fentanyl-related overdoses in Brantford.

At Nelson's behest and in a short eight months, the group that includes a who's-who of front-line service agencies, emergency responders and health-care organizations has tackled and, as the chief put it, "checked the box" next to seven action items in an attempt to spread awareness of the dangers related to fentanyl and other opioids.

Fentanyl, for those unfamiliar, is a powerful painkiller that's estimated to be between 50 and 100 times more powerful than morphine. It has, according to a special report in *Maclean's* in 2015, featured a rise in use that many attribute to the crackdown on OxyContin [oxycodone] in Ontario. Whether laced into other drugs, such as heroin or marijuana, or taken on its own in pill or liquid form, overdose deaths from fentanyl can happen quickly when a user suffers prolonged respiratory depression—or hypoventilation. Without medical intervention, death is sometimes the result.

This is where naloxone comes into the equation, and where a big push from the roundtable for education is focused. Basically, naloxone works quickly to counter the effects of fentanyl and other opioids, reversing the effects of hypoventilation in minutes and possibly saving the life of a user who has overdosed.

The No. 1 action item for the roundtable that was identified at its third meeting in December was information sharing and education. To accomplish this goal ("check the box"), the Brantford Police Service engaged local marketing firm Octopus Red to create a brand and website at FentanylCanKill.ca.

On the website, which has been kept simple and quick-to-navigate on purpose, there is information on fentanyl and naloxone. Perhaps surprising to those with only passing awareness of the drug, such as myself, there is also information on where recreational opioid users can pick up their free naloxone kit. At nine Brantford pharmacies, plus the Brant County Health Unit, the kits can be picked up in advance by users.

"While we advise against using illicit drugs, people who choose to use should be sure to ... have a kit accessible at all times and know how to use it," the website says.

It's a bold and encouraging step not dissimilar from safe needle programs that recognizes that people will abuse drugs, but tries to keep them safe while they do so.

Eliminating the root of the problem takes time, but education about the dangers and options to mitigate the risk are laudable stopgap measures.

It won't be the only bold step. Lucas and Laura Duguid of Octopus Red noticed the happy coincidence of the website's acronym, which will allow for them to create some eye-catching T-shirts and other paraphernalia. A clever design with the letters FCK—for FentanylCanKill—will be sure to turn a few heads if it is displayed out in public (though the local school board representatives on the roundtable were less sure how the T-shirts might play out in their hallways).

The website and awareness campaign came together quickly thanks to the desire and willingness of the roundtable members to take on a problem in the community.

Myself and fellow scribe Vince Ball from the *Expositor* were invited to join to help amplify the message on education. Hopefully this column, and future projects I have in mind for *Brant News*, will be enough to "check another box" for this campaign.

and addiction tend to rise (Wolfe-Wylie, 2014). A 2014 report on world drug prices showed the following, in Canadian prices:

- **marijuana:** $14.98 a gram
- **cocaine:** $99.89 a gram
- **heroin:** $299.66 a gram

FIGURE 5.3 Police-Reported Violations Associated with Drug Violations, Canada, 2013

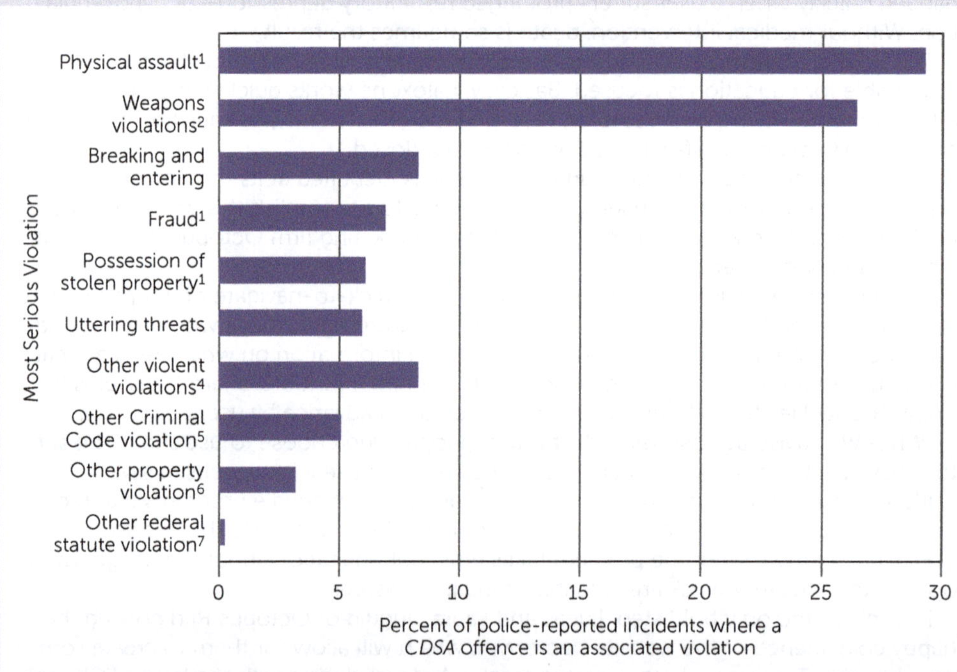

1 Includes levels 1 (common), 2 (with a weapon or causing bodily harm), and 3 (aggravated) assaults, assault against police officers, and other assaults.

2 Includes, for example, violations related to unlawful possession, possession contrary to order, unsafe storage, or improper documentation.

3 Includes identity fraud.

4 Includes sexual assault, use of/discharge/pointing a firearm, robbery, forcible confinement, criminal harassment, and other violent violations.

5 Includes counterfeiting, administration of justice offences, child pornography offences, and other *Criminal Code* violations.

6 Includes motor vehicle theft, theft over $5,000, mischief, and arson.

7 Includes violations against federal statutes other than the *Criminal Code* or the *Controlled Drugs and Substances Act* (i.e., the *Youth Criminal Justice Act*, the *Bankruptcy Act*, the *Firearms Act*, etc.).

Source: Cotter, Greenland, & Karam, 2015.

- **methamphetamine:** $111 a gram
- **opium:** $59.93 a gram (Wolfe-Wylie, 2014)

The *World Drug Report 2016* report prepared by the United Nations Office on Drugs and Crime reminds readers that "market dynamics, reflected by changes in availability, purity or price, can affect the choice of drugs. In such circumstances, people who use drugs can turn to substituting with different drugs; transitioning to alternative routes of drug administration; decreasing their consumption of the drug; or deciding to enter treatment" (United Nations Office on Drugs and Crime, 2016, pp. 2–3).

This is important to note as trends in substance use and abuse may change based on these factors. It is important for first responders and other helping professionals to be aware of the trends and risks associated with substance use patterns in their area.

DISCUSSION QUESTIONS

Usage rates and the cost to society and individuals vary from year to year, but addiction clearly remains a large problem for society generally and justice and helping professionals specifically. Take a look at the questions below and discuss your answers with friends and colleagues in order to help bring more awareness about addiction issues to the fore.

1. In the stats shared in this section of the chapter, what did you find most surprising?
2. With overall crime rates becoming lower but substance-related crimes on the rise, what do you feel are the best ways for justice and helping professionals to combat this trend?
3. What impact might the cost of specific types of substances have on different communities? For example, which illicit drugs might be more prevalent in wealthy communities and which in poorer communities and areas of the country?
4. What are some of the positive and negative effects that might occur with marijuana legalization?

Concurrent Disorders

Concurrent disorders occur when a person experiences addiction issues and mental illness simultaneously. Someone would be classified as having a concurrent disorder if, for example, he or she were abusing alcohol while living with schizophrenia. Another example would be if someone were addicted to cocaine while also experiencing severe anxiety.

Working with or being a person living with a mental health issue can be difficult. When people have more than one difficulty at a time, such as a mental health problem and an addiction, it can be difficult to know where to begin and how to help. The ways in which these problems relate to one other can be difficult to discern. For example, an individual can be traumatized by a pattern of sexual abuse that occurred when the person was a child. That abuse and trauma can result in the person developing an anxiety disorder. The person may then may use alcohol to **self-medicate** to calm their anxious feelings. Perhaps the person was given alcohol as a child to groom them for sexual abuse, so that their relationship with alcohol, the trauma they experienced, and their battle with anxiety creates a very complex problem.

self-medication behaviour in which drugs and/or alcohol are used without the consent or recommendation of a doctor or other professional in order to treat physical or psychological pain; an example of this is when someone drinks alcohol to deal with depression or post-traumatic stress disorder (PTSD) symptoms

Approximately 50 percent of people who have had either a mental health problem or a substance-use problem have had both problems concurrently for some portion of their life (Centre for Addiction and Mental Health & Rush, 2002). Many of our helping systems were originally developed to deal with only one problem at a time, but more recently a movement toward more comprehensive treatments for persons presenting with multiple problems at the same time has begun.

The Centre for Addiction and Mental Health has developed some guidelines to help set limits for individuals who are living with concurrent disorders. The guidelines are meant to help create a sense of security and predictability for both the individuals and their families, as well as others who are working with persons living with concurrent disorders. Families and others associated with an individual suffering from concurrent disorders should try to avoid:

- Making excuses for the person. For example, "He's just upset today." "She'll go to her day program tomorrow." "A few drinks won't hurt him and it may help him calm down." "It's okay if she comes home late. She has such a hard life."
- Paying the person's bills.
- Giving the person extra money, often over and over again, and being surprised when it's used to buy more alcohol or other drugs.
- Bailing the person out of jail.
- Making excuses for irresponsible behaviour.
- Ignoring the problems caused by the person's substance use. For example, mental, emotional, financial, employment, and legal problems.
- Accepting excuses the person makes or lies they tell (O'Grady & Skinner, 2007).

Police may interact with these individuals and their families on a regular basis, as might any number of first responders and helping professionals. In emergency or crisis situations related to self-harm, violence, and/or threats, police and other front-line professionals can offer invaluable services to the public and the individual and his or her family.

In the past, concurrent disorders were categorized using many different labels, including terms such as co-morbid disorders, co-occurring disorders, dual diagnosis, and dual disorders. Dual diagnosis now refers only to persons living with a developmental disability while also living with a psychiatric disorder. Some of these terms are still used internationally. This is important to know if you are a helping professional who works with a diverse population.

DISCUSSION QUESTIONS

1. Based on what you now know about certain addictions and mental health problems, what are some combinations of the two that might be particularly difficult for a person to live with?
2. Why might some families have a difficult time in setting limits for their loved ones who are struggling with concurrent disorders? How might this affect the justice and other helping professionals who are called on to intervene?
3. What advantages would the integrated treatment of multiple problems have?

Behavioural Addictions

Substances are not the only things that people become addicted to. The brain's reward system can be activated by behaviours in much the same way that it is activated by substance abuse. Persons with impulse control issues caused by brain impairment might also be predisposed to addictive behaviours (American Psychiatric Association, 2013). There are a variety of behavioural addictions that are widespread in Canada. Some of these other addictions are illegal, depending on the circumstances (for example, gambling), and while some other addictions are not illegal, helping professionals should be aware of them (for example, Internet gaming).

Other terms used to describe these types of addictions are "soft addictions" (discussed earlier in this chapter) and "process addictions." Activities such as gambling, exercising, eating, sexual activity, playing video games, Internet and social media use, shopping, and even some forms of crime have been theoretically linked to addiction, although the research for all but gambling is not sufficient to include them in the DSM (American Psychiatric Association, 2013).

Behavioural addictions can share some of the traits normally seen in substance-use disorders, such as negative effects on cognition and decision-making, ritualistic behaviour that triggers arousal, low success rates in treatment, an inability to maintain enjoyment levels in the long term, and individuals' perception that they have little to no control over their actions related to the activity (Brown, 1997).

DISCUSSION QUESTIONS

1. Other than the activities outlined above, what are some other activities that have the potential to be considered behavioural addictions?
2. Could behavioural addictions lead to crime? If so, which addictions have this potential, and how would they lead to crime?
3. Do you believe crime itself could be addictive? Why or why not?
4. Do you believe it is possible within a harm-reduction strategy to replace a dangerous substance-use disorder with a less harmful behavioural addiction? What might some of the consequences of this type of treatment be?
5. Could the reverse be true? Could a person trying to "get over" a behavioural addiction try to self-medicate or distract him- or herself from the behavioural addiction and develop a substance-use disorder? Describe how this might occur.

Justice and Helping Professionals: Best Practices for Intervention with Addiction and Concurrent Disorders

A police officer catches a person who is intoxicated in public; a corrections officer finds contraband substances in a prisoner's cell; a group-home worker walks in on a client who is about to smoke some pot: all of these scenarios see the intersection of substance use or abuse and the justice and helping professions.

In fact, slightly over one quarter (26 percent) of all drug crimes reported to police are cleared using departmental discretion; this means that the officer elects to warn the substance user and may refer the person to a community program to deal with the issue. A high proportion (41 percent) of cannabis offences are cleared in this way as well (Cotter, Greenland, & Karam, 2015).

In adult criminal court, cannabis-related charges are often stayed or withdrawn. This happens in 55 percent of cannabis-related cases, but in only 38 percent of cases that involve other drugs (Cotter, Greenland, & Karam, 2015). In this regard, discretion (including confiscation of illicit substances) can save time for the courts and provide quicker access to treatment for substance users. It also means that substance users may not develop or worsen their criminal records, which works in their favour when seeking work and becoming involved in other community activities.

DISCUSSION QUESTIONS

1. What are the positives for the officer and the substance user when departmental discretion is used in substance use cases? What are the drawbacks?
2. Some correctional officers have been known to use discretion to not intervene in substance use in correctional institutions. How do you see this contributing to the inmate culture in places where some substance use is accepted by officers?

Treatment of Concurrent Disorders

The Centre for Addiction and Mental Health (CAMH) provides the following tips in its publication *Concurrent Substance Use and Mental Health Disorders: An Information Guide.*

BOX 5.2 HOW ARE CONCURRENT DISORDERS TREATED?

Special Treatment Situations

During their recovery, people may need specific interventions, such as:

- withdrawal management
- crisis management
- relapse prevention
- hospitalization.

Withdrawal Management

People sometimes need short-term help with withdrawal from substance use. Withdrawal management helps them manage symptoms that happen when they stop using the substance. Withdrawal management helps prepare individuals for long-term treatment. Individuals also learn about substance use and treatment options.

There are three types of withdrawal management:

- In community withdrawal management, the person goes through withdrawal at home. Health care professionals help support and guide the person through this.
- A person may stay in a withdrawal management centre. This is a special facility where the person receives more intensive care and supervision.
- Medical withdrawal management may be needed if an individual has severe withdrawal symptoms, such as seizures or hallucinations. A doctor and nurse supervise the withdrawal. The individual may stay in hospital or visit as an outpatient and may receive medications to replace the drug or ease symptoms.

Crisis Management

There may be times when people who have concurrent disorders are in crisis. For example, the person may be in danger of hurting himself or herself, or other people.

It can be very hard for family members to cope effectively with a sudden crisis. It is useful to plan some emergency strategies when the person is well. This allows everyone to be prepared if anything does happen.

Depending on the situation, a crisis may be managed at home with family, peer, and professional support. Sometimes, the person may need to be hospitalized as a result of a crisis.

After the crisis has passed, the person may need a change in the treatment approach. The person may need to return to therapy if he or she has finished treatment.

Relapse Prevention

In their most severe forms, mental health and substance use problems are chronic and recurring. This means that, even after a person has received treatment, the problems may come back, or elapse.

relapse
a recurrence of use after a period of abstaining from use

Relapse is part of the recovery process. A relapse is not a reason to stop treatment. If the person is taking medications for a mental health problem, he or she needs to keep taking them.

It is important to acknowledge and discuss the relapse. Relapse can be used as:

- a chance to learn
- a chance to review the treatment plan
- a chance to renew a plan of action.

People who have had a relapse of substance use or mental health problems may not need intensive medical care. The relapse may be handled through individual therapy or in a group setting.

Hospitalization

During a severe crisis or relapse, some people may need to be in the hospital. This may be when individuals are at risk of serious consequences, due to:

- aggressive behaviour
- taking dangerous risks
- **overdosing**
- self-harming or suicidal behaviour
- failing to look after their own basic needs.

overdose/overdosing accidental or intentional consumption of a substance in excess of safe parameters

In such cases, the person may stay in the hospital from a few days up to a few weeks.

In hospital, the person may attend group or individual therapy sessions each day.

Individuals should expect to leave hospital when:

- follow-up arrangements are in place
- symptoms have improved
- they are able to function safely and care for themselves at home.

Voluntary versus Involuntary Admissions

People are usually admitted to hospital voluntarily. This means that they

- agreed to enter the hospital
- are free to leave hospital at any time.

However, in most places, the law also allows any doctor to admit a person to hospital involuntarily. This means the person may not agree that he or she needs help, and does not want to be in the hospital. This can happen if the doctor believes there is a serious risk that:

- the person will physically harm himself or herself
- the person will physically harm someone else.

Each province, state, or jurisdiction has its own process for admitting people to hospital involuntarily. For example, in Ontario, if the person doesn't have a doctor, families may ask a justice of the peace to order an examination by a physician. In the examination, the physician will decide if the person needs to be assessed in a hospital with a psychiatric facility. The physician must be able to prove that the person's illness represents a risk of harm.

Laws protect the rights of people who are admitted involuntarily. For instance, a "rights advisor" will visit. The rights advisor will ensure that the individual has the chance to appeal the involuntary status before an independent board of lawyers, doctors, and laypeople.

The police are sometimes needed to help get a person to hospital. Family members may agonize over whether to involve the police. They often feel very guilty about calling the police, even if the police are needed to protect the person's life. Remember, when people threaten suicide, they are usually pleading for help. They are taken seriously. Suicidal thinking is often a temporary feeling. When a person feels suicidal, he or she needs to be kept safe (Centre for Addiction and Mental Health, 2012).

Mental Health Training in the Justice Professions

As one of several Canadian organizations providing specialized mental health training to justice professionals, CAMH created a program to help corrections workers who work with inmates who have mental health issues.

VOICES FROM THE FIELD

CAMH Delivers Mental Health Training to 5,000 Ontario Corrections Workers

Toronto, July 29, 2016—High turnover in provincial corrections facilities can make it tougher to manage inmates' mental health challenges. At the same time, Ministry of Community Safety and Correctional Services (MCSCS) employees' knowledge of, and attitudes toward, mental illness may vary.

CAMH has just completed an ambitious program to train more than 5,000 Ontario Corrections employees on issues of mental health and **human rights**. The training also addresses issues such as trauma, resiliency, forensic practices, and risk prevention.

human rights approach a framework in which respecting a person's rights and his or her value as an individual is the driving principle of care

With its expertise in mental health and addiction, "CAMH was a natural partner for this training," said CAMH Education Operations Manager Laura Mattila. "The goal is to strengthen the Ontario prison system so it can better accommodate and manage mental illness, connect inmates with the right kinds of care, and increase the workplace quality of life for correction employees."

Addressing Complex Needs with Practical Solutions

She notes that inmates are sent to a provincial corrections facility for sentences of less than two years, or in cases where they are awaiting trial or judgment. "With brief sentences and high inmate turnover rates, the MCSCS required a training curriculum focused on practical, short-term interventions to support inmates with complex needs."

Key areas of the curriculum included human rights obligations, accommodating inmates' needs, barriers related to mental health symptoms, the impact of punitive measures, and vulnerable populations (including women, Aboriginal, and LGBTQ inmates).

In response to an earlier human rights case, the Ministry is implementing new measures, including inmate mental health screening, treatment plans, and training for front-line staff and managers on mental health and human rights issues.

MCSCS turned to CAMH's global expertise in mental health and its capacity to deliver required training at the provincial level.

A series of more than 200 two-day training sessions ran from May to July. Each session was delivered by a pair of facilitators, one representing CAMH's mental health expertise, and the other from MCSCS, providing institutional knowledge and context.

Aligning Training with Employee Needs

Mental Health Training Project Lead Grant Hilborn of the Ontario Correctional Services College noted the training content was tightly aligned with needs of employees. "CAMH's curriculum designers toured our institutions and spoke to corrections staff, including many front-line staff, to understand their perspectives and see what they would find most helpful."

"The primary goal was to educate our staff on how to recognize, respond and refer inmates who have a mental health challenge," Grant said. "Another key element was explaining our obligations as they related to human rights."

From the point of view of an inmate, "appropriate mental health response is a human right," said Chief of Forensic Psychiatry Sandy Simpson of CAMH's Complex Mental Illness (CMI) group. "Corrections officers may be challenged at times to know how to address mental health issues—this can affect them personally, as well as affecting the inmate. We are using an evidence-based approach to equip corrections officers with the knowledge they need to provide appropriate responses and better outcomes for inmates."

Tapping into Diverse Expertise

CAMH's effort included a partnership of its CMI Forensic group, CAMH Education, and the Business Development Office. The team developed a specialized curriculum to meet MCSCS learning objectives and conducted a robust evaluation of the Train the Trainer program. The team drew on diverse expertise across CAMH in forensics, education, underserved populations, outpatient services, legal services, health equity, Aboriginal engagement and human resources.

"It's a really great example of how teams across CAMH can contribute to such a large project for a great outcome," said CAMH Business Development Office Manager Michael Shaw.

"We are really pleased to help an important community partner meet a critical need," said CAMH BDO Director Linda Callander. "MCSCS is building capacity to provide high-quality mental health support."

Transforming Lives

"CAMH's objectives to care, discover, learn, and build are a great foundation for this training initiative," said Ivan Silver, Vice-President, Education. "We will continue to partner with MCSCS, and to assist in evaluation as we move forward. This initiative enhances the safety and wellness of both inmates and the dedicated employees in the Ontario corrections field."

Learn More

CAMH is advising Correctional Services Canada and the Canadian Centre on Substance Abuse on a national initiative that aims to break the **cycle of addiction** for offenders when they move between prison and the community: visit http://www.camh.ca/en/hospital/about_camh/newsroom/CAMH_in_the_headlines/stories/Pages/Breaking-the-cycle-of-addiction-for-offenders-CAMH-advises-new-national-project.aspx.

Source: Centre for Addiction and Mental Health, 2016.

cycle of addiction
a circular and often repetitive process in which a person living with addiction uses, tries to stop, relapses, experiences guilt, and is triggered into using again

Discussion Questions

1. How do partnerships such as this improve the health of both individuals (in this case, inmates) and helping professionals?
2. Why is a human rights approach a key element to this training?
3. When a great number of employees are trained in this way, how can management ensure that parts of that new knowledge are disseminated to workers who were unable to attend the training sessions?

POINTS TO REMEMBER

- ✓ Just as there are many types of addiction, there are numerous perspectives—even among professionals—about how best to tackle the disease. Harm-reduction, abstinence, individual therapies, group therapy, peer support, 12-step programs, rehab, criminalization, and legalization are just some of the different responses within the Canadian justice and helping professions.
- ✓ Within our national history we have had distinct phases of response to the overall problem of addiction. In that process we have generally moved from a point of view that viewed addiction as a personal failing to a much broader concern with the many reasons for its occurrence. We have also begun to focus on and develop an understanding of concurrent disorders and how mental health issues interact with addiction, and vice versa.
- ✓ Addiction issues have a significant impact on our economy, our health care system, and our justice system, as well as on the quality of life for all affected individuals and the health of their communities. It has become increasingly important for professionals from across a variety of disciplines to understand the variety of treatment options available.

KEY TERMS

12-step recovery program, 102
adaptive behaviours, 101
addiction, 102
a fix, 107
a high, 101
Alcoholics Anonymous (AA), 102
black market, 100
brain reward system, 101
concurrent disorders, 103
cycle of addiction, 120
fentanyl, 107
harm-reduction strategy, 107
human rights approach, 118
intoxication, 101
naloxone, 107
overdose/overdosing, 117
relapse, 116
self-medication, 112
soft/behavioural/process addictions, 103
substance abuse, 100
substance dependence, 100
substance-induced disorders, 101
substance-use disorder, 100
withdrawal, 101

RESOURCES

Drug Awareness Sheets

The Drug Awareness Sheets are an RCMP-produced resource that helps identify various drugs and informs the general public about their effects. This information is provided as part of the RCMP Drug and Organized Crime Awareness Service. The sheets can be found at http://www.rcmp-grc.gc.ca/qc/pub/sens-awar/drogue-drug/drogue-drug-eng.htm.

REFERENCES

Allen, S. (2017, March 22). Fentanyl can kill [Editorial]. *Brant News*. Retrieved from https://www.brantnews.com/opinion-story/7203982-editorial-fentanyl-can-kill/

American Psychiatric Association. (2013). *Diagnostic and statistical manual of mental disorders* (5th ed.). Washington, DC: Author.

Brown, I. (1997). A theoretical model of the behavioural addictions—Applied to offending. In J.E. Hodge, M. McMurran, & C.R. Hollin (Eds.), *Addicted to Crime?* (pp. 13–65). Chichester, UK: John Wiley.

Canadian Press. (2016, November 17). A province-by-province look at opioid-overdose stats, including fentanyl. Retrieved from http://globalnews.ca/news/3072316/a-province-by-province-look-at-opioid-overdose-stats-including-fentanyl

Centre for Addiction and Mental Health. (2012). How are concurrent disorders treated? In *Concurrent substance use and mental health disorders: An information guide*. Retrieved from http://www.camh.ca/en/hospital/health_information/a_z_mental_health_and_addiction_information/concurrent_disorders/concurrent_substance_use_and_mental_health_disorders_information_guide/Pages/how_cd_treated_infoguide.aspx

Centre for Addiction and Mental Health. (2016, July 29). CAMH delivers mental health training to 5,000 Ontario Corrections workers. In *CAMH in the Headlines, CAMH Stories*. Retrieved from http://www.camh.ca/en/hospital/about_camh/newsroom/CAMH_in_the_headlines/stories/Pages/CAMH-delivers-mental-health-training-to-5,000-Ontario-Corrections-workers.aspx

Centre for Addiction and Mental Health & Rush, B. (2002). *Best practices: Concurrent mental health and substance use disorders*. Ottawa: Health Canada. Retrieved from https://www.canada.ca/content/dam/hc-sc/migration/hc-sc/hc-ps/alt_formats/hecs-sesc/pdf/pubs/adp-apd/bp_disorder-mp_concomitants/bp_concurrent_mental_health-eng.pdf

Cotter, A., Greenland, J., & Karam, M. (2015). Drug-related offences in Canada, 2013. Catalogue no. 85-002-X. *Juristat*, *35*(1). Ottawa: Statistics Canada.

Kirby, M.J.L., & Keon, W.J. (2004). *Mental health, mental illness and addictions: Overview of policies and programs in Canada*. The Standing Senate Committee on Social Affairs, Science and Technology. Ottawa, ON: Parliament of Canada.

Krishnan, M. (2016, March 8). The cost of being a drug addict in Canada. *VICE Canada*. Retrieved from https://www.vice.com/en_ca/article/nn9p3k/the-cost-of-being-a-drug-addict-in-canada

O'Grady, C.P., & Skinner, W.W. (2007). *A family guide to concurrent disorders*. Toronto: Centre for Addiction and Mental Health. Retrieved from http://www.camhx.ca/Care_Treatment/Resources_clients_families_friends/Family_Guide_CD/index.html

Rehm, J., Baliunas, D., Brochu, S., Fischer, B., Gnam, W., Patra, J., … & Recel, M. (2006). *The costs of substance abuse in Canada 2002*. Ottawa: Canadian Centre on Substance Abuse.

Statistics Canada. (2014). Table 252-0051: Incident-based crime statistics, by detailed violations, annual. Retrieved from http://www5.statcan.gc.ca/cansim/a26?lang=eng&retrLang=eng&id=2520051&pattern=&csid

Statistics Canada. (2017). *Canadian tobacco, alcohol and drugs survey (CTADS): Summary of results for 2015*. Ottawa: Government of Canada. Retrieved from https://www.canada.ca/en/health-canada/services/canadian-tobacco-alcohol-drugs-survey/2015-summary.html

Statistics Canada. (2017). Incident-based crime statistics, by detailed violations. CANSIM table 252-0051. Retrieved from http://www5.statcan.gc.ca/cansim/a26?lang=eng&retrLang=eng&id=2520051&pattern=&csid

United Nations Office on Drugs and Crime. (2016). *World drug report 2016*. Sales No. E.16.XI.7. New York: Author.

Wolfe-Wylie, W. (2014, October 13). Interactive: What illegal drugs cost on the street around the world. *O Canada*. Retrieved from http://o.canada.com/business/interactive-what-illegal-drugs-cost-on-the-street-around-the-world

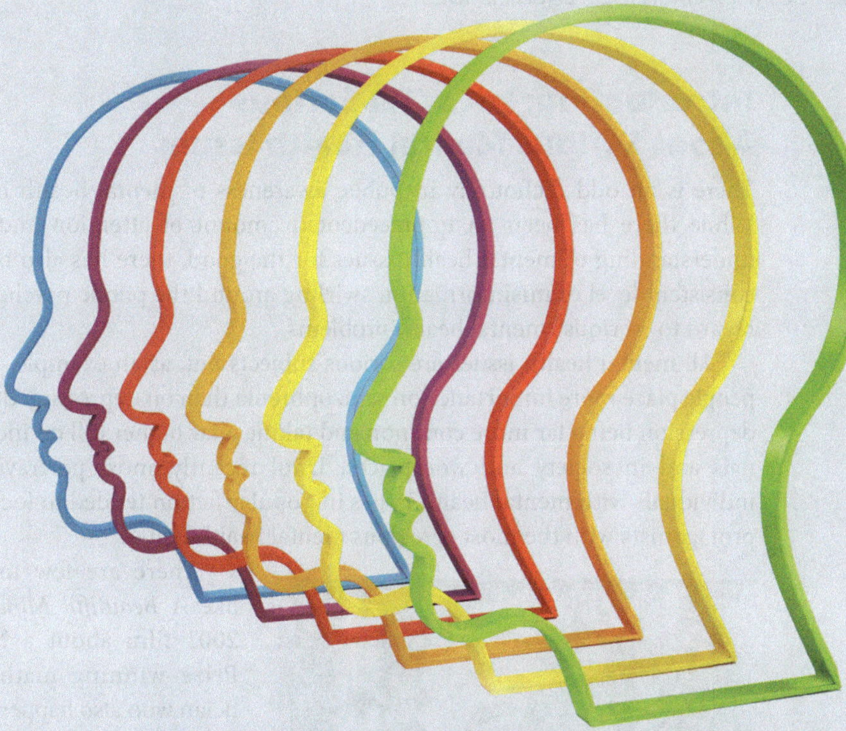

6 PERSONALITY DISORDERS AND SCHIZOPHRENIA

LEARNING OUTCOMES

After reading this chapter, you will be able to:

- Name the most common symptoms of personality disorders and schizophrenia.
- Recognize the disconnect between the popular public portrayal of serious mental illness and the reality of these diseases.
- Classify some of the tactics that can be helpful when working with someone who is living with a serious mental illness.
- Critically assess policy related to the use of "therapeutic quiet" and other incarceration methods used for persons with borderline personality disorder.
- Comprehend some of the difficulties that individuals who are living with a serious mental health issue may experience when connecting with first responders and other helping professionals.

Introduction: Let's Get Serious About Serious Mental Health Issues

There is an odd dichotomy in public awareness of mental health issues. While there has been an unprecedented amount of attention and new understanding of mental health issues for the good, there has also been a consistent level of misinformation swirling around the public psyche with regard to "serious" mental health problems.

All mental health issues are serious subjects but, as an example, many people place more importance on schizophrenia than on depression despite depression being far more common and taking a far higher toll on individuals and in society and workplaces. Until recently, most portrayals of individuals with mental health issues in popular fiction tended to focus on protagonists with the most egregious mental health issues.

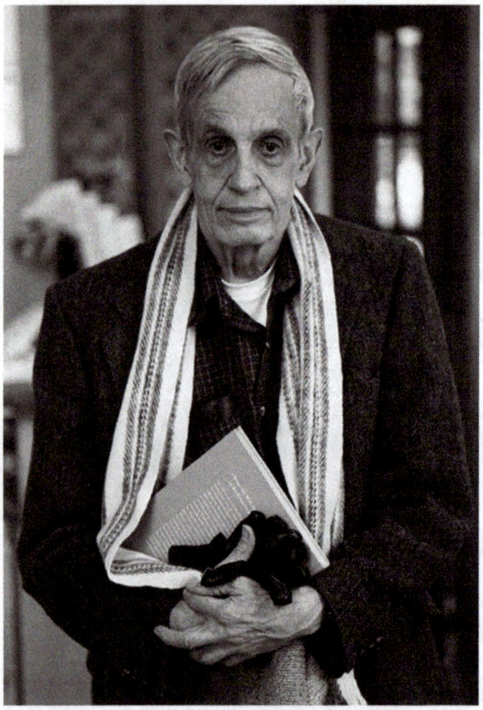

Dr. John Nash won the Nobel Memorial Prize in Economic Sciences in 1994. He also lived with severe mental health issues as popularized in the movie and book *A Beautiful Mind*.

There are few movies like *A Beautiful Mind*, the 2001 film about a Nobel Prize–winning mathematician who also happened to live with schizophrenia. It is rare to see a serious mental health issue portrayed in such a nuanced way. It is even rarer (although circumstances are improving) to see realistic media representations of someone living with a mental health issue who has been cast as the protagonist and capable person rather than a "mad" scientist, super-villain, or serial killer, which is the type of characterization that has tended to dominate in fiction and popular culture.

Similarly, we can all name numerous real-life examples of violent, trou bled persons with mental

BOX 6.1 ACTIVITY

Work on your own or in a group. Divide a piece of paper into four sections, and follow these steps:

1. In the top left box: Take two minutes to write down every portrayal in fiction of a villain or antagonist you can think of with mental health issues.
2. In the top right box: Take two minutes to write every portrayal in fiction of a hero or protagonist you can think of living with mental health issues.
3. In the bottom left box: Take two minutes to write down every major news story you can think of seeing, reading, or hearing about that showed a person living with mental health issues in a negative light.
4. In the bottom right box: Take two minutes to write down every major news story you can think of that showed a person living with mental health issues in a positive light.

Discussion Questions

Which box has the most examples? Which side has a longer list: the left or the right? Why might this be the case? What does this suggest about how mental health is portrayed in fiction and non-fiction in our media? What effect would this have on individuals who are living with mental health issues? What about its effect on society as a whole?

health issues who made national news headlines rather than advocates who made the same headlines because of their determination, strength, and poise while living with mental health issues.

This chapter uses recent data and research on mental health issues such as personality disorders and schizophrenia to help readers gain a more accurate perception of these issues and allow them to work successfully in environments where they will come into contact with individuals who have been diagnosed with these illnesses.

Personality Disorders

Personality disorders exist in a variety of forms and the effects they have on the individuals living with them range from slight to serious. These disor-

rigidity resistance to adaptation and change

ders usually first appear in adolescence or the early stages of adulthood, and can be marked by a kind of **rigidity** in thinking that manifests itself in the individual's life through unhealthy and enduring patterns of behaviour. Most individuals develop the foundational skills for adulthood in and around adolescence and in the very late teen years and early adult years. These crucial years tend to be very important for the development of relationships, attaining education, and the beginning stages of a career. Personality disorders that take root during this time in an individual's life can have "implications that extend for a lifetime" (Stewart, Lips, Lakaski, & Upshall, 2002, p. 73).

An individual living with a personality disorder may become so accustomed to these thoughts and behaviours that he or she doesn't see them as problematic even if they cause significant difficulties in his or her social, professional, and educational pursuits.

maladaptive behaviour behaviour that hinders a person's capacity to adjust to situations in a healthy manner

Personality is made up of thoughts, feelings, and behaviours and is influenced by our experiences, our environments, and through inherited genetic characteristics. When one has a personality disorder, the **maladaptive behaviour** associated with the disease creates long-term difficulties for the person in question (American Psychiatric Association, 2013).

Individuals with personality disorders will experience life in ways that differ from what is socially accepted in their culture. Some potential markers of these disorders include poor impulse control, sudden shifts in attitude from admiration of loved ones to dislike and anger, unstable emotionality, and issues that develop because of an inability to pick up on social cues, among many others (American Psychiatric Association, 2013; Langlois, Samokhvalov, Rehm, Spence, & Connor Gorber, 2012).

Health Canada describes personality disorder symptoms as follows:

- Difficulty getting along with other people. May be irritable, demanding, hostile, fearful, or manipulative.
- Patterns of behaviour deviate markedly from society's expectations and remain consistent over time.
- Disorder affects thought, emotion, interpersonal relationships, and impulse control.
- The pattern is inflexible and occurs across a broad range of situations.
- Pattern is stable or of long duration, beginning in childhood or adolescence (Stewart, Lips, Lakaski, & Upshall, 2002, p. 70).

Health Canada also provides the following table, which gives a brief synopsis of the ten major personality disorders:

TABLE 6.1 Types of Personality Disorders

TYPE	PATTERNS
Borderline personality disorder	Instability in interpersonal relationships, self-image and affects, and marked impulsivity.
Antisocial personality disorder	Disregard for, and violation of, the rights of others.
Histrionic personality disorder	Excessive emotionality and attention seeking.
Narcissistic personality disorder	Grandiosity, need for admiration, and lack of empathy.
Avoidant personality disorder	Social inhibition, feelings of inadequacy, and hypersensitivity to negative evaluation.
Dependent personality disorder	Submissive and clinging behaviour related to an excessive need to be taken care of.
Schizoid personality disorder	Detachment from social relationships and a restricted range of emotional expression.
Paranoid personality disorder	Distrust and suspiciousness in which others' motives are interpreted as malevolent.
Obsessive-compulsive personality disorder	Disorder preoccupation with orderliness, perfectionism, and control.
Schizotypal personality disorder	Acute discomfort in close relationships, cognitive or perceptual distortions, and eccentricities of behaviour.

Source: Stewart, Lips, Lakaski, & Upshall, 2002, p. 71.

Even with training, working with persons who have a personality disorder can be very taxing, confusing, and difficult. Helping professionals, including those who work with clients in the criminal justice system, must be aware of their status and perceived authority when working with an individual with a personality disorder. For example, if a police officer is responding to a nuisance call such as a noise complaint, the situation can escalate if the call is made to a person living with paranoid personality disorder. The person may become agitated if he or she perceives the officer as being there for nefarious reasons. In other examples, an individual with dependent personality disorder may display an uncomfortable closeness toward a particular group home or halfway house worker with whom they had some positive interactions, whereas someone with a schizotypal personality disorder could have a poor relationship with a group home worker or halfway house worker despite having worked with the person for months.

Correctional workers tend to deal with a high number of inmates who have personality disorders that co-occur with at least one other mental health disorder such as depressive disorder, substance abuse disorder, or an anxiety disorder. A recent study of incoming federal offenders in the Atlantic, Ontario, and Pacific regions of the country saw an overall prevalence of a 51.6 percent occurrence of anti-social personality disorder and an 11.6 percent occurrence of borderline personality disorder (BPD). When rating impairment levels using the Global Assessment of Function scale, offenders with borderline personality disorder were among those with the highest degree of impairment (Beaudette, Power, & Stewart, 2013).

When exploring borderline personality disorder, it is evident that someone living with that diagnosis could see himself or herself in conflict with the law and in contact with first responders more often than an average member of the population. Sudden changes to one's **affect**, instability with self-image and interpersonal relationships, elevated substance abuse rates, self-harming behaviour, and anti-social and possibly violent behaviour are all characteristics of borderline personality disorder (Conn et al., 2010). In a criminal justice service setting, "awareness of the behavioural manifestations of BPD, and the dysfunctional emotions and cognitions behind these behaviours, can lead to more effective strategies for managing and treating these individuals" (p. 2).

affect
how a person expresses emotions or feelings physically; for example, through a change in facial expression, body language, and/or tone of voice

According to the latest *Diagnostic and Statistical Manual of Mental Disorders* (DSM-5), someone with borderline personality disorder would have five or more of the following traits:

- frantic efforts to avoid real or imagined abandonment.
- a pattern of unstable and intense interpersonal relationships characterized by alternating between extremes of idealization and devaluation.
- identity disturbance: markedly and persistently unstable self-image or sense of self.
- impulsivity in at least two areas that is potentially self-damaging (for example, spending, sex, substance abuse, reckless driving, binge eating). (Note: Do not include suicidal or self-mutilating behaviour.)
- recurrent suicidal behaviour, gestures, or threats or self-mutilating behaviour.

- affective instability due to a marked reactivity of mood (for example, intense episodic dysphoria, irritability, or anxiety that usually lasts a few hours and only rarely more than a few days).
- chronic feelings of emptiness.
- inappropriate, intense anger or difficulty controlling anger (for example, frequent displays of temper, constant anger, recurrent physical fights).
- transient, stress-related paranoid ideation or severe dissociative symptoms (American Psychiatric Association, 2013).

When a helping professional is working in the field or in the community with someone who is living with borderline personality disorder, there are some options available to help improve communication. The following strategies can be implemented: use active listening, pay attention to nonverbal cues that the person is using to show his or her emotions outside of the words he or she is speaking, ask open-ended questions, move away from arguments or scenarios that involve a winner and a loser, validate the individual's feelings, **depersonalize**, distract, and stay calm.

Dialectical behavioural therapy is a common treatment for borderline personality disorder and it was specifically designed in the 1980s to treat the disorder. Dialectical behavioural therapy focuses on reducing suicidal behaviour, reducing behaviour that interferes with therapy, improving quality of life, and reducing post-traumatic stress symptoms. This is done through individual therapy, around-the-clock access to telephone intervention to deal with any crisis, and group therapy that focuses on a number of skills (mindfulness, interpersonal relations, **emotional regulation**, and **distress tolerance**). Therapeutic teams that work with borderline personality disorder clients in this way also have therapeutic consultation teams to support the therapists because of the difficult nature of this type of work for even highly trained mental health practitioners (Gonidakis, 2014). This is similar to the peer support teams that first responders have been using to prevent burnout. If you work with even a few individuals who are living with borderline personality disorder, it is imperative that you have strong professional peer support networks to help you fend off burnout and secondary trauma.

depersonalize
make something impersonal; for example, helping an individual who is troubled by the actions of another understand that it is not because of or directed at him or her

emotional regulation
a person's ability to manage his or her emotions when responding to experiences that are emotional

distress tolerance
skills developed in dialectical behavioural therapy when a situation that causes distress cannot be changed by the person experiencing distress

VOICES FROM THE FIELD

This article is reproduced here because it relates to some of the potential consequences of not addressing borderline personality disorder in a correctional or criminal justice setting and the authors of this text want to give representation to the voices of family members. For more on suicide, please refer to Chapter 7.

Ashley Smith's Sister Disappointed by Federal Solitary Confinement Bill

By Patrick White

Thursday, Jun. 22, 2017, *The Globe and Mail*—For over a year, Dawna Ward has been sending encouraging notes to Prime Minister Justin Trudeau about prison reform.

"We're counting on you," she recalls writing. "What's your plan and when do you plan to do it?"

Her requests are similar to the notes the Prime Minister receives from average Canadians every week—with one stark difference. Ms. Ward is the sister of Ashley Smith, the New Brunswick teenager who drew her last breath on the floor of a solitary-confinement cell in Ontario almost 10 years ago. She had spent at least 1,065 days in solitary.

As of this week, Ms. Ward wonders whether it's all been in vain – the letters and the inquests and the investigations that preceded them. On Monday, Public Safety Minister Ralph Goodale evoked her sister's name in touting Bill C-56, a proposal to change the federal solitary-confinement regime. When Ms. Ward read the bill for herself, she felt the reference dishonoured her sister's name.

"The fact that the minister mentioned Ashley's name is so disappointing and so upsetting," she told The Globe and Mail. "Solitary confinement is a horrific, torturous, inhumane practice. This bill will not change that."

The suicide of 19-year-old Ashley Smith as guards watched launched numerous inquests, investigations and news stories examining how the correctional system places mentally ill prisoners in cells the size of hotel bathrooms for 23 hours a day with no external oversight.

A rough consensus emerged from many of those probes.

The federal government needed to prohibit vulnerable inmates from being sent to solitary confinement, place hard limits on the duration inmates can languish in segregation and appoint an independent adjudicator to make sure the Correctional Service of Canada follows the law.

Ottawa insists that C-56, along with some internal rule changes at Correctional Service Canada, will address those points. Ms. Ward feels differently.

"I do not believe this bill would have changed the outcome [for Ashley]," she said.

Her sister was first sentenced to prison at the age of 15 for breaching probation, assault and causing a disturbance. At the time, Ms. Ward knew a much different Ashley Smith from the one who would become classified as dangerous, aggressive and self-harming in the federal correctional system.

"I was quite a bit older than her, but my children were very close with her," said Ms. Ward, whose children were 12, 17 and 23 years old at the time of the death. "I can't imagine a more close-knit family, really. The kids attended daycare together. They swam together every day in the summertime. Sledding, ice skating, tobogganing, all of those things."

For the next two years, Ms. Smith would be in and out of youth custody. Once, she was charged for throwing an apple at a postal worker. On another occasion, she did time for pulling a fire alarm.

In custody, she racked up hundreds of institutional infractions and new charges for assaulting staff and damaging property. She was routinely sent to segregation, or "therapeutic quiet," as it was termed.

She turned 18 in 2006 and was transferred to adult custody under Correctional Service Canada. There, she exhausted correctional officers by continually tying strands of fabric around her neck and physically resisting staff attempts to remove them. She was diagnosed with borderline personality disorder, a condition typified by fear of abandonment, self-harm, and mercurial temper.

The Correctional Service kept her in near-continuous solitary confinement, transferring her 17 times between seven institutions in four provinces over 11 months.

"Fortunately, my parents had the means to travel all over the country," Ms. Ward said. "Everywhere they moved Ashley, my mom would visit. But she wasn't allowed a contact visit. She couldn't hold her hand, couldn't touch her hair, she couldn't hug her, she couldn't do anything. For a kid to go from a caring, conservative upbringing to being caged like an animal—how could anyone cope with that?"

On Oct. 19, 2007, Ms. Smith told a correctional officer of a recent nightmare wherein her mother had died while she was still in prison. She felt like tying something around her neck. "Just let me do it," she told the concerned officer, who had been ordered not to intervene. "I won't die. I know what I'm doing."

By then, guards had been ordered not to intervene unless Ms. Smith stopped breathing. They followed orders on that day and entered her cell too late to save her.

The jury in that 2013 inquest deemed the death a homicide and recommended a prohibition on keeping inmates in segregation beyond 15 days.

"That was the first time we started to feel closure," Ms. Ward said. "With the homicide designation, we expected change would happen, that no family would ever have to go through this again."

Days after taking office, Mr. Trudeau instructed cabinet to implement the recommendations from inquest. Bill C-56 would create a presumptive segregation time limit of 21 days, dropping to 15 days a year-and-a-half after taking effect. But it also proposes to give any warden the power to override those time limits.

Under the proposed legislation, independent reviewers would be appointed to examine all solitary placements extending beyond the presumptive limits, but would be granted no power to release inmates from segregation. The bill doesn't mention mentally ill prisoners.

"It's too discretionary," Ms. Ward said. "It still allows for the use of solitary confinement. I think if this legislation were in place years ago, Ashley would have received the same treatment."

The family received an undisclosed settlement in 2011.

Ms. Ward still has trouble erasing the dreadful images from the inquest. She holds on to hundreds of hours of home movies showing Ms. Smith laughing and playing.

"That's the Ashley I think of on a good day," Ms. Ward says. "We are starting to have good days, but the dark cloud of her demise is always going to overshadow the good we have in our collective memory."

Discussion Questions

1. What dynamics exist in prisons that would exacerbate symptoms of borderline personality disorder for an inmate? What about in other contact with first responders, such as the police or in an emergency room situation?
2. Why might correctional officers want to be able to use their discretion with regard to extending the use of solitary confinement time? Do you agree or disagree that they should have this power?
3. Helping professionals other than corrections personnel may use "therapeutic quiet" for shorter periods of time in a place such as a quiet room in a residential care facility or a child-proof safe room in a youth home. Do you think "therapeutic quiet" can be an effective therapeutic tool when used for one hour or less?

Schizophrenia

According to DSM-5, schizophrenia exists on a spectrum (American Psychiatric Association, 2013). This is a change from the outdated titles that were previously attached to schizophrenia as subtypes. In the past, a number of these subtypes became part of popular usage when discussing schizophrenia and were often misused by non-professionals. Terms such as paranoid schizophrenia, disorganized schizophrenia, and others such as catatonic, undifferentiated, and residual schizophrenia are no longer in use (Tandon et al., 2013).

The schizophrenia spectrum includes schizophrenia; other psychotic disorders such as **delusional disorder**, **schizophreniform disorder**, and **schizoaffective disorder**; and schizotypal personality disorder. The disorders on this spectrum exist when at least one or more of the following abnormalities are present: delusions, hallucinations, disorganized thinking, grossly disorganized or abnormal motor behaviour, and negative symptoms (American Psychiatric Association, 2013).

Delusions on the schizophrenia spectrum can take on a range of themes. Individuals may believe that they are being persecuted or are someone of religious significance. They may have grandiose thoughts or be fixated on a belief that they are the reincarnation of Jesus, an alien, or

delusional disorder a mental health issue in which delusions exist for at least one month without the other symptoms of schizophrenia or mood disorders

schizophreniform disorder shares the symptoms of schizophrenia for more than one month but less than six months

schizoaffective disorder shares the symptoms of schizophrenia as well as mood disorder symptoms such as those seen in depressive disorders

someone with powers beyond human capacity. Individuals living with delusions may believe that someone they barely know is in love with them, that the government is watching their every move through cameras installed in smoke alarms, that they are pregnant and have been for years, or that naturally occurring phenomenon such as flooding is directed at them.

Hallucinations involve perception; for example, affected individuals may "see" something that does not exist or hear something that is not there. This is not a vivid imagining, but a non-voluntary hallucination that appears real to the affected person. Auditory hallucinations are most common (American Psychiatric Association, 2013) and involve hearing someone or something that is not there, such as water dripping or a voice outside of their own that is saying derogatory things to them.

It is important when working with someone who is experiencing delusions or hallucinations to not state that you believe them, to not "play along" with the delusions. However, it is also important to not dismiss what the person is thinking and feeling. Minimizing the person's experience or arguing about it will not help.

Active listening skills can be used. State that you are not seeing or hearing what the person is describing, but you understand that to him or her the experience is real. A first responder can be empathetic and state that he or she is concerned and want to help, that he or she is there for support.

The first responder should avoid speculation about diagnosis. Instead, ask the individual whether he or she is seeing any professionals or has had a mental health diagnosis. Ask for the names and contact information of these professionals.

Ask the person whether other distractions such as a television or radio that is on can be turned off, speak clearly and in short sentences that are easy to follow, and do not touch the person unless you have his or her permission or because you need to ensure safety.

Note that the use of humour and sarcasm or laughing with or whispering to others in the vicinity of the person affected by these delusions or hallucinations can be misinterpreted and can break trust. Avoid these behaviours.

Disorganized thinking is usually inferred when someone communicates verbally in ways that seem odd and hard to follow. Scenarios that involve this behaviour can be difficult for a first responder or helping professional who is trying to assess a situation and gather information from an individual. It may also be difficult to decide which information is a sign of disorganized thinking that is clinically significant, and what might be communication errors due to age or medical issues such as a stroke or hearing impairment, and even cultural and language differences. One sign of disorganized thinking can be when the individual switches rapidly from topic to topic and goes on odd tangents that may be incomprehensible (American Psychiatric Association, 2013).

Grossly disorganized or abnormal motor behaviour might appear similar to the behaviour of a child who is acting out and can include silliness and being quick to anger. It might also involve a person who is living with schizophrenia becoming catatonic, that is, not reacting to his or her environment (American Psychiatric Association, 2013).

The DSM-5 describes the phenomena of catatonia as follows:

> This ranges from resistance to instructions (negativism); to maintaining a rigid, inappropriate or bizarre posture; to a complete lack of verbal and motor responses (mutism and stupor). It can also include purposeless and excessive motor activity without obvious cause (catatonic excitement). Other features are repeated stereotyped movements, staring, grimacing, mutism, and the echoing of speech. Although catatonia has historically been associated with schizophrenia, catatonic symptoms are nonspecific and may occur in other mental disorders (American Psychiatric Association, 2013).

Negative symptoms include symptoms that make it difficult to control emotions, behaviours, and ability to relate to others. Canada's Public Policy Forum created a report on schizophrenia in Canada in 2014 and listed negative symptomology as typically presenting in the following ways:

- flattened mood and poor interaction with others,
- difficulty with volition and motivation (apathy),
- alogia (difficulty speaking),
- an absence of motivation,
- lack of pleasure in life, and
- social withdrawal and isolation (Canada's Public Policy Forum, 2014, p. 6).

brief psychotic disorder
shares at least one of the symptoms of schizophrenia but for less than one month; can occur as a response to an extreme life stress

While **brief psychotic disorder** lasts more than a day and less than a month and schizophreniform disorder lasts more than a month but less than six months, schizophrenia lasts for at least six months and has at least one month of active symptomology. Schizophrenia is not the same as a drug-induced psychosis. Some symptoms may be similar but schizophrenia is not acute and not created by the physiological effects of substances and medication (American Psychiatric Association, 2013).

It is typically believed that about 300,000 individuals in Canada (1 percent of Canadians) are affected by schizophrenia (Canada's Public Policy Forum, 2014, p. 5). Treatment can be effective; however, barriers to treatment exist and include issues with ongoing need for medication, adherence and treatment compliance, isolation, discrimination, and caregiver burnout (pp. 8–9; Chandra, 2017; García et al., 2016).

VOICES FROM THE FIELD

This article was chosen in an effort to impress on first responders and other helping professionals that persons with a lived experience of mental health should be listened to and heard. Although not directly written by Sean Clifton, his quotes here provide a great deal of personal insight on what it is like to live with schizophrenia, and especially doing so after involvement with the justice system.

Sean Clifton's Search of Forgiveness: Followup Film Tracks Notorious Cornwall "NCR" Case

By Blair Crawford

November 20, 2016, *Ottawa Citizen*—The woman he almost killed forgives Sean Clifton, but Clifton, it seems, can't forgive himself.

"I don't see much positive that came out of this disaster," Clifton says to filmmaker John Kastner near the end of Kastner's follow-up to his extraordinary 2013 documentary *NCR: Not Criminally Responsible*.

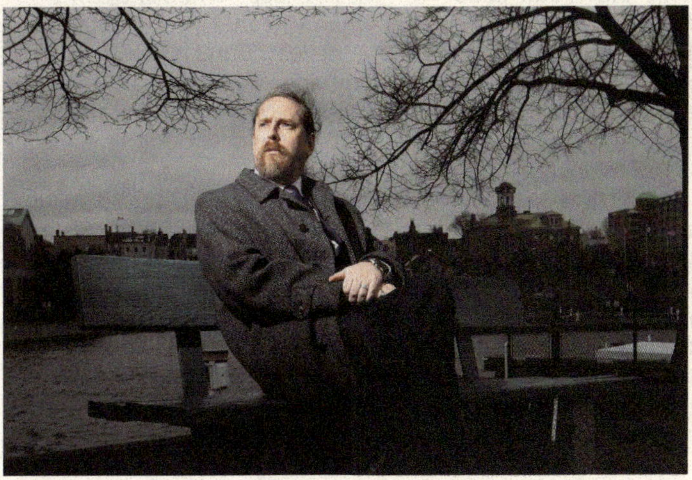

Pictured here is Sean Clifton, who has had first-hand experience with both the mental health system and the justice system.

The follow-up, *Not Criminally Responsible: Wedding Secrets*, examines Clifton's life since he was released after nine years of treatment at the Brockville Mental Health Centre, where he had been committed after he stabbed Julie Bouvier, a woman he chose at random in a Cornwall parking lot in October 1999.

It's a remarkable story: Clifton meets Bouvier for the first time since the attack and apologizes. He is reunited with a son he and his then girlfriend had given up for adoption when Clifton was just 15, and two key players in the story, meet, fall in love and marry.

But for Clifton, it all seems hollow.

"I can't really, I can't forgive myself for that," he tells Kastner.

"Part of the cruel irony of sufferers with schizophrenia who commit terrible acts of violence like this is that as they get better, it's a two-edged sword," says Kastner. "On the one hand, they begin to function better as normal people. On the other, the more normal they become, the more it hits them what the terrible thing is that they have done.

"It's that sad paradox of getting better when you have this cruel, devastating disease."

The disease is paranoid schizophrenia and Clifton was in the throes of delusion when he saw Bouvier in a Walmart parking lot and stabbed her six times. He was charged with attempted murder but was found not criminally responsible when the court ruled he was too mentally ill to have formed an intent to commit a crime. Instead, Clifton was sent for treatment in Brockville. He was one of the sickest patients staff in the hospital's secure forensic ward had ever seen.

Kastner and his cameras spent more than 3½ years filming NCR. The crew was given unprecedented access to the patients, but operated under strict guidelines imposed by the hospital's ethics committee. His intention was to shine a light "in the belly of the beast" at where and how NCR individuals are treated.

"I was spooked when I went in there," Kastner says. "I've done a lot of films on prison, I know a lot of people who've done unspeakable things to other people. But I had the same prejudices as most people do when I walked in the door. I saw all these people sitting around and I thought, 'Are they going to attack me?'"

But Kastner says the public knows little about NCR cases, except in rare and sometimes shocking high-profile events. Like last February, when Vincent Li was granted unsupervised access to the community seven years after he was found not criminally responsible for beheading and partially cannibalizing another passenger on a Greyhound bus in Manitoba. In September, an Ottawa judge found Jeffrey Weber NCR for attacking a man with a hammer on a Centretown street corner in 2014. It is the fourth time Weber has been found NCR for a violent incident.

Incidents like that give the public a distorted view of NCR rulings, Kastner said. In fact, a 2015 study by the Canadian Mental Health Commission—*The National Trajectory Project*—found that less than one percent of individuals found NCR repeat a violent offence within three years of their release. Their recidivism rate for any type of offence is 17 percent, half the recidivism rate of those released after a criminal conviction.

The first film premièred just a few months after the previous Conservative government of Stephen Harper introduced legislation to tighten the laws around NCR rulings. Kastner feared the sudden attention to NCR cases could put Clifton at risk.

"When the film was conceived in 2010, nobody knew what NCR was or even what the initials meant. It was a much quieter time and we thought it would be safe to put a patient's face out there for the first time. Then there was the ugly backlash began in Canada.

"In a small town like Brockville, suddenly everybody knew where to find this guy. ... We were terrified."

To the surprise of Kastner—and Clifton—the reaction was overwhelmingly positive. He was recognized, but people came up to show their support. At one screening, the audience gave Clifton a standing ovation.

"Can you imagine Vincent Li getting a standing ovation?" Kastner says.

In *Not Criminally Responsible: Wedding Secrets*, we see Clifton in the basement apartment where he lives in Brockville. We learn how his son, Jon McMahon, 31, decided to reconnect with his birth father after watching Clifton in the original documentary. The "wedding secret" is the instant attraction between McMahon and Kastner's associate producer, Nicole Rogers. McMahon and Roger's marriage in August of this year is the stage for the film's finale.

But most extraordinary is the face-to-face meeting between Clifton and Bouvier for the first time since the attack. Bouvier said she forgave Clifton in the first film, but Clifton had waited 16 years to apologize to Bouvier in person. The meeting between he and Bouvier and her parents is short and awkward and does little to ease his guilt.

"I think Julie came out of that meeting happier than Sean did," Kastner says.

"Julie is almost a saint. She's such a sweet, good, good person. The whole Bouvier family is. Where do you find such decent people who would react this way?

"But partly it made it harder for Sean. He was so anxious to meet with her. We found records in the hospital going back 15 years saying, 'I want to apologize. I want to apologize.' I think, come the actual moment, it even made it harder for him because she was such a wonderful person."

Clifton's discomfort intensifies a few weeks later at the wedding, which the Bouviers attended. Kastner says he could see it happening, Clifton withdrawing into himself even as those around him laugh and celebrate.

"There are people out there who say, 'These guys are getting away with murder. Send them to prison. A forensic psychiatric hospital is a walk in the park compared to going to prison.'" Kastner said.

"But look at the torment of that guy at the end of this film and tell me if you think his life was a walk in the park. He's in a kind of hell."

Source: Crawford, 2016.

Discussion Questions

1. For a person who is living with schizophrenia, what are some of the negative aspects of the fact that schizophrenia is such a rare disease?
2. Are you aware of three service providers in your region to whom you could refer someone living with schizophrenia? If not, please research this and share with your class what you discover.
3. What effect might negative media portrayals and sensationalized coverage of violent news stories involving individuals who are living with schizophrenia have on self-reporting rates? How can this be overcome?

POINTS TO REMEMBER

- ✓ Serious mental health issues such as personality disorders and schizophrenia are often focused on in sensational ways in today's pop culture. This creates issues around shame and fear of exposure for people living with these mental illnesses.
- ✓ It is important to have an understanding of the dynamics of personality disorders, including the types of disorders and how symptoms may manifest. This is important in part because of the higher rate of justice system contact and incarceration that can occur for persons living with these issues.
- ✓ Likewise, the same is true with regard to the importance of understanding how individuals with disorders on the schizophrenia spectrum may interact with first responders, the justice system, and helping professionals.
- ✓ The development and maintenance of strong, active listening skills, empathy, peer support networks, and suicide prevention skills is important for first responders and other helping professionals so that they can provide the best help and treatment to individuals with mental health issues.
- ✓ When first responders, helping professionals, and organizations work with people who are living with serious mental health issues, it is recommended that they take the time to listen to them and their families and include their input in organizational policy decisions. Lived experience should be respected as a source of knowledge in addition to what is provided by mental health and policy experts.

KEY TERMS

REFERENCES

American Psychiatric Association. (2013). *Diagnostic and statistical manual of mental disorders* [DSM-5]. (5th ed). Washington, D.C.: Author.

Beaudette, J., Power, J., & Stewart, L.A. (2013). Prevalence of mental health disorders among incoming federal offenders: Atlantic, Ontario, and Pacific regions. Ottawa: Correctional Service of Canada.

Canada's Public Policy Forum. (2014, February 19). Schizophrenia in Canada: The social and economic case for a collaborative model of care. Retrieved from http://www.ppforum.ca/publications/new-report-examines-social-and-economic-costs-schizophrenia-canada

Chandra, P.S. (2017). [Review of the book *Mental illness and caregiving: Challenges, concerns and complications* by Amrit Bakhshy.] Pune, India: Schizophrenia Awareness Association.

Conn, C., Warden, R., Stuewig, J., Kim, E.H., Harty, L., Hastings, M., & Tangney, J.P. (2010). Borderline personality disorder among jail inmates: How common and how distinct? *Corrections Compendium*, *35*(4), 6.

Crawford, B. (2016, November 21). Sean Clifton's search of forgiveness: Followup film tracks notorious Cornwall "NCR" case. *Ottawa Citizen*. Retrieved from http://ottawacitizen.com/news/local-news/sean-cliftons-search-of-forgiveness-followup-film-tracks-notorious-cornwall-ncr-case

García, S., Martínez-Cengotitabengoa, M., López-Zurbano, S., Zorrilla, I., López, P., Vieta, E., & González-Pinto, A. (2016). Adherence to antipsychotic medication in bipolar disorder and schizophrenic patients: A systematic review. *Journal of Clinical Psychopharmacology*, *36*(4), 355-371. http://doi.org/10.1097/JCP.0000000000000523

Gonidakis, F. (2014). Dialectical behavior therapy for borderline personality disorder. In Soldatos, C., Ruiz, P., Dikeos, D., & Riba, M. (Eds.), *Pluralism in psychiatry* (pp. 145–148). Bologna, Italy: World Psychiatric Association.

Langlois, K.A., Samokhvalov, A.V., Rehm, J., Spence, S.T., & Connor Gorber, S. (2012). *Health state descriptions for Canadians: Mental illnesses*. Catalogue No. 82-619-M—No. 004. Ottawa: Statistics Canada. Retrieved from http://www.statcan.gc.ca/pub/82-619-m/82-619-m2012004-eng.pdf

Stewart, P., Lips, T., Lakaski, C., & Upshall, P. (Eds.). (2002). A report on mental illnesses in Canada [Report]. Ottawa: Health Canada. Retrieved from http://www.phac-aspc.gc.ca/publicat/miic-mmac/pdf/men_ill_e.pdf

Tandon, R., Gaebel, W., Barch, D.M., Bustillo, J., Gur, R.E., Heckers, S., & Van Os, J. (2013). Definition and description of schizophrenia in the DSM-5. *Schizophrenia Research, 150* (1), 3–10.

White, P. (2017, June 22). Ashley Smith's sister disappointed by federal solitary confinement bill. *The Globe and Mail.* Retrieved from https://www.theglobeandmail.com/news/national/ashley-smiths-sister-disappointed-by-federal-solitary-confinement-bill/article35442553/

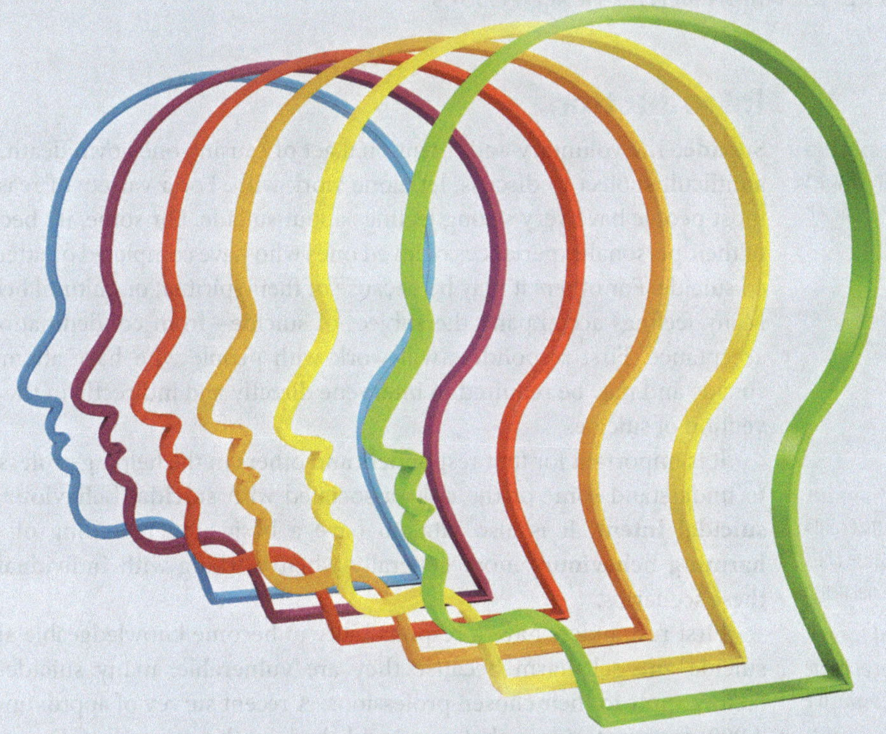

7 SUICIDE INTERVENTION

LEARNING OUTCOMES

After reading this chapter, you will be able to:

- Name a variety of terms associated with suicide and self-harm.
- Recognize that while suicide can affect anyone, there are specific demographics that have been disproportionately affected in the Canadian context.
- Classify various risk and protective factors as well as stages of response to suicide within a suicide prevention continuum.
- Critically assess the dynamics that make first responder a high-risk occupation for suicidal thoughts and suicide completion.
- Use or refer others to a variety of services that are available to prevent suicide and promote life.

Introduction

suicide
voluntary and intentional act causing the death of oneself

Suicide. The voluntary and intentional act of causing one's own death. It is a difficult subject to discuss, let alone work with. For a variety of reasons, most people have very strong feelings about suicide. For some, it's because of their personal experiences of loved ones who have completed or attempted suicide. For others it may be because of their spiritual or cultural beliefs. Many feelings accompany the subject of suicide—from condemnation to acceptance. First responders will work with people who have attempted suicide and may be required to intervene directly and indirectly in the prevention of suicide.

suicidal behaviour
any action that could reasonably cause one's own intentional death

suicidal intent
conscious aim or desire to end one's own life

self-harming behaviour
deliberate harm or risky behaviour that can lead to physical harm of oneself; sometimes called self-injury

It is important for first responders and others in the helping professions to understand some of the risks associated with **suicidal behaviour** and **suicidal intent**. It is also vital to have a basic understanding of **self-harming behaviours** more generally when working with individuals in these scenarios.

First responders have a responsibility to become knowledgeable about suicide and self-harm because they are vulnerable: many suicide-risk factors apply to their chosen professions. A recent survey of approximately 4,000 first responders that was published in the *Journal of Emergency Medical Services* found that 6.6 percent of first responders—10 times the national average—have attempted suicide in the United States. The same survey also found that 37 percent of first responders had contemplated suicide—again, 10 times the average of the general population in the United States (Newland et al., 2015).

While Canadian suicide statistics for first responders are difficult to find, a charitable group called the Tema Conter Memorial Trust (TEMA) has been keeping count and posits that over 200 Canadian public safety and military personnel have died by suicide since 2014.

Canadian public safety personnel suicides by year, according to TEMA:

2014	48
2015	68
2016	68
2017 (Jan 1–Sept 12)	42

Source: TEMA, 2017b.

That's a total of 226 suicides at the time of writing. These statistics include Corrections, police, and military personnel as well as firefighters and paramedics.

You can visit TEMA's website (TEMA, 2017a) to see updated numbers and yearly breakdowns of this information and learn more about TEMA and the issue of first-responder suicide in the Voices from the Field feature in this chapter. For more preventive measures for first responders you can consult the *Mental Health Awareness: Self-Care for First Responders* handbook that pairs with this text (Laferriere & Miloknay, 2018).

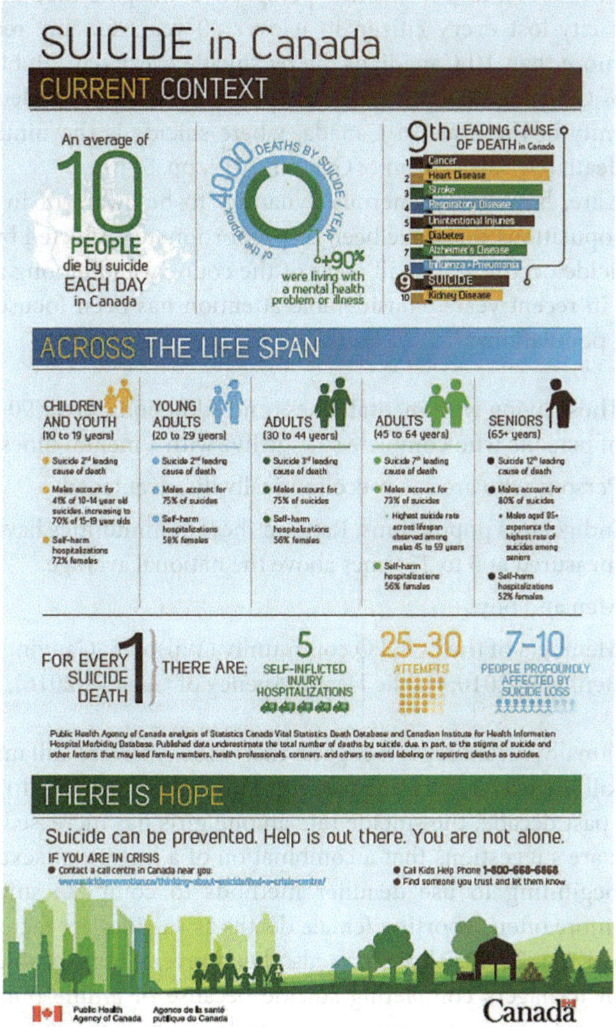

This Suicide in Canada infographic was created by the Public Health Agency of Canada as part of its effort to educate the public on the issue of suicide.

Source: Public Health Agency of Canada, 2016a.

Suicide: History and Statistics

In Canada, intentional self-harm is responsible for approximately 11 deaths for every 100,000 persons. It is known that in 2013 over 4,000 persons took their own lives; 2013 is the latest date for which these statistics are available (Statistics Canada, 2017). For comparison purposes, data suggest that within a period of 30 years in Canada over 100,000 persons have completed suicide (Rae, 2011): to put this into perspective, imagine that a mid-sized Canadian city lost every citizen in it over 30 years for any reason. On average, more than 10 Canadians die by suicide every day (Public Health Agency of Canada, 2016a, p. 6; 2016b, p. 2). These statistics demonstrate the enormity of the issue in Canada, where suicide is the ninth leading cause of death overall (Wilson & Gauvin, 2012, pp. 5, 10).

There are, however, numerous dynamics to be aware of in terms of specific populations that have been disproportionately affected by suicide. While suicide occurs across all areas of the country and among all demographics, in recent years, considerable attention has been focused on the following populations:

- Those living with mental illness and addictions. Over 90 percent of persons who complete suicide live with a mental illness.
- Persons who are socio-economically disadvantaged.
- Indigenous populations. Rates in these communities have been measured at 5 to 25 times above the national average.
- Men and boys.
- Members of the LGBTQ community (Wilson & Gauvin, 2012; Benibgui, 2010; Public Health Agency of Canada, 2016).

Additionally, recent reports suggest that while "men are still much more likely to kill themselves in Canada, young women are starting to catch up. Over the past decade, the suicide rate among girls has increased by 38%," and there are suggestions that a combination of a history of sexual abuse, women beginning to use deadlier methods to complete suicide, and coroners more often reporting female deaths as suicides are factors in this (Levinson-King, 2017). There have also been several high-profile cases in Canada of teenagers completing suicide because of online bullying and organized sextortion—a process where girls are tricked, encouraged, or shamed into sending sexually explicit photos that are then shared widely and used to mentally torment and bully the victim.

A 2016 report from **Kids Help Phone** on a survey of teens found that 22 percent of them had seriously considered suicide over the 12 months of the study. The report also noted that of those who had seriously considered suicide, 47 percent did not speak to others about their feelings and 46 percent had a **suicide plan** (Russell, 2016).

The topic of Indigenous suicide has received a great deal of media and government attention in recent years. A study published in the *Canadian Journal of Psychiatry* in 2017 showed evidence that "exposure of one previous familial generation to the **Indian residential school (IRS)** experience was associated with increased risk for lifetime **suicide ideation** and attempts compared with those with no IRS history. Having two generations of IRS familial history was associated with greater odds of reporting a suicide attempt compared with having one generation" (McQuaid et al., 2017). Furthermore, it has been argued that Indigenous youth suicide rates higher than the general national average could "be understood as an expression of societal, historical, cultural and familial trauma" (Barker, Goodman, & Debeck, 2017).

There has been a demand for federal action to prevent suicide, but responses as of yet have "underwhelmed" community members and experts alike (Eggertson, 2017). One part of a recently announced federal

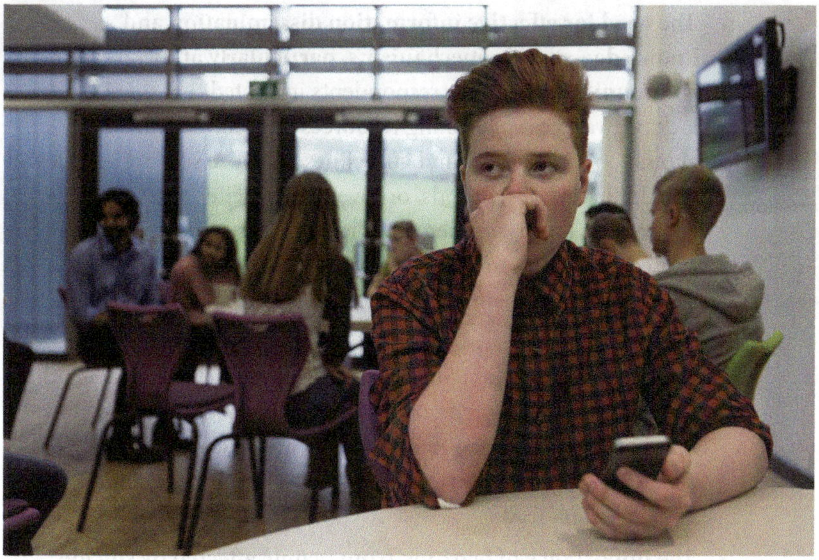

Contact Kids Help Phone by calling 1-800-668-6868, through their Always There app, or at kidshelpphone.ca.

Kids Help Phone
Canadian organization established in 1989 initially for children to report abuse and access telephone counselling 24-hours a day; now also provides web counselling and referrals for children and youth

suicide plan
specific plan a person may have to end his or her life

Indian residential schools (IRS)
system of federally run boarding schools that was forced upon Indigenous children and operated in Canada into the late 1990s; more than 150,000 children were removed from their families and communities; spiritual, emotional, physical, cultural, and sexual abuse was widely reported to have occurred

suicidal ideation
suicidal thoughts, be they momentary and transitory, or longer-lasting and detailed

framework discusses plans to create a national phone, text, and online chat portal that will link existing crisis services to a single toll-free number across the country. At the time of publication, this framework was not coupled with a national suicide prevention strategy, funding, goals, and timelines for implementation or other specific activities to reduce and prevent suicide (Eggertson, 2017).

Part of the process for creating the recent suicide prevention framework was public consultation, which included over 376 organizations and individuals from "government departments, non-governmental organizations, national Indigenous organizations, officials from provinces and territories and community stakeholders" who are involved with suicide prevention work across the country (Public Health Agency of Canada, 2016b, p. 4). The themes that emerged from this consultation process are shared verbatim below for analysis:

- **Public perception as a barrier to suicide prevention.** Both the stigma of suicide and the fear of contagion when talking about suicide challenge efforts to raise awareness and disseminate information about suicide. Increased awareness of suicide in the general population to support open dialogue would help advance suicide prevention efforts.
- **The need for effective information dissemination and knowledge-sharing mechanisms, particularly at the community level.** Many respondents indicated that there is a lack of awareness of existing resources or that it is difficult to access tools, resources, and guidelines for those seeking services to help themselves, friends, or loved ones. Better access to support for those experiencing thoughts of suicide or suicide-related behaviour and for survivors grieving a loss due to suicide would be beneficial.
- **The need for a centralized, credible source of data and research information.** Suicide information, including data and research results, is fragmented, complex, sometimes costly, and often difficult to access. Access to data and research about suicide, in a range of formats appropriate for diverse audiences, could be enhanced.
- **The importance of learning from people affected by suicide.** The knowledge and lived experience of Canadians who have

been affected by suicide should inform the development of guidelines and resources and should be included in prioritizing suicide prevention research. In addition, the perspectives of survivors of suicide loss and survivors of suicide attempts should inform dissemination strategies to ensure resources are reaching those who need them most.

- **The need to bring evidence into front-line practice, such as through partnerships between researchers and practitioners.** Priorities should be established for suicide prevention research, including both a traditional focus on risk and **etiology** as well as emerging science on protective factors and what works in which contexts and for whom. Enhancing knowledge exchange and transfer across sectors and effective collaborations could help result in better outcomes for those affected by suicide. (Public Health Agency of Canada, 2016b, pp. 4–5)

etiology
the cause of a condition

Those consulted strongly recommended a **multi-sectoral approach** to suicide prevention that includes populations who are at greatest risk for suicide. Traditional Indigenous knowledge and cultural relevance should inform best practices. Changing public perceptions through comprehensive and sustained public awareness campaigns, prioritizing research and its dissemination, sharing best practices, and improving collaboration and coordination across sectors are critical in improving suicide prevention in Canada and will require a collaborative approach between all levels of government, across sectors, and within communities across Canada (Public Health Agency of Canada, 2016b, pp. 4–5).

multi-sectoral approach
approach to solving systemic problems where collaboration between governments, not-for-profits, non-governmental organizations, communities, and individuals occurs

Clearly another pan-Canadian study of the dynamics and trends of suicide with up-to-date statistics and a concrete national prevention strategy is required because there is evidence of changing demographics and the need for specific preventive action to be bolstered throughout the country.

While these statistics are of interest, it is important to note that suicide can affect anyone, even if certain risk factors are missing from his or her profile. Table 7.1 provides an excellent resource that includes both **risk factors** and **protective factors** for suicide-related behaviours. The table is from McMaster University in Hamilton, Ontario, and is adapted from a US suicide prevention strategy.

risk factors
variety of factors that may increase the risk of someone completing suicide

protective factors
variety of factors that may decrease the risk of someone completing suicide

TABLE 7.1 Risk and Protective Factors for Suicide-Related Behaviours (Adapted from the 2001 US National Suicide Prevention Strategy)*

RISK FACTORS			PROTECTIVE FACTORS
BIOPSYCHOSOCIAL	**ENVIRONMENTAL**	**SOCIOCULTURAL**	
Sex, gender, and sexual orientation	Job or financial loss	Lack of social support and sense of isolation	Effective clinical care for mental, physical, and substance use disorders
Mental disorders (particularly mood disorders, schizophrenia, anxiety disorders, and certain personality disorders)	Negative life transition and stressful events	Stigma associated with help-seeking behaviour	Easy access to a variety of clinical interventions and support for help-seeking
Low levels of serotonergic neurotransmission	Relative poverty	Barriers or lack of access to health care and/or mental health and substance abuse treatment	Restricted access to lethal means of suicide
Alcohol and other substance use disorders	Relational or social loss	Certain cultural and religious beliefs (for instance, the belief that suicide is a noble resolution of a personal dilemma)	Strong connections to family and community support
Impulsive and/or aggressive tendencies	Easy access to lethal means	Exposure to and influence of others who have died by suicide (including through the media)	Support through ongoing medical and mental health care relationships
History of trauma and abuse	Local clusters of suicide that have a contagious influence		Skills in problem solving, conflict resolution, and nonviolent handling of disputes
Some major physical illnesses, functional impairment, or having a terminal condition	Poor family environment and low level of parental monitoring		Cultural and religious beliefs that discourage suicide and support self-preservation
Previous suicide attempt			Cultural continuity (e.g., activities toward preserving and rehabilitating culture through different means such as self-government, land claims, education, health services delivery, cultural facilities, and police and fire services)
Family history of suicide			

* The factors listed in each column are not rank ordered in a specific way.

Source: Wilson & Gauvin, 2014, p. 13.

DISCUSSION QUESTIONS

1. Describe the differences between suicidal behaviour, suicidal intent, and self-harming behaviours.
2. Public perception of suicide is a barrier to suicide prevention. What are some of the stigmas that exist around the topic of suicide?
3. List three ways that a first responder can support someone he or she suspects is suicidal.

Programs for Prevention

Although a national strategy is still highly recommended to help with the crisis of suicide, there are many programs operating in Canada to help those who may be contemplating suicide or practising self-harm.

Recommendations and referrals to counselling are a primary tactic to help persons who are struggling with suicidal thoughts and/or practising self-harm. Working through underlying trauma, feelings of depression, isolation, and hopelessness are just some of the ways a positive counselling relationship can help.

There are numerous resources across the country that offer help, including crisis lines, Kid's Help Phone, drop-in counselling services, reporting to the emergency room of a local hospital, and other options, depending on the mental health support infrastructure in a particular community.

The Public Health Agency of Canada has developed a suicide prevention continuum that provides early prevention, intervention, and postvention recommendations. The continuum will serve as a good reference sheet, and is shown in Table 7.2.

For specific interventions with Indigenous communities there is a case to be made for strengthening your knowledge of Indigenous cultures and customs as a way to help prevent and intervene in suicide and self-harm.

A growing body of research argues that conventional interventions, largely rooted in Western individual-level behavioural change frameworks, are culturally discordant with Indigenous paradigms. In response, some Indigenous communities are turning to cultural revitalization as a holistic community-driven response to suicide prevention and treatment. [There is an] emerging evidence base for "culture as treatment"—a novel approach to suicide that emphasizes the significance of interconnectedness in healing, alongside the revitalization of traditional values to reclaim community wellness (Barker, Goodman, & Debeck, 2017).

TABLE 7.2 Suicide Prevention Continuum

<table>
<tr><th colspan="3">SUICIDE PREVENTION CONTINUUM</th></tr>
<tr><th>EARLY/PRIMARY PREVENTION (BEFORE SUICIDE RISK)</th><th>INTERVENTION</th><th>SUPPORT FOR SURVIVORS (POSTVENTION)</th></tr>
<tr><td>Prevention works to build protective factors and promote mental health and well-being and reduce risk factors that could lead to suicide.</td><td>Intervention works to address risk of suicide. It focuses on how best to respond early when someone has thoughts of suicide or suicide-related behaviours.</td><td>Postvention works to help support and heal those affected after the loss or experience of suicide, as well as providing follow-up education/ prevention to reduce the risk of future crises.</td></tr>
<tr><td>Population
• Everyone</td><td>Population
• Individuals in crisis, at high risk for suicide
• People seeking help for someone else
• Survivors of suicide attempt</td><td>Population
• Survivors of suicide loss (e.g., family, friends, classmates, colleagues, and communities of those lost)
• Survivors of suicide attempt</td></tr>
<tr><td>Types of Activities
Aimed at promoting mental health and well-being and building stronger, more resilient individuals and communities.
• Social/emotional learning programs in schools
• Mental health literacy programs
• Peer, family and (culturally-safe) community programs
• Stigma reduction and safe messaging campaigns
• Media guidelines
• Online resources and helpful information
• Training for gatekeepers and first responders</td><td>Types of Activities
Aimed at intervening and preventing the onset of suicide.
• Crisis and distress line services (via telephone and Internet)
• Support and treatment
• Mental health services
• Emergency medical or social services
• Means restriction
• Employee assistance programs
• Training and counselling for gatekeepers, first responders, and primary caregivers</td><td>Types of Activities
Aimed at providing support and promoting mental health and well-being for those affected by suicide.
• Peer support (e.g., groups)
• Individual and family counselling
• Follow-up services (including new technologies to connect people with support)
• Online support groups and information
• Employee assistance programs
• Counselling and crisis interventions in schools, workplaces, and communities to prevent suicide contagion
• Training and counselling for first responders</td></tr>
</table>

Source: Public Health Agency of Canada, 2016b, p. 14.

Additionally, a number of training and educational programs exist that front-line professionals should consider using as part of their professional development that include but are not limited to the following:

- **Applied Suicide Intervention Skills Training (ASIST):** A two-day workshop that specializes in suicide first aid. This program helps persons recognize when individuals are having thoughts about suicide and focuses on supporting the vulnerable person's immediate safety. See https://www.livingworks.net/programs/asist/.
- **safeTALK:** A half-day training course that helps individuals become aware of the subtle invitations that persons who may be contemplating suicide use to make others aware of their thoughts. The safeTALK-trained helpers are able to connect struggling individuals with helpful resources. See https://www.livingworks.net/programs/safetalk/.
- **Suicide Prevention Resource Centre:** This US organization offers a number of free online courses that individuals can take on their own time and at their own pace to develop a greater knowledge about suicide and suicide prevention. See http://training.sprc.org/.
- **The Centre for Suicide Prevention:** Workshops and resources to help equip persons to respond when an individual is at risk of suicide are available here. Specific workshops focus on a range of topics that include intervention, prevention, postvention, and Indigenous dynamics of suicide and grief. See https://www.suicideinfo.ca/.
- **The Jack Project:** A Canadian network of young leaders that has over 100 chapters across the country. Its aim is to enable young leaders to improve mental health systems and reduce youth suicide rates. See https://www.jack.org/.
- **The Mental Health Commission of Canada:** This organization offers Mental Health First Aid, which has a component that trains individuals to help keep those who are living with serious mental health issues alive. The Commission has also created online modules, webinars, and toolkits on suicide prevention, intervention, postvention, and life promotion as well as resources for those who are mourning the loss of someone to suicide. See https://www.mentalhealthcommission.ca/English/.

These and many other resources exist to help fight stigma, increase awareness, and support life-saving measures that both everyday people and helping professionals can use to keep people safe.

VOICES FROM THE FIELD

Canada's Lack of First-Responder Suicide Stats is a National Disgrace

By Mack Lamoureux and Alex MacPherson, Vice News

March 6, 2015—On the morning of April 10, 2012 Sgt. Douglas Marshall, a 22-year veteran of the Ontario Provincial Police (OPP) entered the Highway 12 detachment for the start of his shift and found it empty. The 45-year-old father of two drew his weapon, turned it on himself, and pulled the trigger.

Sgt. Marshall had been acting erratically since the summer of 2011. After responding to a number of traumatic calls, including a suicide and the death of a four-year-old, the veteran officer began suffering from nightmares and insomnia. Once a proud athlete and competitor, Marshall stopped running, missing the annual Terry Fox run for the first time in six years. He became impulsive, waking his son up late at night to ask about school or his hockey team. He also started suffering from flashbacks to previous trauma.

Sgt. Marshall was diagnosed with PTSD and briefly sent to a clinic for treatment in October 2011, but by mid-January, he was back on the job, and had his service weapon returned to him by February. It was that pistol he used to kill himself.

Sgt. Marshall's story is a tragedy, but it isn't a rare one in Canada. First responders across the country struggle with PTSD and suicide every day. Just how widespread this trend was remained unknown for years because no one was keeping track of the numbers. Furious at the lack of record keeping, one group is starting to shed some light on first responders' struggle with PTSD.

In 1988, Toronto paramedic Vince Savoia was called to the brutal rape and murder of Tema Conter. That call changed his life. Conter's body was covered in stab wounds; however, she looked exactly like Savoia's fiancée, so much so that his partner asked if it was her. He left the profession after that and suffered from the memory for 12 years before being diagnosed with PTSD.

Recognizing he wasn't the only one struggling, Savoia founded the Tema Conter Memorial Trust (TEMA) in 2001 to raise awareness for PTSD. Frustrated with the lack of available numbers, TEMA began keeping track of suicides in the first-responder community on Apr. 28, 2014 and releasing them to the media.

"We felt that this needed to be done because we felt that this needed to be on the radar," Savoia told VICE. "Whether or not provincial governments are keeping track, again, we haven't been made aware. If they are smart they should be keeping track of what's happening in their provinces because it is an issue."

The numbers that TEMA reports are tragic. Every month, first responders all over the country are hurting themselves, sometimes fatally, to escape their PTSD. While the majority of media outlets have recently been reporting this information as a shocking spike in suicides, the reality is far more unsettling.

This isn't a spike. It is an ongoing trend in Canada that has been quietly accepted as the norm in the first-responder community. In 2014, there were more suicides among police, fire, and paramedic divisions (22) than in the military (19). Since TEMA began keeping track of first-responder suicides in April of 2014, that number has risen to 26, including six paramedics, five firefighters, and 15 police officers. All but one of these were men, and the majority (17) happened in Ontario. What's more shocking is that those numbers would have gone unreported if it wasn't for TEMA.

If Savoia hadn't started recording and distributing these statistics, the public would still be ignorant of the actual price our first line pays for PTSD. The organizations that should have been keeping these numbers, and keeping Canada's uniformed safe, have failed to do so. According to Alberta Health Services, employee suicides "haven't been a statistic [that AHS] has tracked since it began providing EMS service in 2009. We don't believe the previous providers tracked that either." WSIB keeps the number of PTSD claims approved in Ontario but not who filed them or what department they came from. The OPP did not to respond to numerous requests to talk about this story and their policies.

We have a responsibility to the men and women in uniform to keep them safe, because they would do the same for us. By not keeping the numbers, we haven't kept our side of the deal. Accurate statistics on first-responder suicides could have been used to implement better policies and protect more members, but no one in government is recording these numbers. TEMA, with their limited resources, is effectively doing someone else's job.

Roméo Dallaire, retired lieutenant-general and the honorary head of the Post Traumatic Stress Disorder Association of Canada, agreed with Savoia that accurate statistics need to be kept. Dallaire led United Nations peacekeepers in Rwanda during the brutal genocide of the Tutsis by the Hutus and his experience there left him suicidal and depressed. Dallaire struggled with his PTSD for years, attempting suicide four times, and has since become an outspoken advocate for better mental health treatment in the armed forces.

"There was this philosophy for a long time that the less you talk about suicide the better," Dallaire says." You didn't want to give the give the impression it might be OK or even glorify it.

"That, to me, was one of the most horrific mistakes we made. We have to tell people that good people are killing themselves and that there is a reason for it. We had better get at it and make sure others don't suffer the same fate."

He says the military had come a long way since he started advocating for better PTSD treatment in 1997. Dallaire believes the treatment of first responders in Canada is still years behind the military's practices.

"First responders are still at stage one," Dallaire explains. "They've just made the realization that these people are vulnerable, that they are being taken for granted, and that they won't be able to carry on."

Despite the shockingly underreported statistics TEMA has collected, Dallaire remains optimistic that changes are coming in first-responder organizations.

"In police forces, firefighters, medical, even teachers, there's a desire to provide much more," he says. "The difficulty is convincing people that the injured aren't sick, they're injured, and that you don't get rid of them, you support them and you can bring them back."

It's a small but significant difference. Dallaire explains that first responders and military personnel exist in an atmosphere that is, "in essence, Darwinian." The men and women in uniform are proud of their responsibilities. In those organizations, admitting to mental health issues can be seen as showing weakness. He compares the stigma of reporting PTSD as a first responder today to the stigma faced by military personnel 18 years ago.

"PTSD is tolerated even less in these organizations than it is in the general population because they demand such a high standard. It makes it hard for these guys to feel like they're being supported," says Dallaire. "One of the things we did in the military was we called it an 'operational stress injury.' An injury. These people aren't sick, they don't have a disease—it's an injury. So how do you treat an injury? You treat it with the same sense of urgency as a physical injury. You get in there early and you take care of it.

"Secondly, you treat it as honourable. There's no shame in being injured psychologically. It took a lot of work to convince people who said, 'You know, I was injured, I've lost an arm.' This guy has lost his mind, he's injured too."

The stigma is real and it is dangerous. In 2012, Ontario Ombudsman André Marin released a report that investigated suicide and depression in the OPP. The 158-page document, titled *In The Line Of Duty*, found that 23 OPP officers had committed suicide from 1989 to 2012. Excerpts from "Over The Blue Wall," the personal memoir of an officer named "Henry," were published in the report:

"Everything from picking up people's parts from under subway trains, to kids' pieces from under cars, to checking dead and suicide victims for identification or evidence ... I had seen and done it all, and like a good policeman, putting personal feelings up on the emotional shelf where it belonged, to be dealt with later, much later, when that time would be ... no one, including me, knew ..."

Officer Henry applied for and successfully received benefits from the Workplace Safety and Insurance Board (WSIB) to treat his psychological injuries, but in 2005 his benefits were challenged by fellow officers.

"We respectfully point out that this case once more illustrates the urgent need for review of entitlement for traumatic mental stress benefits, and demands that the WSIB stop wasting the taxpayers' money in this fashion," a unit commander wrote to the WSIB after Henry began attending community events again. Prior to this, Henry had spent months alone in his bedroom, only leaving when recommended by his doctor. He kept his benefits, but the accusations hurt.

Officer Henry killed himself in 2009.

Marin supplied the OPP with 28 recommendations in 2012. Echoing Dallaire and Savoia, Marin called for accurate statistics to be kept regarding officer suicides and slammed the OPP for not keeping them sooner. Unfortunately, the majority of Marin's recommendations have not been followed.

As noted above, the OPP did not respond to requests to talk about this story.

On January 26 of this year, Greg Turner, husband, father of two, and paramedic of 16 years took his own life after a shift at Edmonton's Kildale neighbourhood dispatch station. He was 41. It was the fourth first-responder suicide in Canada that month.

"I am broken," wrote his wife, Bridget, in an emotional Facebook post. "I know in my heart that this was not a choice. He did not choose death over us. Depression made that choice for him and it was a battle he was too sick to fight. It is a disease that kills without the right treatment, just like cancer."

An anonymous letter from an Edmonton first responder published online by the *Edmonton Sun* in February brutally reinforces the fact that this problem is widespread in the community. In it, the author struggles with his own PTSD and praises Turner for his bravery.

"I wish I could tell you today that after all I've gone through with the mental health system (I've barely scratched the surface of my experience of the system in this letter) that I've been cured but the honest truth is that I will never be cured," the letter read.

"I will live with my depression and other mental illness until the day I die, I will forever be plagued by the thoughts that I should have done my wife and kids a favour and went out like Greg did long ago instead of subjecting them to a life lived with a person who no longer has emotion happy or sad thanks to depression and/or the drugs that treat it. I will continue to feel a bit of jealousy each time a news story airs of a first responder who has committed suicide or was killed in the line of duty, and I'll continue to wish that I too could have been killed in the line of duty so my family would have the memory of all the uniforms at my funeral and they could be proud of how I left earth.

"Instead even though the real me died at work years ago my family is stuck with an empty shell of the man I was, and even though I try my best to be the man they deserve I always feel they deserve more."

Stress injuries cause tremendous strain on the victim and their family. But experts point out that support from those closest to the victim—their family and peers—is critical to treating the injury. Dallaire explains the relationship between professional treatment and peer support.

"If you have a meeting with a psychiatrist once a week, and you are feeling the hurt during the week, the peers are there to listen, to respond, to fight those urges to self-destruct because a lot of people forget that those urges, and PTSD, can be terminal."

Dallaire goes on to explain the stigma from the point of view of someone who had battled with mental health injuries in the past.

"Those who are in uniform, they wear that uniform because they want to be distinctive and do a job," he says. "They feel they are part of an organization and that they have a responsibility to that organization. That they have a responsibility to perform."

That sense of responsibility drives first responders to do brave and heroic things every day. But that same sense of responsibility, that determination to keep working and keep saving and keep ignoring the psychological damage, is killing them.

Twenty-six first responders that we know of have taken their own lives between April 29, 2014, and today. That statistic isn't cherry picked. It's currently the only number we have, and it's an average of one suicide every two weeks.

There will be more. And most won't be reported. There is an officer, a paramedic, a firefighter, who is struggling right now to hide their injuries. They are suffering and will not survive the year.

Tomorrow, all over the country, Canadians will dial 911 and call for help.

And even though it's killing them, help will come.

DISCUSSION QUESTIONS

1. Which resources or programs might you refer a fellow first responder or other helping professional to if they were feeling suicidal?
2. What are some ways to prevent or treat PTSD and thus prevent the suicides related to it?
3. Develop in one to two paragraphs a personal plan that would fit you if you were to develop PTSD and/or suicidal thoughts from front-line work. Include resources you would connect with, specific people in your life you would speak to about your plan, and some self-care activities. Then share with a partner and discuss each other's plans.

Intervention Strategies

In addition to the numerous strategies for first responders that are detailed in *Mental Health Awareness: Self-Care for First Responders*, the handbook that pairs with this text, there are other widely used strategies for assessing risk and intervening with those who may be contemplating suicide.

One of the most well-known strategies is "IS PATH WARM." This acronym has been designed to help individuals recollect some of the most common warning signs of suicide risk.

Below you will find the original explanation for IS PATH WARM, with the corresponding letter of each part of the acronym highlighted.

- Suicide **I**deation: Does the client report active suicidal ideation or has she written about her suicide or death? Does the client report the desire to kill herself? Does she voice a desire to purchase a gun with the intention of using the gun to kill herself? Does she voice the intention to kill herself with a gun, weapon, or car that she currently has in possession or can gain access to?
- **S**ubstance Abuse: Does the client excessively use alcohol or other drugs, or has she begun using alcohol or other drugs?
- **P**urposelessness: Does the client voice a lack or loss of purpose in life? Does she see little or no sense or reason for continued living?
- **A**nger: Does the client express feelings of rage or uncontrolled anger? Does she seek revenge against others whom she perceives have wronged her or are at fault for her current concerns or problems?
- **T**rapped: Does the client feel trapped? Does she believe there is no way out of her current situation? Does the client believe death

is preferable to a pained life? Does the client believe that no other choices exist except living the pained life or death?

- Hopelessness: Does the client have a negative sense of self, others, and her future? Does the future appear hopeless with little chance for positive change?
- Withdrawing: Does the client indicate a desire to withdraw from significant others, family, friends, and society? Has she already begun withdrawing?
- Anxiety: Does the client feel anxious, agitated, or unable to sleep? Does the client report an inability to relax? Just as important, does the client report sleeping all the time? Either can suggest increased risk of suicide or self-harm.
- Recklessness: Does the client act recklessly or engage in risky activities, seemingly without thinking or considering potential consequences?
- Mood Change: Does the client report experiencing dramatic mood shifts or states? (Juhnke, Granello, & Lebrón-Striker, 2007.)

When working as a first responder you may be required to intervene in a potential suicide situation with a member of the public or a colleague. Intervention is not counselling. It may involve skills borrowed from that field, including active listening, but the goal of intervention is to keep the person alive—not to explore his or her deep-seated trauma. When intervening, remember the following:

1. **Ensure your own safety:** This is key and must be addressed. Do not take risks with your own safety in order to build rapport with a person who may wish to harm themselves or others. No one will be helped if a first responder or helping professional is seriously injured or killed in an intervention.
2. **Check in with yourself:** Although it will be difficult, you must remain rational and calm in these situations. It is an effective means of seeing a positive end result.
3. **Engage the person about his or her feelings:** Use non-judgmental listening skills to engage the person in discussing the situation. Ask whether the person is thinking about ending his or her life. Ask about previous suicide attempts and what happened that brought the person to this point.
4. **Engage the person about his or her supports:** Ask about other care providers, such as doctors or mental health professionals, loved

ones, and other community services and supports that the person may have access to. Be aware of supports in your region so that you can refer the person to supports that he or she may not be aware of.

5. **Do not make promises that you cannot keep:** Do not promise someone 24/7 attention if that is not something you can provide. Offer help, help him or her create a safety plan, offer to go with him or her to another professional who can help, but do not promise things that are unrealistic or not possible under your professional mandate.

For further guidance, the World Health Organization suggests the following for a first responder who is engaging with someone who may be actively suicidal:

- Approach all situations involving someone who is suicidal as a psychiatric emergency and act accordingly. Never assume that suicidal ideas or gestures are harmless bids for attention or an attempt to manipulate others.
- Clear the scene and keep yourself and others who may be present safe.
- Give physical space. Don't get too close to the person too soon. Sudden movements, attempts to touch the person, or the introduction of others into the scene, may be misunderstood.
- Express acceptance and concern. Avoid sermonizing, arguing, problem-solving, giving advice, or telling someone to "forget about it." It is important to convey an attitude of concern and understanding.
- Engage the individual. Encourage the person to talk. Most suicidal people are ambivalent about dying. Asking someone if he or she is suicidal or otherwise talking about suicide will not tip him or her over the edge, but will provide a sense of relief and a starting point for a solution. To assess intent, ask if the individual has a plan, access to lethal means, or has decided when to act.
- Remove access to all lethal means of self-harm, particularly firearms, and toxic substances (such as large supplies of psychotropic medications or pesticides).

- Suicide may be averted if people receive immediate and appropriate mental health care. If the individual fulfills *Mental Health Act* criteria, take immediate action to ensure that the individual is committed to a hospital for psychiatric assessment and treatment. If the individual does not appear to meet *Mental Health Act* criteria, it is still important to ensure that he or she has prompt access to mental health and substance abuse treatments. As most individuals are ambivalent about suicide, they will agree to receive treatment. Pre-arranged agreements with local hospitals and community mental health and addictions agencies will facilitate this process.
- Never leave a potentially suicidal individual alone based on his or her promise to visit their mental health worker or the hospital. Ensure that family members or significant others are on the scene and accept responsibility for seeking help (World Health Organization, 2009).

POINTS TO REMEMBER

- ✓ Suicide can be a loaded concept for many people, with notions of stigma, shame, and hurt surrounding it. This, unfortunately, has perpetuated misinformation about the issue and prevented numerous individuals from speaking openly about suicide.
- ✓ While suicide can affect anyone and is prevalent across Canada, numerous populations have been disproportionately affected by it. Two of those groups are first responders and military personnel, because they are often exposed to traumatic events.
- ✓ The good news is that in the absence of a tangible national strategy to prevent suicide, there are numerous ways to access help for yourself or other individuals who are at risk of suicide. Training programs and resources are readily available to first responders, police, and other helping professionals to help bolster interventions along the suicide prevention continuum.

KEY TERMS

REFERENCES

Barker, B., Goodman, A., & Debeck, K. (2017). Reclaiming Indigenous identities: Culture as strength against suicide among Indigenous youth in Canada. *Canadian Journal of Public Health*, *108*(2), E208.

Benibgui, M. (2010). *Mental health challenges and resilience in lesbian, gay, and bisexual young adults: Biological and psychological internalization of minority stress and victimization* (Doctoral dissertation). Retrieved from Spectrum Research Repository, Concordia University. (979282).

Eggertson, L. (2017). Federal suicide prevention framework underwhelms. *Canadian Medical Association Journal*, *189*(2), E96-E97. doi:10.1503/cmaj.109-5367

Juhnke, G.A., Granello, P.F., & Lebrón-Striker, M. (2007). IS PATH WARM? A suicide assessment mnemonic for counselors. ACAPCD-03. Alexandria, VA: American Counseling Association.

Laferriere, M., & Miloknay, S. (2018). *Mental health awareness: Self-care for first responders.* Toronto: Emond.

Lamoureux, M., & MacPherson, A. (2015, March 6). Canada's lack of first responder suicide stats is a national disgrace. Vice News. Retrieved from https://www.vice.com/en_ca/article/kwkxdx/canadas-lack-of-first-responder-suicide-stats-is-a-national-disgrace-263

Levinson-King, R. (2017, March 13). Teen suicide on the rise among Canadian girls. British Broadcasting Corporation News. Retrieved from http://www.bbc.com/news/world-us-canada-39210463

McQuaid, R.J., Bombay, A., McInnis, O.A., Humeny, C., Matheson, K., & Anisman, H. (2017). Suicide ideation and attempts among First Nations peoples living on-reserve in Canada: The intergenerational and cumulative effects of Indian residential schools. *Canadian Journal of Psychiatry*, *62*(6), 422–430. doi:10.1177/0706743717702075.

Mental Health Act, RSO 1990, c M.7.

Newland, C., Barber, E., Rose, M., & Young, A. (2015). Critical stress: Survey reveals alarming rates of EMS provider stress and thoughts of suicide. *JEMS: Journal of Emergency Medical Services*, *40*(10), 30–34.

Public Health Agency of Canada. (2016a). Working together to prevent suicide in Canada: The 2016 progress report on the federal framework for suicide prevention. Ottawa: Government of Canada, Minister of Health [Report]. Retrieved from http://www.healthycanadians.gc.ca/publications/healthy-living-vie-saine/framework-suicide-progress-report-2016-rapport-d-etape-cadre-suicide/alt/64-03-15-1430-suicideprev-progressreport-eng.pdf

Public Health Agency of Canada. (2016b). Working together to prevent suicide in Canada: The federal framework for suicide prevention. Ottawa: Government of Canada, Minister of Health [Report]. Retrieved from https://www.canada.ca/content/dam/canada/public-health/migration/publications/healthy-living-vie-saine/framework-suicide-cadre-suicide/alt/framework-suicide-cadre-suicide-eng.pdf

Rae, Hon. B. (2011). Opposition motion—National suicide prevention strategy. 41st Parliament, 1st Session, *Edited Hansard*, Number 026. Ottawa: Parliament of Canada. Retrieved from http://www.parl.gc.ca/HousePublications/Publication.aspx?Mode=1&Parl=41&Ses=1&DocId=5155242&Language=E - SOB-4342018

Russell, A. (2016, September 8). 22% of Canadian teens considered suicide this past year: Kids Help Phone study. Global News. Retrieved from http://globalnews.ca/news/2925079/22-of-canadian-teens-considered-suicide-this-past-year-kids-help-phone/

Statistics Canada. (2017). Table 102-0551. Deaths and mortality rate, by selected grouped causes, age group and sex, Canada, annual. CANSIM (database). Retrieved from http://www5.statcan.gc.ca/cansim/a26?lang=eng&retrLang=eng&id=1020551&&pattern=&stByVal=1&p1=1&p2=37&tabMode=dataTable&csid

Tema Conter Memorial Trust [TEMA]. (2017a). How can we help you today? Retrieved from https://www.tema.ca/

Tema Conter Memorial Trust [TEMA]. (2017b). [Infographic]. *Reported Canadian Public Safety Suicides*. Retrieved from https://infogram.com/reported_canadian_first_responder_suicides

Wilson, M.G., & Gauvin, F.P. (2012). Evidence brief: Preventing suicide in Canada. Hamilton, ON: McMaster Health Forum. Retrieved from https://macsphere.mcmaster.ca/bitstream/11375/14862/1/fulltext.pdf

World Health Organization. (2009). Preventing suicide: A resource for police, firefighters and other first line responders. Geneva, Switzerland: WHO Press. Retrieved from http://www.who.int/mental_health/prevention/suicide/resource_firstresponders.pdf

PART 3

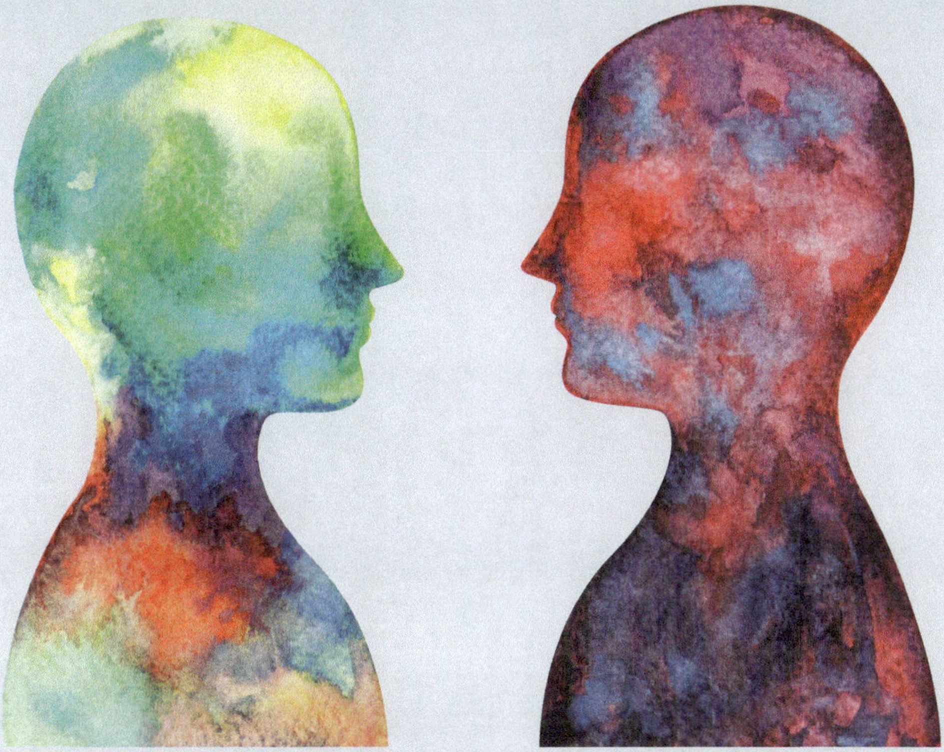

MENTAL HEALTH INTERVENTIONS FOR THOSE IN CRISIS

CASE STUDY 3

William is a 49-year-old male living in London, Ontario. He grew up in a relatively stable environment with both parents and two younger siblings. During his teen years he experienced bouts of depression and anxiety but was never formally diagnosed or treated.

When he was in his early 20s, William married Sandra, who was an alcoholic and also suffered from bouts of depression and anxiety. William gradually withdrew from his family and focused intensely on Sandra and supporting her needs. William continued to suffer from depression and anxiety and began abusing alcohol and drugs. His behaviour toward his family began to grow more and more peculiar, but he refused to be assessed or have any treatment. He eventually isolated himself entirely from his family and became unemployed, which left Sandra as his only source of social contact. Sandra was also unemployed and had no family or friends.

William and Sandra, now in their late 30s, were living life in isolation, with very few social and financial supports. They were living in subsidized housing and preferred to keep to themselves, rarely even leaving their home. Sadly, after a night of drinking, Sandra fell asleep with a cigarette in her hand, setting herself on fire. William awoke to the horror of seeing his wife on fire, and he called 911. Sandra was rushed to the hospital, but later died. William blamed himself for not being able to save her.

William's life spiralled downward following this tragedy. Witnessing his wife's death caused him to display symptoms of PTSD, but he refused to receive treatment. William frequently called 911 for events that were not occurring, with the result that he became very familiar to the police for his abuse of dialling 911 for no good reason, as well as for his odd behaviour. He was frequently seen walking around downtown, and local shop owners and residents could easily identify him. He quickly became known as a nuisance to the police and public because of his loitering and reporting of fictitious events.

QUESTIONS

1. What are the factors that contributed to the deterioration of William's life over the years?
2. What role could the police have in providing support to William?
3. What community services are available to William?

4. What effects could labelling William "a nuisance" have on police response?
5. How can the various mental health resources connect to provide overall care and support to William?
6. Should William be forced into treatment? Why or why not?

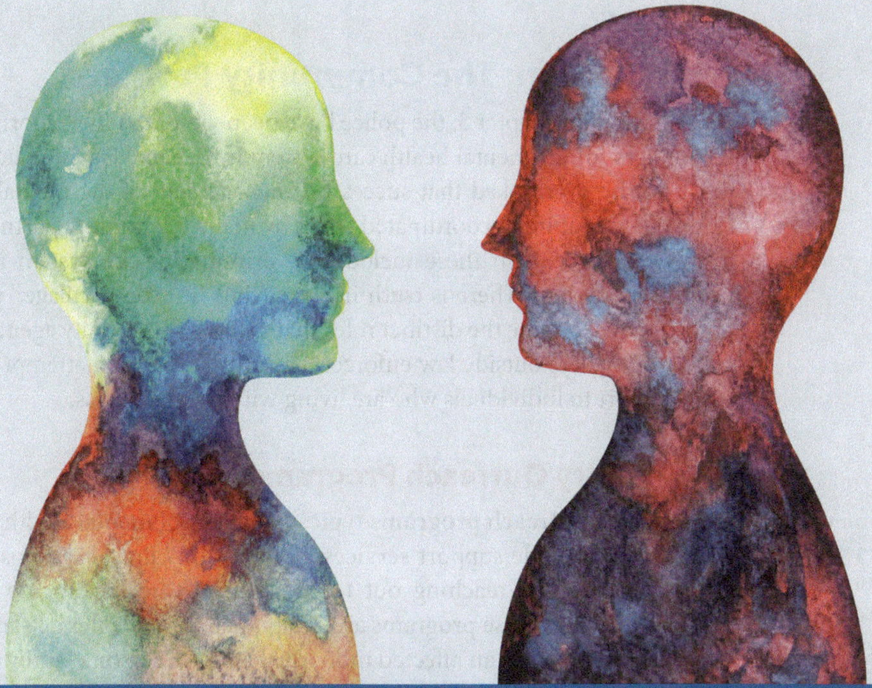

8 SKILLED LABOUR
Helpful Skills Across the Fields for Crisis Intervention

LEARNING OUTCOMES

After reading this chapter, you will be able to:

- Distinguish between the various services available to individuals with mental illness.
- Identify the specific role each agency or service provider is responsible for in the arena of mental health.
- Understand the complexities of mental health issues and recognize the need to have various services available to provide support to individuals living with mental illness.

Introduction: The Community Partners

As discussed in Chapter 3, the police have been viewed as the "informal first responders" of the mental health care system in Canada. Having said this, it must not be overlooked that successful management of the mental health care system requires a coordinated effort by many community partners, not just law enforcement: these include the criminal justice system and the health care system. There is truth in the saying "it takes a village," and the following will outline the distinct roles that various community agencies and service providers outside law enforcement undertake in an attempt to provide support to individuals who are living with mental illness.

Community Outreach Programs

community outreach program program designed to provide flexible and individualized mental health services for people living with mental illness in their home or community

Community outreach programs typically consist of mental health professionals who provide support services, both within clinical settings and in the community, by reaching out to individuals who have acute mental health problems. These programs are designed to provide flexible and individualized services to an affected individual and the person's family in their home community. A community outreach program's aim is to improve an individual's coping skills and provide support to him or her and his or her family. While doing this, the program continues to engage the individual and the family by involving them in building relationships with other mental health providers in their community.

Community outreach programs provide intensive mental health services with the goal of stabilizing an individual's condition and making appropriate referrals. The treatment offered is similar to what an individual would receive in a hospital setting or medical office, but it is provided in the person's home. Individuals participating in this type of program are visited by a mental health professional who assesses the individual's problem, and a treatment plan is developed jointly between the mental health professional and the individual. The plan will include items such as ongoing counselling/therapy, couple or family support, educational or support groups, and medication information. When required, referrals to other community services are arranged prior to the individual being discharged from the program.

Referrals for community outreach programs must be made by a psychiatrist or a staff member of an in-patient unit or a crisis intervention team (for example, see Crisis Outreach and Support Team (COAST) in Chapter 3).

Distress Centres and Crisis Lines

Distress centre crisis lines are confidential helplines that are available 24 hours a day, 365 days a year to any person experiencing emotional distress. These programs are operated through trained volunteers who provide emotional support, crisis intervention, suicide prevention, and links to emergency services when needed. Since many calls are received after-hours, crisis lines are viewed as "backup" for many mental health and social service programs.

distress centre crisis lines
confidential helplines that are available 24 hours a day, 365 days a year to any person experiencing emotional distress

Distress centres enable individuals to continue functioning in the community when it is possible for them to do so. Volunteers working at these centres refer individuals to appropriate community support and professional resources, intervene in life threatening situations, and provide support to individuals living in the community who have chronic mental health problems. A helpline volunteer will respond to the immediate needs of a caller, taking into account the individual's culture, perspective, and problem-solving abilities.

Distress centres and crisis lines work collaboratively with mental health professionals to ensure that those at risk are made aware of this 24-hour service. Several agencies, counsellors, and psychiatrists leave crisis line numbers on their voicemail to provide after-hours support.

Addiction Programs

Addiction programs are either long- or short-term; however, most treatment programs require an individual to be sober, which means the person has to go through a detoxification process and be medically managed through withdrawal before commencing with any therapeutic treatment. Detoxification is the process by which the physical body clears itself of drugs and/or alcohol. The detoxification process does not address the psychological, social, and behavioural problems associated with addiction; without additional counselling, the process will not likely produce the long-lasting results that are necessary for recovery. Detoxification is often managed by a physician who administers medication in an in-patient setting. This is commonly referred to as "medically managed withdrawal."

long-term treatment program (residential)
type of program that provides 24-hour care in a non-hospital setting and lasts from 6 to 12 months—the focus is on "re-socialization" of an individual living with addiction and substance abuse issues

A **long-term (or residential) treatment program** provides around-the-clock care, generally in a non-hospital setting. This type of program involves planned lengths of stay between 6 and 12 months. The focus of this type of treatment program is on the "re-socialization" of the individual through the involvement of the program's staff and other residents. Addiction is examined in the context of the individual's social and psychological deficits, with treatment focusing on helping the individual develop personal responsibility and accountability. This type of program is highly structured and designed to assist individuals by examining destructive patterns of behaviour and then developing constructive ways for the person to interact with others. Other services are usually available to assist the individual with reintegration into society (for example, employment training). These programs can be tailored to meet the needs of various groups of people, such as adolescents, women, the homeless, people with mental illness, and individuals who are within the criminal justice system.

short-term treatment program type of program that provides intense yet brief treatment based on a 12-step approach

Short-term treatment programs provide intense yet brief treatment based on a 12-step approach. This type of program was designed to treat alcohol abuse problems, but it is also used to treat other substance abuse problems. This treatment model typically consists of a three- to six-week hospital-based in-patient treatment phase, followed by an extended outpatient therapy program that includes participation in a self-help group such as Alcoholics Anonymous (known as "AA"). Following residential programs, it is important for individuals to remain in aftercare programs to reduce the risk of relapse.

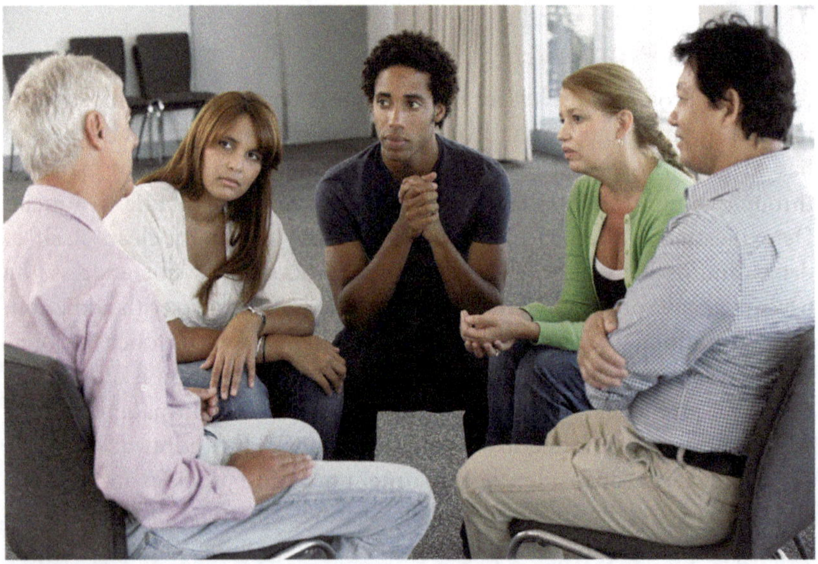

A group treatment session.

Housing and Support for the Homeless

Housing is not just having a place to sleep. It is tied to an individual's physical, emotional, and social well-being. Decent, safe, and affordable housing is an important factor in an individual's physical, mental, and social well-being.

According to the United Nations' *Universal Declaration of Human Rights*, the right to housing is protected under international law, and Canada has endorsed such rights, guaranteeing "a standard of living adequate for ... health and well-being ... , including adequate food, clothing, [and] housing" (The United Nations, 1948, art. 25). Similarly, *The Ottawa Charter for Health Promotion* identifies shelter as a basic prerequisite for health (World Health Organization, 1986).

BOX 8.1 WHY ARE PEOPLE HOMELESS?

Two trends are largely responsible for the rise in homelessness over the past 20 years: (1) a growing shortage of affordable rental housing and (2) a simultaneous increase in poverty. Homelessness and poverty are linked. Poor people are frequently unable to pay for housing, food, child care, health care, and education. Difficult choices must be made when limited resources cover only some of these necessities.

There are numerous reasons why an individual finds himself or herself homeless. Some possible reasons are:

- inability to afford rent,
- low vacancy rate for renters,
- poverty/inadequate income,
- long wait lists for subsidized housing,
- loss of employment, and
- mental illness and addiction conditions.

In response, there are a variety of shelters and transitional residences in place to support various groups of individuals: families, refugees, women and children, single men, Indigenous men and women, and youth. There are also shelters and housing available for individuals living with substance abuse issues and mental illness. These shelters provide support to individuals to assist and connect them with appropriate community agencies based on individual needs.

What Constitutes Homelessness?

- Individuals who reside in places that are not intended as, or are unfit for, human habitation, including in cars, abandoned buildings, bus or train stations, under bridges, or in garbage or recycling dumpsters, parks, or other places lacking basic amenities.
- Individuals sharing housing at the whim of other persons on an interim or emergency basis.
- Individuals whose primary nighttime place of abode is a supervised publicly or privately operated shelter designed to provide temporary living accommodations, including shelters for victims of domestic violence, welfare hotels, short-term family housing (congregate shelters), and transitional housing.

Affordable Housing

According to the organization Canada Without Poverty, an estimated 235,000 Canadians were homeless in 2016. Additionally, approximately 3 million Canadians are living in unaffordable, below-standard, or overcrowded housing. It is also estimated that of the homeless population, approximately 45 percent are individuals living with a disability and/or mental illness. Many individuals with mental illness are on social assistance and a majority of them do not have access to affordable housing (Canada Without Poverty, 2017).

Housing and Mental Health

Housing is a basic human right and requirement for good physical and mental health. Adequate housing leads to increased personal safety and decreased stress. If a person living with mental illness resides in a place that is rundown and overcrowded, it can make his or her recovery from mental illness or substance abuse problems more challenging. Good housing can help a person living with mental illness rebuild and maintain his or her independence and confidence, and create a structured daily routine, all of which can lead to an overall higher quality of life. Housing is more than shelter; it is a pathway to safety, security, and connectedness.

People living with mental health and addiction conditions are disproportionately affected by homelessness. While many factors can lead to homelessness, mental illness plays a significant role. The consequences of homelessness tend to be more severe when coupled with a mental health condition. Individuals with mental illness tend to remain homeless for longer periods of time and have less contact with family and friends. They encounter more barriers to employment and tend to be in poorer health than other homeless people.

> Many studies show that people who are homeless are more likely to experience compromised mental health and mental illness than the general population. For some, these issues can precede the onset of homelessness or, through their interaction with other determinants such as income and employment influences, contribute to homelessness. They also worsen with continued homelessness or contribute to the duration of homelessness (Canadian Institute for Health Information, 2007).

For individuals living with mental illness and/or addiction conditions, safe and affordable housing can provide a place to live in dignity and move toward reintegration and recovery. Housing with supports gives individuals access to a range of housing options: supportive housing, supported housing, and rent supplements. **Supportive housing** provides assistance by staffing housing units with 24-hour support services. **Supported housing** may be appropriate for individuals who live in the larger community and receive supports such as homecare and counselling when they need it.

supportive housing an individual receives 24-hour assistance within a housing unit

supported housing an individual lives in the community and has supports such as homecare and counselling when required

Supports within housing include:

- up to 24-hour support for individuals living with mental illness and/or addictions and their significant others to ensure a stable housing environment.
- individualized assessment and planning, hands-on assistance with activities of daily living, coordination and support, crisis management, facilitating peer and group support, and resident input to their housing environment.
- support services provided to individuals who are homeless, or at risk of being homeless.
- support services such as connecting with landlords, matching people to housing, housing advocacy, and teaching life skills.

Service providers have also identified the following factors that support successful housing arrangements: rent geared to income, community support services, a strong personal support network, and availability of case management.

Residential care and permanent supported housing approaches appear to yield the greatest reduction in hospitalizations. People living in housing with support are less likely to be institutionalized in jails and prisons. Individuals in supported housing report a higher quality of life because they have more choice and control over their housing and the quality of their housing (Canadian Mental Health Association, 2014, p. 3).

Rent supplements or rent-geared-to-income housing are two strategies that can provide individuals with the financial resources they need to access desirable housing in their community.

The challenges of poverty, stigma, and discrimination that individuals with mental illness face directly affect their ability to access, find, and keep housing. Many individuals are often denied housing in the private market as a result of their mental health and addiction conditions. Furthermore, many supportive housing projects also encounter a "not-in-my-backyard" response from neighbours, businesses, politicians, and so on. This type of behaviour may include discriminating and slanderous comments in person, by email, or through flyers and posters that protest a new local supportive housing development.

DISCUSSION QUESTIONS

1. In what ways does suitable housing impact the lives of people living with mental illness?
2. What can be done to reduce the stigma surrounding mental illness and supportive housing developments?
3. Supportive housing lessens the impact on the health care system. In what ways can it reduce the impact on the criminal justice system?

Corrections

The responsibility for Canada's health care system is shared between the federal and provincial governments under the legal framework of the *Canada Health Act* (CHA). The CHA is the federal legislation for publicly funded health care insurance. The CHA sets out the primary objective of Canadian health care policy, which is "to protect, promote and restore the physical and mental well-being of residents of Canada and to facilitate reasonable access to health services without financial or other barriers" (CHA, s. 3).

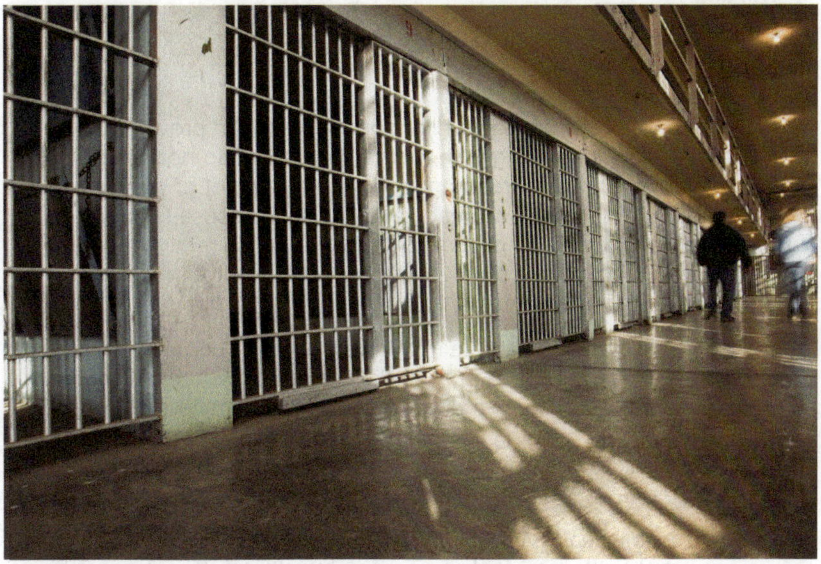

The interior of a corrections facility.

Under the CHA, the federal and provincial governments are responsible for the management and delivery of health services to the residents of their provinces and territories—including those incarcerated in correctional institutions and all individuals serving sentences in the community; however, inmates in federal penitentiaries are excluded. In relation to federal inmates, the Correctional Service of Canada is required by statute "to provide essential health care, including medical, dental, and mental health care, and reasonable access to non-essential mental health care that will contribute to the inmate's rehabilitation and successful reintegration into the community" (MCSCS, 2016). All federal, provincial, and territorial correctional jurisdictions have the responsibility to provide care to individuals in their facilities who are living with mental health illnesses. There are safeguards in place for individuals in the correctional system to ensure that they are provided with adequate access to essential services and supports.

POINTS TO REMEMBER

- ✓ There are several ways in which communities can provide support to individuals living with mental illness that do not necessarily involve law enforcement being the first point of contact. There are community outreach and substance abuse support groups, agencies, and programs that offer help directly in the individual's home or community and do not involve in-patient or residential treatment.
- ✓ Housing plays a crucial role in the well-being of people who are living with mental illness. It is hard to determine whether mental illness contributes to an individual becoming homeless or if the lack of suitable housing and a stable environment contributes to the breakdown of a person's physical, emotional, and mental wellness.
- ✓ The *Canada Health Act* ensures that all Canadians receive appropriate health care, including mental health treatment, regardless of where an individual lives or what his or her circumstances are. This includes individuals who are incarcerated and serving a sentence in a provincial correctional facility. Inmates serving a federal sentence are protected under section 86 of the *Corrections and Conditional Release Act* to receive suitable mental health support and treatment while under the care and control of the Correctional Service of Canada.

KEY TERMS

community outreach program, 170

distress centre crisis lines, 171

long-term treatment program (residential), 171

short-term treatment program, 172

supported housing, 175

supportive housing, 175

REFERENCES

Canada Health Act [CHA], RSC 1985, c C-6.

Canada without poverty. (2017). Just the Facts. Retrieved from http://www.cwp-csp.ca/poverty/just-the-facts/

Canadian Institute for Health Information. (2007). *Improving the health of Canadians: Mental health and homelessness*. Ottawa: Author.

Canadian Mental Health Association. (2014). Backgrounder: Housing and mental health. Retrieved from https://ontario.cmha.ca/documents/housing-and-mental-health/

Corrections and Conditional Release Act, SC 1992, c 20.

Ministry of Community Safety and Correctional Services [MCSCS]. (2016). *Mental health strategy for corrections in Canada: A federal-provincial-territorial partnership*. Retrieved from http://www.mcscs.jus.gov.on.ca/english/publications/MCSCS_pubs_mental_health.html

The United Nations. (1948). *The universal declaration of human rights*. Retrieved from http://www.un.org/en/universal-declaration-human-rights/

World Health Organization. (1986, November 21). *The Ottawa charter for health promotion*. Geneva, Switzerland: Author. Retrieved from http://www.phac-aspc.gc.ca/ph-sp/docs/charter-chartre/

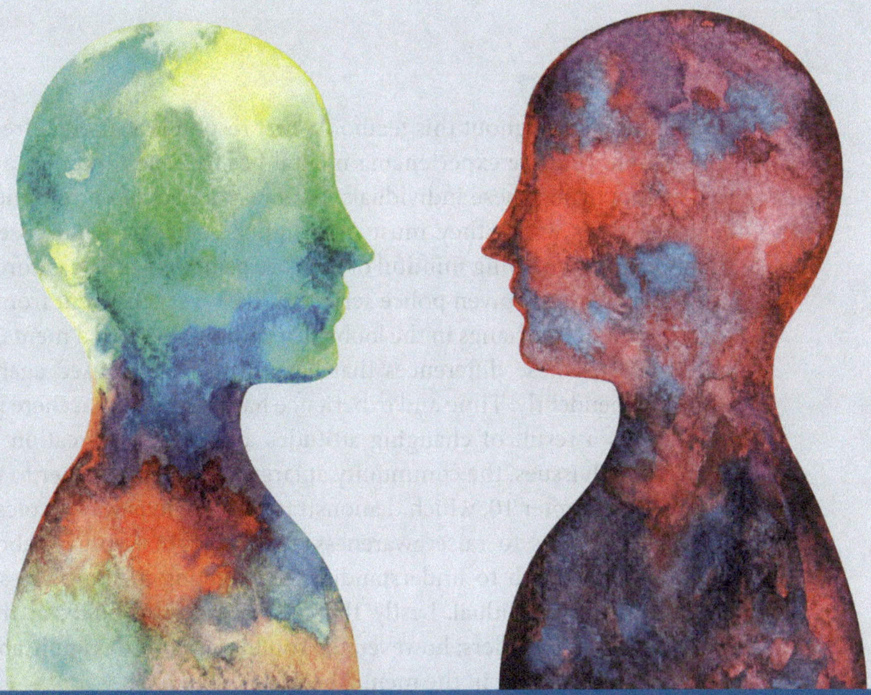

9 IT TAKES A COMMUNITY

Connecting and Collaborating for Service Delivery that Focuses on the Individual

LEARNING OUTCOMES

After reading this chapter, you will be able to:

- Identify the fundamental principles and expectations of contemporary policing.
- Identify helpful ways to communicate with an individual with mental illness to encourage disclosure.
- Understand the role of police discretion and ethical decision-making within the context of the mental health system.
- Critically analyze the role stigma plays in service delivery.
- Differentiate the broader mandates of law enforcement and mental health professionals.
- Identify non-police programs aimed at educating mental health professionals
- Recognize barriers to mental health services in the community.
- Understand what community capacity and community mobilization are.

Introduction

As discussed throughout this textbook, first responders interact frequently with people who are experiencing mental health issues and play a crucial role in supporting these individuals. First responders often respond to urgent situations where they must make quick decisions while assessing a situation and remaining mindful of the core principles of law enforcement. The mandate of any given police service is likely very different from a mission statement that hangs in the lobby of a community-based mental health provider. It is these differences that have historically caused agencies to work independently. Time and experience have revealed that there is a better way. As a result of changing attitudes and greater education around mental health issues, the community at large is coming together to work as a team; see Chapter 10, which demonstrates the various ways professionals have joined forces to raise awareness, reduce stigma, and collaborate to achieve an approach to understanding and treating mental illness that is centred on the individual. Lastly, this chapter refers to police as the most common first responders; however, the content discussed is applicable to all professionals working in the mental health field.

Centre Procedural Justice on the Individual

It is fair to say that all Canadians expect to be treated equitably and with respect. This expectation does not change if an individual is living with a mental illness.

Police are called on every day to assess and manage a variety of situations, many of which require officers to de-escalate and mediate situations, rather than enforce the law. These situations require exceptional interpersonal and communication skills in addition to a service-oriented focus. This focus is what led Canadian police organizations to replace the term "police force" with "police service" for referral to their formal title. This change also reflects the fundamental principles and expectations of contemporary policing.

Interacting Effectively with People with Mental Illness

The ability to interact and communicate effectively and in a caring and compassionate manner benefits interaction between first responders and any member of the public. When police respond to a call involving a person with mental health issues, the initial contact will set the tone that leads to

TABLE 9.1 The Fundamental Principles and Expectations of Contemporary Policing

• Due process, equity, and fairness (procedural justice); • Ethical practice; • Community confidence and trust; • Responsive to the environment; • Focus is on the individual; • Consultation and collaboration with the community; • Quality and valued individual service; • Continuous evaluation, continuous improvement, and change;	• Teamwork; • Decentralization of authority and decision-making; • Total involvement; • Participative leadership; • Increased communication; • Internal and external alignment; • Outcome-focused.

Source: Adapted from Coleman & Cotton, 2014, p. 16.

either a positive or negative experience. Watson, Angell, Vidalon, and Davis (2010) indicate that the literature is clear about the outcome of positive and respectful behaviour by the police. When police exercise their authority in a procedurally just manner (**procedural justice**), the community responds with cooperation and respect. On the other hand, if police act disrespectfully, cooperation and respect are diminished.

procedural justice refers to due process, equity, and fairness in policing

Additionally, the impact of a poor initial response could exacerbate the distress the individual is already experiencing and it could mean that he or she does not get the assistance he or she needs. It could also prevent the individual from contacting police when he or she requires help in the future. Also, as with most negative experiences, the consequences are often difficult to reverse, especially when it comes to lasting impressions. If an officer has a negative initial experience with an individual, any follow-up interactions may not be positive.

Key Factors in Interaction

A number of key factors shape the quality of interactions between police and individuals.

Response to Disclosure of Mental Health Issues

When an individual discloses a mental health issue, his or her experience is likely to be more positive if police show empathy and understanding, respond in a sensitive manner, and make necessary adjustments where appropriate, as the situation unfolds. Negative experiences can include police making insensitive or judgmental remarks, responding poorly to an individual's distress, and not providing appropriate support after becoming aware of the person's mental health issue.

Validation and Being Taken Seriously

Having their experiences acknowledged and believed by law enforcement is important to individuals who are experiencing a mental health crisis. When individuals tell officers that they are living with a mental illness, it is important for officers to not deny, challenge, or minimize individuals' concerns.

Centre Support on the Individual

It is valuable to all parties involved when an individual is asked about his or her needs, involved in decision-making, and kept informed. For example, a small yet respectful gesture is to provide the name of the attending officer as a main point of contact to help foster a trusting relationship.

Collaborative Approach

A collaborative approach involves police, as first responders, making contact with services that are already in place to support an individual or putting that person in touch with helpful services. It is not beneficial when agencies work in isolation or when an individual is rapidly referred from one agency to another. According to Watson, Angell, Vidalon, and Davis (2010), the important factor in this collaborative approach is the building of police relationships with mental health resource agencies and organizations and the "[s]hifting of police roles and organizational priorities from an exclusively traditional law-enforcement model, which reluctantly deal[s] with persons with mental illness, to a more service-oriented model that responds to mental illness as a community safety and public health concern" (Watson et al., 2010).

Key Points to Remember During an Interaction

When an individual with a mental health issue comes into contact with the police, it is likely that the person has already been through a distressing experience. The individual may also be wary about interacting with the police because of fear or previous negative experiences with law enforcement.

Keep the following in mind when you are interacting with an individual:

1. Introduce yourself and explain your role. The use of first names in an introduction may lessen any perceived power differential. For example, "Hi, I'm Steve. I'm with the Toronto Police Service and I'm here to help you."
2. Acknowledge and respect the individual and his or her feelings.
3. Actively listen with sensitivity.
4. Use responsive body language.
5. Use a calm and reassuring tone.
6. Ask short, simple, and open-ended questions.
7. Be mindful that the individual may be unable to effectively communicate what he or she is experiencing. Be patient, compassionate, and understanding.
8. Reflect information given back to the individual and summarize issues to demonstrate active listening.
9. Be honest and transparent about what is going on.
10. Provide the name of an officer the individual can contact directly.
11. Provide regular updates and explain why certain decisions have been made.
12. Remain aware that the individual's level of functioning/ability to comprehend may fluctuate with each follow-up interaction. This means that maintaining contact may require continued encouragement and support.

Mental Illness and Victimization

As mentioned in Chapter 3, 5 percent of all calls that police respond to involve individuals who live with mental health issues. It is important to keep in mind that some of these interactions involve the individual as the victim of a crime and not a person who is in crisis or who has committed a criminal offence. Mentally ill individuals are at risk of being victimized by people who want to take advantage of their circumstances. For example, a person with mental illness may be targeted because the perpetrator feels the victim will have no credibility when disclosing the crime and therefore will not be believed by law enforcement. Additionally, the offender may feel the victim simply does not have the resources or capacity to report the crime committed against him or her. Because of this, individuals with mental illness are vulnerable to all types of offences, ranging from property crimes (theft and fraud) to crimes against the person (assault and sexual assault).

VOICES FROM THE FIELD

Study Shows Mentally Ill More Likely to Be Victims, Not Perpetrators, of Violence

by Matt Shipman, NC State News

February 25, 2014—New research shows that almost one-third of adults with mental illness are likely to be victims of violence within a six-month period, and that adults with mental illness who commit violence are most likely to do so in residential settings. The study also finds a strong correlation between being a victim of violence and committing a violent act.

The work was done by researchers at North Carolina State University; RTI International; the University of California, Davis; Simon Fraser University; and Duke University.

"We hear about the link between violence and mental illness in the news, and we wanted to look not only at the notion that the mentally ill are a danger to others, but the possibility that they are also in danger," says Dr. Sarah Desmarais, an assistant professor of psychology at NC State and lead author of a paper describing the work.

The researchers compiled a database of 4,480 mentally ill adults who had answered questions about both committing violence and being victims of violence in the previous six months. The database drew from five earlier studies that focused on issues ranging from antipsychotic medications to treatment approaches. Those studies had different research goals, but all asked identical questions related to violence and victimization.

The researchers found that 23.9 percent of the study participants had committed a violent act within the previous six months. The majority of those acts—63.5 percent—were committed in residential settings, not in public. Only 2.6 percent of the violent acts were committed in school or workplace settings.

The researchers found that a significantly higher percentage of participants—30.9 percent—had been victims of violence in the same time period. And of those who said they were victimized, 43.7 percent said they'd been victimized on multiple occasions.

"We also found that participants who had been victims of violence were 11 times more likely to commit violence," Desmarais says. "This highlights the need for more robust public health interventions that are focused on violence. It shouldn't just be about preventing adults with mental illness from committing violent acts, it should also be about protecting those at risk of being victimized.

"For one thing, it's the right thing to do," Desmarais adds. "In addition, while correlation is not necessarily causation, preventing violence against the mentally ill may drive down instances of violence committed by the mentally ill."

The paper, "Community Violence Perpetration and Victimization Among Adults With Mental Illnesses," is published online in the *American Journal of Public Health*. The paper was co-authored by Dr. Richard Van Dorn of RTI International; Kiersten Johnson, a graduate student at NC State; Dr. Kevin Grimm of University of California, Davis; Dr. Kevin Douglas of Simon Fraser University; and Dr. Marvin Swartz of Duke University.

Source: Shipman, 2014.

Discussion Questions

1. The study indicates that most violent acts committed by individuals with mental illness are committed in residential settings and not in public. What conditions may contribute to this?
2. This research relied on *self-reporting*. What are the benefits and limitations of this type of data gathering?
3. What factors may influence a person who is a victim of violence to also commit violent acts?

Barriers to Reporting

Several barriers affect whether people with mental illness who have been victimized will disclose an offence. The following points outline some significant barriers that should be considered by police and other first responders as well as mental health professionals when interacting and working with these individuals.

- **Discrimination:** Stigma and discrimination are common barriers to reporting crime. Many victims with mental health issues fear they will not be perceived as credible because of their diagnosis or condition. They may even fear that their ability to recount events accurately is impaired by the state of their mental health.
- **Accessing support:** Once a crime has been reported to the police, additional follow-up interviews and documentation can overwhelm a victim, especially if the person does not have additional support and assistance. Required practical tasks, such as completing a victim impact statement and providing medical information, may also create barriers to accessing support in the criminal justice system; a certain level of literacy and comprehension is required for many of these tasks. Further, the preparation of these documents can be invasive and may require information and documentation from a physician. Be aware that there is limited support available to help people maintain mental health and self-care throughout the court process. More commonly, they will need to access community mental health care through their physician or mental health team.
- **Fear of retaliation:** A common barrier for victimized individuals when reporting offences is the fear of retaliation. As previously

mentioned, offenders may deliberately target people with mental illness because they see them as vulnerable and less likely to report an incident to the police. Further, if illegal drugs are involved, a victim is less likely to report it to police. The individual may not want to disclose the fact that he or she has addiction issues and may fear being subjected to a criminal investigation.

- **Protecting the offender:** It often happens that when a crime is committed against an individual and the offender is known to that person (the offender may be a family member or a friend), the victim may feel a sense of loyalty to the offender. The victim may feel confused as to why someone close to him or her would do such a thing and may want to protect the offender. It may also happen that the offender has threatened the victim with death or bodily harm if he or she reports the incident, or may simply have told the victim to keep it a secret.
- **Daunting court process:** The court process is intimidating and can produce anxiety. Anxiety and fear are further complicated by the fact that the victim must see the accused in court. Further, the victim may have to interact with police in uniform, which can be difficult for the victim if he or she has had a negative past with law enforcement, or delusions or paranoia related to authority systems.

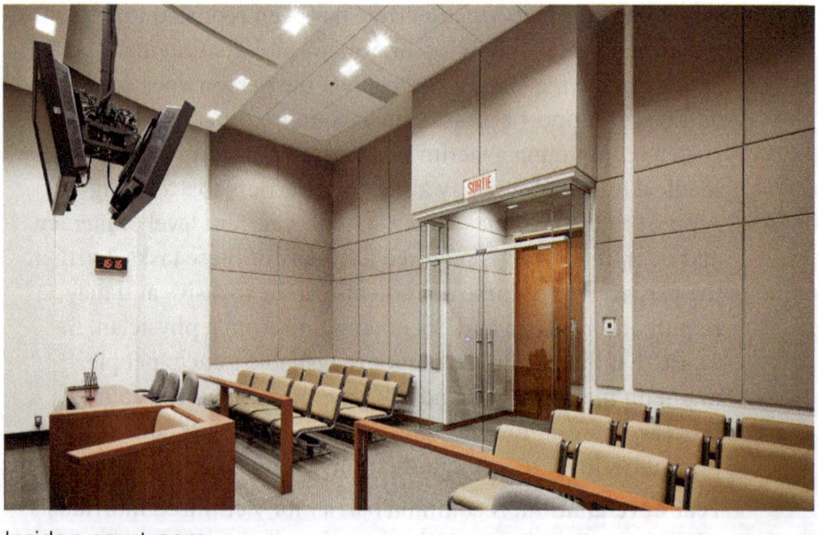

Inside a courtroom.

Factors that Encourage Reporting

In order to reduce the barriers outlined above, there are factors that can assist or encourage a victim to report. Some helpful strategies are:

- easy accessibility to police officers (visibility in the community).
- support of family and friends.
- support of professionals to assist in navigating the various community and social service processes.
- public education in relation to certain crimes (for example, sexual assault and domestic violence).
- court support programs (for example, see Box 9.1 below).

Box 9.1 outlines Ontario's Victim/Witness Assistance Program, which is an important service offered to individuals who have to take part in the criminal process.

BOX 9.1 VICTIM/WITNESS ASSISTANCE PROGRAM

What Is the Victim/Witness Assistance Program?

If you are a victim or witness of a violent crime, it is likely that you will need to go to court. This can be a difficult and confusing experience. You may have a lot of questions about the criminal court system, and what will be expected of you.

The Victim/Witness Assistance Program is here to help. We will talk to you and provide assistance based on your specific case and needs.

Our services begin once police have laid charges and will continue until the court case is over.

Who Can Receive Help?

Services are provided on a priority basis to vulnerable victims and witnesses of violent crimes, such as domestic violence, child abuse, sexual assault, elder abuse, homicide, and hate crimes.

In addition, we offer help to:

- victims with special needs,
- families of victims of homicide,
- families of victims of traffic fatalities resulting in criminal charges.

Age-appropriate information and services are available for children.

How Do I Get Help?

After charges have been laid, the police or Crown attorney refers victims and witnesses to the program for help. If you are a victim of violent crime, you can also call to access the program on your own or have someone in the community call on your behalf. Staff will try to contact you as soon as possible to offer support and to respond to any safety concerns.

How Much Does It Cost?

The services are free across Ontario.

What Kind of Help Is Available?

The Victim/Witness Assistance Program can:

- answer your questions about the criminal justice system, courtroom procedures and your role in court.
- help you understand what to expect at each court date, and help you prepare for your appearance in court.
- provide you with copies of court papers, such as bail conditions and probation orders.
- contact the Crown attorney or the police officer in charge of your case on your behalf.
- offer ongoing emotional support throughout the court process.
- refer you to community agencies for other services you may need, such as counselling and safety planning.
- arrange for language interpreters in domestic violence cases and/or accommodate any special needs.
- help you understand and complete a victim impact statement.

The program cannot:

- receive or discuss your evidence,
- withdraw charges,
- provide or arrange for childcare,
- provide transportation to and from court.

How Do I Contact the Program?

The Victim/Witness Assistance Program is offered by the Ministry of the Attorney General in all 54 court districts.

To find the office nearest you, call the **Victim Support Line** toll free at 1-888-579-2888 or at 416-314-2447 in the Greater Toronto Area or visit www.ontario.ca/victimservices.

Source: Ontario, Ministry of the Attorney General, n.d.

Ethical Practice

As previously mentioned, police, as first responders, are permitted (in most cases) to use discretion when enforcing the law. With this power, ethical decision-making plays a critical role in effective and acceptable standards of practice.

Officers can best apply this discretion when equipped with accurate information and knowledge about the circumstances they may face on a day-to-day basis. For example, if police are contacted when someone is in crisis, discretion is required to decide whether the person should be apprehended under the *Mental Health Act* or if he or she is able to seek assistance voluntarily. Being able to understand both the parameters of the law and the signs and symptoms of mental illness is crucial to making informed, lawful, and ethical decisions. Further, the type of action chosen must be based on sound reasoning and good judgment while balancing the individual's safety as well as public safety. Best practices are supported when an officer determines the level of force required in order to respond to a person in crisis, which can range from verbal communication to lethal force.

mission statement
brief summary of the goals and values of an organization

core values
foundation upon which an organization makes decisions, plans strategies, and interacts with its own members and external groups, organizations, and stakeholders

Police Working with Mental Health Professionals

Now that the role of the police in relation to their interactions with people who have mental health issues has been reviewed, it should be compared to the various mandates that other mental health professionals are responsible for when providing service to individuals with mental illness.

Police service **mission statements** often include phrases such as

- protect and serve the public,
- enforce federal, provincial, and municipal statutes,
- partner with the community, and
- reduce, deter, and prevent crime.

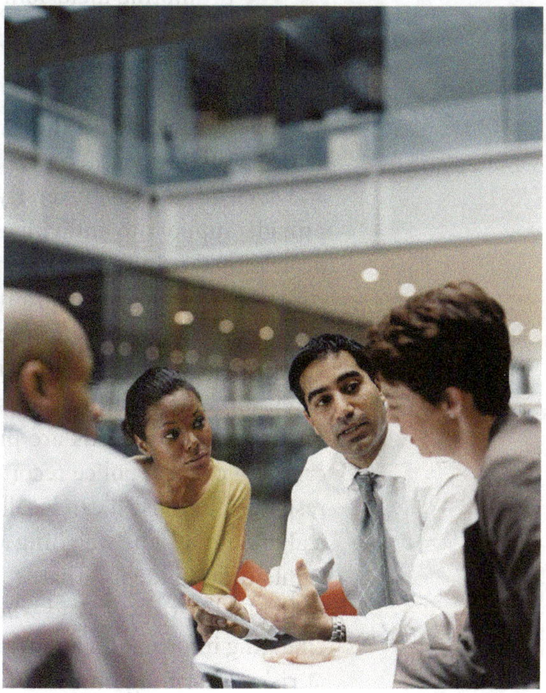

Police working collaboratively with a mental health professional.

Additionally, statements about the **core values** of police services often include words such as

- honesty,
- fairness,
- accountability,
- reliability,
- integrity,
- respect, and
- teamwork.

In comparison, in describing their mandates and/or mission statements, mental health agencies use phrases such as

- advocating for people with mental illness,
- influencing policy,
- providing services,
- developing resources,
- building capacity,
- promoting inclusion, and
- being transparent and accountable.

On review, there are some clear differences between the mandates held by police services and those held by mental health agencies. In a broad sense, police services' responsibility is primarily focused on community and societal safety. Conversely, the role of mental health professionals is to provide support to individuals. With these differences embedded in the professional cultures, each service and agency should be mindful of the occupational and legal constraints of the other.

These professions and other agencies (including Canada Border Services Agency) often face dilemmas in sharing information. For example, when a mental health professional is treating an individual, that person's medical/health records are protected. In the same way, if a person has a criminal or local police record, the information contained in that record is restricted to those it can legally be disclosed to. Therefore, the ongoing ethical dilemma is the weighing and balancing of public safety and the privacy rights of individuals. That is, at what point does public safety override an individual's privacy? And when should these various organizations be exchanging information about an individual with mental illness who could be at risk of harming himself or herself or others? Box 9.2 highlights privacy issues that must be considered prior to organizations sharing an individual's personal information.

BOX 9.2

Toronto Police to Restrict Mental Health Record Sharing

July 12, 2016, Canadian Civil Liberties Association (CCLA)—CCLA supports today's announcement that the Toronto Police Service (TPS) will restrict the entry of some suicide-related mental health flags into national databases, but cautions that more action on this front is needed to properly protect privacy.

The announcement today from the Information and Privacy Commissioner and the TPS confirms that many suicide-related police interactions will no longer be automatically shared with US officials; it remains unclear, however, whether other mental health-related police records, beyond alleged or actual suicide attempts, will receive similar protection. We recommended that this information not be shared with the United States, and will continue to engage with police services across the country to put in place procedures that will protect individuals from discrimination at the US border.

Frequently we are contacted by individuals who are concerned about travelling to the United States because of a mental health-related interaction they have had with Canadian police. In some cases, individuals have even been stopped mid-transit by border officials, completely unaware that private information has been shared. This is why we have consistently advocated for police to stop sharing mental health-related police records across the border, including via submissions to the Information and Privacy Commissioner in 2014 and through involvement in lawsuits challenging the constitutionality of these practices.

Source: Canadian Civil Liberties Association, 2016.

Discussion Questions

1. What could be the benefit of sharing these records specifically with border officials?
2. What impact could this type of information sharing have on an individual?
3. Could information sharing contribute to further stigmatization of the individual and the larger mental health community?
4. When could information sharing with outside agencies be beneficial or even necessary?

Stigma and Its Impact on Service Delivery

Stigma can be defined as a social process that has the intent to exclude, shame, and devalue individuals. Some belief still exists that people with mental illness are incompetent and dangerous. The members of society who believe these stereotypes are predisposed to behaving unproductively and even harmfully toward individuals who live with mental health issues. This very same stigma is embedded in the rules, policies, and practices of some organizations. With this social construct, some individuals who live with mental illness are conditioned to believe the stereotypes. Livingston and Boyd (2010), referring to **self-stigma**, say that when people with mental illness are socialized into believing that they are devalued members of society, and this belief impacts their opinions and feelings about themselves, it affects their relationships with others and their overall perception of their place in the world.

self-stigma
socialization of individuals with mental illness that leads them to the belief that they are devalued members of society

There are several ways that stigma can negatively influence interactions between the police and individuals with mental illness. Some researchers speculate that stereotyping by police contributes to the overrepresentation of individuals with mental illness who are involved in police shootings, incidents where conducted energy weapons are discharged, and interactions that result in fatalities. Research in Canada (Brink et al., 2011) indicates that individuals with mental health issues report numerous experiences in which they believed that their mental health status contributed to unfair treatment by police. Overall, however, individuals with mental illness tend to have mixed feelings in relation to the quality of interaction between themselves and law enforcement. An example of this was shown in a study conducted in Vancouver that had 60 participants—all individuals with mental illness. It was found that despite prevalent experiences of police use of force, the majority of participants maintained positive attitudes in their interactions with police (Brink et al., 2011). The positive perceptions that arose from these interactions were the result of officers engaging in procedural justice-related skills, such as active listening, empathy, and respect, rather than manipulation and excessive use of force.

Keep in mind that stereotypes and attitudes held by some members of law enforcement in relation to mental illness may also be held by other professionals and members of the general public—that is, stigma is not restricted to the police; however, because of the power given to police, actions taken by officers that are the result of a limiting belief system can have damaging consequences for people with mental illness.

Community Programs

The following are examples of programs that focus specifically on **community engagement** in relation to mental illness.

community engagement
process with the specific purpose of working with identified groups of people, whether they are connected by geographic location or special interest, to address issues that affect their well-being

Mental Health First Aid

Mental Health First Aid (MHFA) was first developed in Australia and is now used worldwide. In Canada, the program has been used by a number of police organizations. The mandate of the program is "[t]o improve mental health literacy and provide the skills and knowledge to help people better manage potential or developing mental health problems in themselves, a family member, a friend or a colleague" (Mental Health Commission of Canada, 2011). Those who engage in MHFA training can

- increase their knowledge of the signs, symptoms, and risk factors of mental health problems;
- decrease the social distance between themselves and those with mental health problems;
- increase their confidence to help individuals who are experiencing mental health crises; and
- identify professional and self-help resources for individuals with mental health problems.

The basic MHFA course is 12 hours long and includes techniques that are effective for a number of mental health problems, including:

- depression,
- suicidal thoughts and behaviours,
- panic attacks,
- psychosis,
- non-suicidal self injury,
- child trauma,
- adult trauma, and
- substance abuse.

Applied Suicide Intervention Skills Training Program

Applied Suicide Intervention Skills Training (ASIST) is a 14-hour workshop held by Living Works Education (n.d.). The goal of the workshop is to give participants the tools they need to assist individuals who may be at risk of suicide. The program is well-established in Canada and other countries, and there is evidence to suggest that it is effective in heightening suicide awareness and increasing intervention skills.

The goal of ASIST is to re-establish community connections and supports by focusing on the quality of interactions between the community and individuals at risk. A number of police services across Canada use ASIST as part of their training. The program is best described as skills-acquisition training, rather than simply suicide awareness training.

International Association of Chiefs of Police: Alzheimer's Initiative

The Alzheimer's Initiative of the International Association of Chiefs of Police (IACP) is geared specifically toward managing interactions with people with Alzheimer's disease. This initiative includes training workshops, podcasts, videos, handouts, and structured questionnaires. The purpose of the initiative is to assist police to:

- better understand Alzheimer's disease,
- identify the different situations first responders might encounter when interacting with persons with Alzheimer's disease,
- distinguish the symptoms of Alzheimer's disease from those of other conditions,
- learn techniques to effectively question and interview persons with Alzheimer's disease to determine the most effective response,
- communicate and collaborate with caregivers,
- engage community resources, and
- establish protocols for search-and-rescue specific to this population (IACP, n.d.; IACP, 2010).

community capacity relates to the resources (physical and intellectual) that exist within a community to solve a community problem

community mobilization process whereby a group of professionals meet on equal terms in order to facilitate a participatory decision-making process

Connection: Community Capacity and Mobilization

When examining a multi-agency approach to mental health, two terms in particular capture the essence of this type of engagement: **community capacity** and **community mobilization**.

Community capacity relates to the resources that already exist within a community. These can include concrete assets required to address particular issues, as well as the expertise, knowledge, and leadership to make things happen. The underlying assumption of community capacity is that all members in the community have something to offer in terms of problem solving and strategies to undertake collective concerns.

Community mobilization is best defined as a process for which a group of professionals have transcended their differences to meet on equal terms in order to facilitate a participatory decision-making process. In other words, it is a process that begins a dialogue among members of the community to determine who is involved, what issues are in question, and how those issues can be identified in order to work toward a successful approach for resolution of a problem or problems.

Often when community agencies come together under the umbrella of community mobilization, common areas of concern are addressed. Frequent topics include:

- collaboration,
- service gaps,
- service accessibility,
- resources and sustainability, and
- collaboration.

The importance of collaboration is acknowledged and supported by the organizations committed to the community mobilization framework. When attempting to build and maintain effective partnerships, the following issues should be addressed:

- working in a **silo**,
- information sharing, and
- community empowerment.

silo
service providers who work in isolation from one another are said to be working in a silo; working in a silo contributes to a lack of teamwork, collaboration, and information sharing

Some service providers (for example, individual counsellors and therapists) often work in isolation, which is otherwise known as "working in a silo." This creates divisions not only between sectors, but also between providers working within the same sector. In some circumstances, silos are reinforced by funding systems that compel agencies to compete with one another, making them less likely to initiate partnerships or share information. When community agencies choose to collaborate, working in isolation must be avoided, while information sharing is encouraged to facilitate community empowerment.

Service Gaps

Community mobilization sessions are excellent opportunities to identify gaps in service that are particular to the needs of each agency. Some examples of common service gaps involve the following sectors:

- mental health,
- poverty and homelessness, and
- youth.

Once service gaps are identified, the problem-solving process can begin in an attempt to reduce gaps that are unique to or shared among the various sectors taking part in the community mobilization session.

Service Accessibility

Service accessibility is an important consideration in addressing a community's service gaps. Many community organizations share common accessibility issues such as:

- lack of knowledge, awareness, and coordination,
- wait-lists, and
- inconvenient locations and insufficient public transportation.

Lack of public awareness of programs available in the community serves as a barrier to access, as do long wait-lists and inconvenient locations that are not accessible by public transportation.

Resources and Sustainability

A contributing factor to the overall availability and accessibility of services may be related to challenges with ensuring the sustainability of the programs and services offered. Resources may be found to be insufficient or unsustainable due to challenging funding structures and funding criteria.

Obtaining funding, either privately or through a government grant, is an ongoing challenge for many not-for-profit organizations that provide services. In relation to grants, there are often specific criteria that outline the areas in which funding can be spent. In some instances, funding may only be used for program start-up costs, rather than for ongoing operations such as staffing or evaluation.

The input received at community mobilization meetings highlights the many common challenges experienced by participants, across various sectors and communities, when they strive to improve community safety and well-being. The framework of community mobilization has shown that organizations can effectively work together in partnership to shrink service gaps, increase service accessibility, and use existing resources in more innovative ways to create sustainable responses. When developing community safety and well-being practices, communities are encouraged to be proactive in considering the challenges outlined above in order to mitigate and/or avoid them if possible. Most importantly, the framework allows communities the opportunity to share and celebrate their successes, and identify promising practices.

POINTS TO REMEMBER

- ✓ In contemporary policing, a shift from decentralization of authority and decision-making to procedural justice has occurred, leading to the creation of a service and approach that focuses on the individual. With this focus on service, additional training has led to increased awareness of mental health issues.
- ✓ Individuals with mental illness do not necessarily become involved with the criminal justice system because they have committed an offence, but rather because they have been victimized. With this in mind, organizations must assist in reducing barriers to reporting for people who are living with mental illness.
- ✓ In all interactions between law enforcement and individuals with mental illness (and all members of society), ethical decision-making is crucial to achieving acceptable standards of practice.
- ✓ It is also important for law enforcement and all mental health service providers to be aware of the role that stereotypes play in interactions while services are being provided, and they must avoid embedding stigmatizing concepts in rules, policies, and practices.
- ✓ And finally, community mobilization is an effective framework to encourage and facilitate a collaborative approach among agencies and organizations in a community.

KEY TERMS

REFERENCES

Brink, J., Livingston, J.D., Desmarais, S.L., Greaves, C., Maxwell, V., Michalak, E., … & Weaver, C. (2011). A study of how people with mental illness perceive and interact with the police. Calgary: Mental Health Commission of Canada. Retrieved from https://www.mentalhealthcommission.ca/sites/default/files/Law_How_People_with_Mental_Illness_Perceive_Interact_Police_Study_ENG_1_0_1.pdf

Canadian Civil Liberties Association. (2016). Toronto police to restrict mental health record sharing. Retrieved from https://ccla.org/toronto-police-restrict-mental-health-record-sharing/

Coleman, T., & Cotton, D. (2014). *Tempo: Police interactions: A report towards improving interactions between police and people living with mental health problems*. Ottawa and Calgary: Mental Health Commission of Canada. Retrieved from https://www.mentalhealthcommission.ca/sites/default/files/2016-05/TEMPO Police Interactions 082014.pdf

International Association of Chiefs of Police [IACP]. (n.d.). IACP's alzheimer's initiatives [Brochure]. Retrieved from http://www.theiacp.org/Portals/0/documents/pdfs/IACP-AlzhBrochure42514.pdf

International Association of Chiefs of Police [IACP]. (2010). IACP initiative: Building safer communities: Improving police response to persons with mental illness. Retrieved from http://www.theiacp.org/Building-Safer-Communities-Improving-Police-Response-to-Persons-with-Mental-Illness

Living Works Education. (n.d.). Applied suicide intervention skills training (ASIST). Retrieved from https://www.livingworks.net/programs/asist/

Livingston, J.D., & Boyd, J.E. (2010). Correlates and consequences of internalized stigma for people living with mental illness: A systematic review and meta-analysis. *Social Science & Medicine*, *71*(12), 2150-2161. doi:10.1016/j.socscimed.2010.09.030

Mental Health Act, RSO 1990, c M.7.

Mental Health Commission of Canada. (2011). Mental health first aid. Overview. Retrieved from https://www.mentalhealthcommission.ca/English/focus-areas/mental-health-first-aid

Ontario, Ministry of the Attorney General. (n.d.). The victim/witness assistance program. Retrieved from https://www.attorneygeneral.jus.gov.on.ca/english/ovss/VWAP-English.html#content

Shipman, M. (2014, February 25). Study shows mentally ill more likely to be victims, not perpetrators, of violence. *North Carolina State University News*. Retrieved from https://news.ncsu.edu/2014/02/wms-desmarais-violence2014/

Watson, A.C., Angell, B., Vidalon, T., & Davis, K. (2010). Measuring perceived procedural justice and coercion among persons with mental illness in police encounters: The police contact experience scale. *Journal of Community Psychology*, *38*(2), 206–226. doi:10.1002/jcop.20360

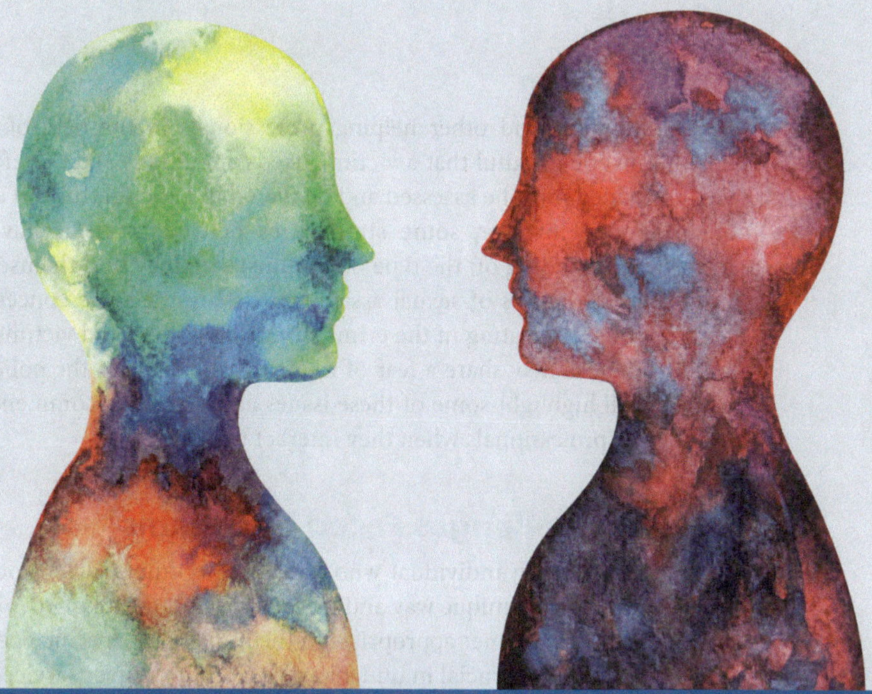

10 WORKING WITH VICTIMS

LEARNING OUTCOMES

After reading this chapter, you will be able to:

- Distinguish between the various groups of victims and the unique challenges they encounter.
- Identify effective strategies when interacting with victims in a professional setting.
- Locate appropriate resources that can provide support to victims.

Introduction

First responders and other helping professionals in the field of mental health must be mindful that a victim's needs are unique and therefore services provided must be assessed and delivered in a thoughtful and deliberate manner. However, some similarities between victims have been identified depending on the type of circumstance they find themselves in. For example, victims of sexual assault may share the same concerns and fears about participating in the criminal justice system, and victims of domestic violence may share a fear of reporting incidents to the police. This chapter will highlight some of these issues and provide recommendations for helping professionals when they interact with victims.

Unique Challenges Faced by Victims

As mentioned, each individual who has been victimized will process the event or events in a unique way and, because of this, must be provided care and support in a manner appropriate to the individual's specific needs. The assessment phase is crucial in understanding how to deliver services. What follows will discuss the signs and symptoms to look for when working with various victim groups.

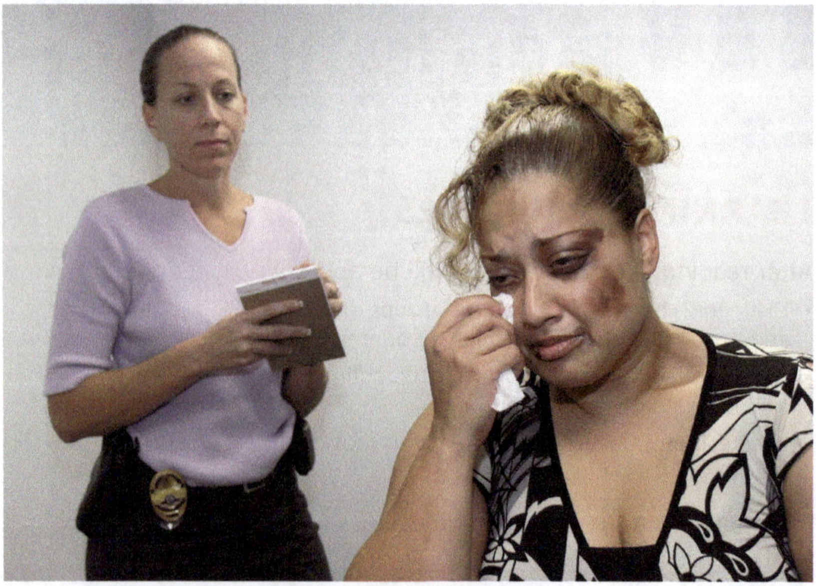

Police detective speaking to a victim of domestic violence.

Victims with Mental Illness

As mentioned in the previous chapter, individuals with mental health issues are at risk of being victimized by those who view them as an easy target. Regardless of an individual's level of functioning, being a victim of a crime is traumatic and may trigger symptoms and behaviours of mental illness. First responders should watch for these signs:

- incoherent conversation and accelerated speech,
- hallucinations or delusion and paranoia,
- signs of depression,
- exaggerated or inappropriate emotional responses,
- memory loss, and
- anxiety and panic.

While being alert to the above potential symptoms, use these strategies when engaging with the identified victim:

- Approach from the front and maintain eye contact.
- Introduce yourself and your role.
- Remove the victim from noisy or chaotic environments (for example, crowds).
- Include the victim in all conversations.
- Explain your actions before proceeding.
- Be calm, reassuring, patient, and honest.
- Contact someone in the victim's support network.
- Find out what he or she needs to feel safe.
- Keep interviews one-on-one, simple, and brief.

Remember that despite the behaviour being displayed by a victim with mental health issues, he or she may still be able to provide accurate details about an incident or crime. Witnesses to and victims of crime may experience shock, anger, confusion, guilt, and humiliation. These feelings may be intensified if the victim also suffers from mental illness. It may appear that the individual is exaggerating the incident, so it is important as a first responder to be sensitive, patient, and compassionate while filtering out the most reliable information (McBratney, 2007). Additionally, understanding the social history of the victim will assist in navigating him or her through the criminal justice or mental health systems. For example, if the victim has experienced abuse and violence in the past, he or she may not trust individuals or the justice system, making it paramount to establish a transparent and honest relationship while providing services and support.

Victims of Trauma

trauma
injury to the body or mind

crisis
acute emotional reaction to a powerful stimulus

It is critical for first responders and other helping professionals who work with victims of trauma to be informed about traumatic stress because these individuals are in an ongoing process of healing and recovery. Put simply, **trauma** is defined as injury to the body or mind. This injury can occur when an individual experiences a **crisis**—an acute emotional reaction to a powerful stimulus. There are many examples of traumatic events, a few of which are: physical assaults, sexual assaults, domestic violence, natural disasters, motor vehicle accidents, and industrial accidents. First responders and other helping professionals must remain mindful that even witnessing these events or hearing about them can have a significant impact on an individual.

When interacting with an individual who has been exposed to trauma, it is important to approach him or her with genuine respect and concern, while understanding the impact of traumatic stress. If this is done, there is an increased ability for the first responder to achieve the following:

- Be able to answer questions in relation to what the individual may be experiencing.
- Assist in normalizing the individual's distress by advising him or her that what he or she is experiencing is normal.
- Assist the individual in learning effective coping strategies.
- Bring awareness of possible symptoms that may require additional assistance.
- Be mindful of any potential interaction that may be perceived as insensitive to the individual while attempting to provide support.
- Achieve the goal of making the experience a positive one for the individual so that there is an increased chance he or she will seek further assistance soon after the incident and in the future, if required.

Symptoms of Trauma

While there are various causes and symptoms of trauma, there are some basic signs that first responders and other helping professionals can watch out for. Individuals who have experienced a traumatic event will often appear shaken and disoriented. They may not respond to conversation as they normally would and may appear withdrawn or unfocused.

An additional sign of a trauma is **anxiety**. Anxiety caused by trauma may manifest in problems such as irritability, poor concentration, mood swings, and sleep disturbances. While these symptoms of trauma are common, this short list is not exhaustive. At times a victim's behaviour may even seem inappropriate given what has happened to him or her. For example, a victim of a sexual assault may appear happy or even laugh when he or she discusses the incident. It is important not to judge or to draw conclusions based on a victim's demeanour and to always remain aware that individuals respond to trauma in different ways. Sometimes trauma is virtually unnoticeable even to the victim's closest friends and family. The following explanations of symptoms of trauma illustrate the importance of talking to someone after a traumatic event has occurred, even if he or she shows no initial signs of disturbance. Trauma can manifest days, months, or even years after the actual event.

anxiety
state of excessive unease and apprehension

Emotional symptoms of trauma: Emotion is one of the most common ways in which trauma manifests. Some common emotional symptoms of trauma include anger, sadness, denial, and emotional outbursts. Victims of trauma may redirect the overwhelming emotions they experience toward other people, such as friends or family members. This is one of the reasons that trauma is difficult for the victim's loved ones. It can be a challenge as a first responder or other helping professional to engage with a victim if he or she rejects assistance, but understanding the emotional symptoms that emerge after a traumatic event can help ease the process.

Physical symptoms of trauma: Trauma often manifests physically as well as emotionally. Some common physical signs of trauma include lethargy, fatigue, poor concentration, and an accelerated heartbeat. A victim may have anxiety or a **panic attack** and be unable to cope in certain circumstances. The physical symptoms of trauma can be as real and alarming as those of physical injury or illness, and care should be taken to manage stress levels after a traumatic event. If a victim is exhibiting concerning symptoms, encourage him or her to be assessed by a medical professional.

panic attack
sudden onset of disabling anxiety

Victims of Domestic Violence

Unfortunately, domestic violence is an all too common occurrence in society. Unlike violence that involves strangers, domestic violence often involves secrecy, embarrassment, and humiliation. What also sets domestic violence apart from other forms of violent crimes is that the victim and abuser are often in a co-dependent relationship with each other, making this type of crime especially difficult to disclose to family, friends, and law enforcement.

Given the complex nature of this crime, first responders and other helping professionals must be aware of the cycle of violence and interpersonal dynamics that have an impact on whether the victim discloses the abuse and whether he or she will be open to receiving community support and participating in the criminal process (if a criminal offence has been committed).

Domestic violence is a crime of power and control. To be an effective support to the victim, first responders and other helping professionals must be aware of the power the abuser exerts over the victim Figure 10.1 outlines common sources or methods that abusers use to maintain control over their victims.

To further appreciate the complexities of this crime, first responders and other helping professionals must keep in mind that the victim may have deep emotional bonds to his or her abuser. The victim may be in a committed relationship and may deeply love the person who is abusing him or her. In cases of domestic violence, it can be particularly challenging to provide support to a victim who may want to remain connected to an abuser and even protect him or her. The victim may even blame himself or herself for the abuse.

Cultural factors may also have an impact on whether a victim discloses abuse. For example, a victim may not understand Canadian immigration law and may fear being deported if the crime is reported. Bringing shame and/or disgrace to the family is a very real concern for some individuals because risk to their safety may be heightened. “Honour killings” have occurred in Canada, which makes this a very real concern for some new Canadians.

Remaining mindful of the complex nature of domestic violence and educating victims in relation to the dynamics of power and control and the cycle of violence can be helpful in assisting the victim regain his or her power to make informed decisions about how to proceed.

Figure 10.2 illustrates the cycle of abuse that is characteristic of domestic violence.

FIGURE 10.1 Power and Control

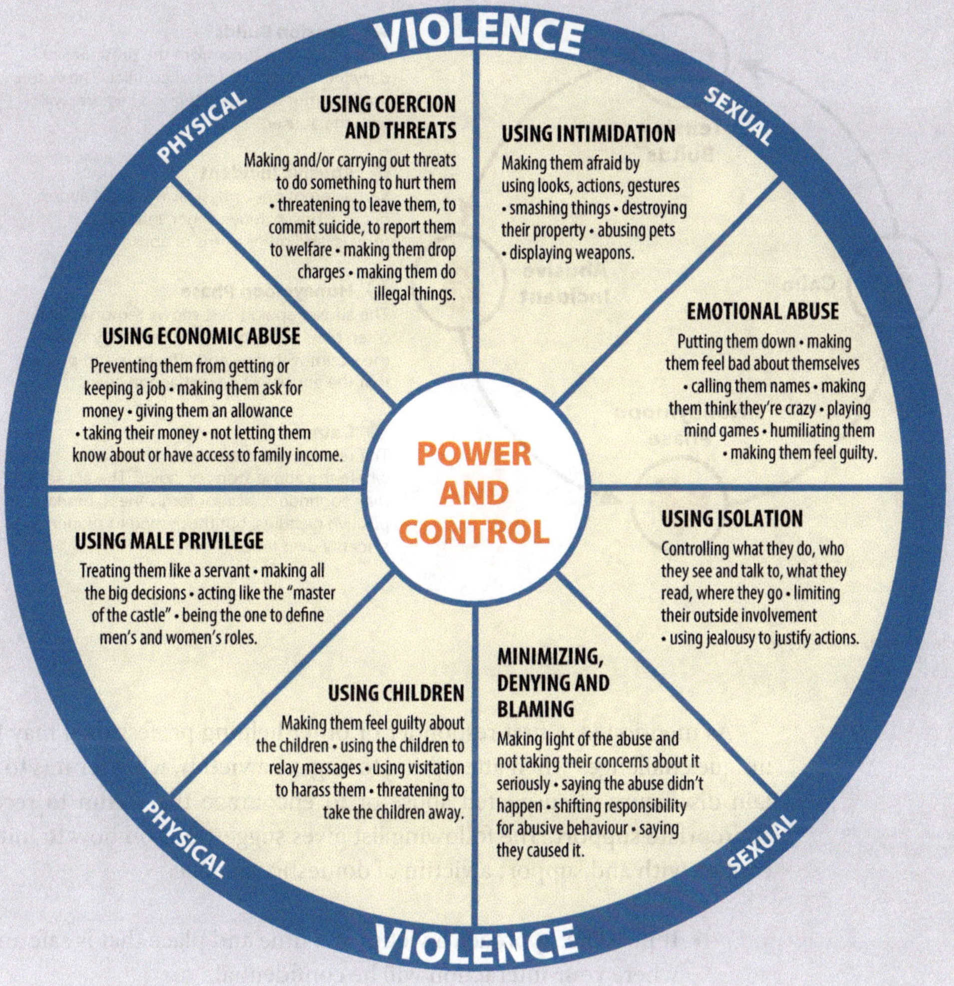

Source: Women's UN Report Network, 2016.

FIGURE 10.2 The Cycle of Abuse

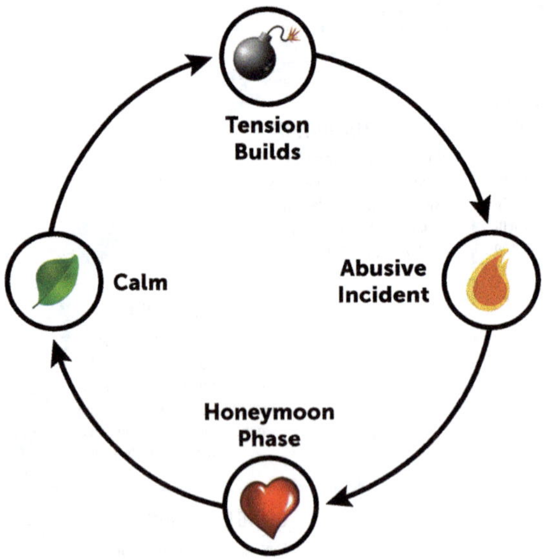

Tension Builds
Stress begins to grow from the pressures of daily life, or other points of conflict. The victim may attempt to reduce tension by complying with the abuser.

Abusive Incident
Verbal, emotional, physical, or sexual abuse occurs. This includes anger, intimidation, threats, and other forms of abuse.

Honeymoon Phase
The abuser apologizes, shows remorse, and often begs for forgiveness. They may shower the victim with love and affection, and promise that the abuse will never happen again.

Calm
The relationship enters a period of calm where the abuse stops or slows. The abuser may continue to ask for forgiveness, or make positive gestures, but these tend to reduce in sincerity over time.

Source: Therapist Aid, 2016.

As mentioned, a first responder or other helping professional may face unique challenges when attempting to engage a victim, whether it is to obtain disclosure of suspected abuse or to encourage the victim to receive appropriate support. The following list gives suggestions on how to initiate contact with and support a victim of domestic violence:

- If possible, approach a victim at a time and place that is safe and where your interaction will be confidential.
- Begin the conversation by expressing concern. For example, you can say, "I am concerned that someone may be hurting you, and I am worried about your safety."
- Communicate that you care about the individual's safety and that you are there to provide information and support.
- Advise the victim that the abuse is not his or her fault.

- Inform the victim that it is normal to feel upset, depressed, confused, and/or scared.
- Be mindful that the abuser may have caused the victim to have low self-esteem. Identify and highlight the victim's strengths to help him or her make confident choices.
- Respect the victim's choices, whether you agree with him or her or not.
- Encourage the victim to build a wide support system and assist in connecting him or her with appropriate community resources.
- Be patient. Empowering the victim may be a slow process. Proceed at the victim's pace, not yours.
- Connect the victim with domestic violence resources. Most Canadian communities provide services through various government programs, women's shelters, court and victim services, and police organizations.
- If there are immediate safety concerns, call 911.

And here is a list of what should *not* be done when initiating contact and attempting to support a victim of domestic violence:

- Do not make accusations.
- Do not judge the victim's choices, or draw conclusions about what he or she may be experiencing or feeling.
- Do not judge or criticize the abuser.
- Do not pressure the victim to leave the relationship. There are many reasons he or she may choose to stay. It is possible the abuser has threatened to harm or kill the victim or his or her children if the victim tries to leave. The abuser may control the victim's finances and may have isolated the victim from friends and family, leaving the victim with very few resources of his or her own. The offender may have promised to change, and the victim may still love him or her. It is never as simple as encouraging a victim to "just leave." However, be sure to communicate that help and community resources are available to keep him or her safe.
- Do not feel the need to be an expert. Do not try to provide counselling or advice, but do connect the victim with trained professionals who can help.

VOICES FROM THE FIELD

Honour Killings in Canada: Even Worse Than We Believe

by Gerald Caplan (Canadian academic, commentator, policy analyst, and political activist)

Friday, Jul. 23, 2010, *The Globe and Mail*—If you are already sufficiently appalled knowing there've been 12 despicable "honour killings" in Canada since 2002, don't read any further. This is only the tip of a nightmarish iceberg, I'm afraid.

For some reason, the term honour killings seems to be reserved for murders committed by male family members against daughters or sisters in South Asian or Middle Eastern communities. These unimaginable crimes have been receiving much high-profile notoriety in the Canadian media, as they surely deserve. All Canadians must now know of the tragic murder of 16-year-old Aqsa Parvez of Mississauga, strangled to death three years ago by her brother and father.

But I'm confident that not one in a million is aware that in Ontario alone, from 2002 until only 2007 (the latest data), 212 women have been killed by their partners. That's 42 every year, compared with 12 so-called honour killings in all of Canada in the past eight years. Women killed by partners are known as domestic homicides, and, unless especially gruesome, are barely worth a mention in the media. Maybe there's just too many of them to be newsworthy.

The data comes from the Ontario Domestic Violence Death Review Committee, which I didn't even know existed until it was recently cited in the Canadian Centre for Policy Alternatives' *Monitor*. I've never come across these figures anywhere else.

Let me rush to be clear here. I don't for a moment minimize the horror of 12 girls and women in Canada murdered by members of their immediate family. To steal a phrase, one would be far too many.

Terrible things still happen to women everywhere, as the domestic violence figures for Canada demonstrate. No nation, religion, class or ethnic group has the monopoly on misogyny.

There is no conceivable excuse or justification for doing anything but condemning such murders in the most unequivocal way. There is no cultural tradition, no sensitivity to the different values of other societies, that can ever justify or even "understand" how a father or brother can kill their daughter or sister, or how a mother can be a sympathetic witness to such a savage act. It is beyond any rational understanding.

What accounts for the high profile of these relatively small number of murders in Canada? Why do we know little or nothing about the larger epidemic of women killed, almost routinely it sometimes seems, by boyfriends or husbands? Is it less terrible to be strangled to death or shot or have your throat slit by them than by family members? Is it just too commonplace to bother paying attention to? Do we still harbour that sneaking suspicion that women murdered by partners have somehow brought it on themselves?

Yet both kinds of murders have a common root. Both are honour killings, reflecting a twisted, pathological male sense of honour. Both are executed by men who feel they haven't received their due deference, men who consider "their" women, whether daughter or partner, to be their chattel, to do with as they choose. Have we smug white Canadians forgotten that you don't have to be a Muslim or South Asian to regard women this way?

Or do we focus on so-called honour killings precisely because the victims are Muslims, or South Asians, or Middle Easterners? By giving such prominence to these communities and their cultures, are we not denigrating them? For all our ostensible acceptance of multiculturalism, are we not feeding our lingering prejudices against certain specific minorities among us? Look at it purely statistically. If so-called honour killings are in fact culturally approved by their communities, as is often charged, shouldn't we expect far more than 12 in the entire country in eight years? And if the rest of us truly embrace a culture that repudiates violence against women, why are so many of them still being murdered?

Let me again emphasize that I have no illusions about these dark issues. According to the United Nations, there are a staggering 5,000 instances annually of women and girls being shot, stoned, burned, poisoned, buried alive, strangled, smothered or knifed to death by family members. I can barely write the sentence without getting sick to my stomach. The killers are fathers, brothers, sons, uncles, and yes, even mothers. The disgusting deeds are carried out in the name of preserving or protecting family honour. Most such murders are indeed carried out in the Middle East or in the countries of South Asia—India, Bangladesh, Pakistan—or by South Asians or Middle Easterners living elsewhere. These terrible crimes can never be "understood," justified or condoned. They must be stopped, wherever they happen.

But terrible things still happen to women everywhere, as the domestic violence figures for Canada demonstrate. No nation, religion, class or ethnic group has the monopoly on misogyny. Honour killings should be seen not as uniquely evil but as the most extreme and perverse proof of this truth. That's why it's encouraging that women's equality groups have been so vocal in their denunciations of all violence against women and are supporting women in minority communities to give them the strength to stand up for their rights.

Despite the remarkable progress women have truly made in the past half-century, clawing for every inch of it, the struggle for women's equality can never rest. It simply has too many enemies, always fighting to keep women in their place, where they belong, dead or alive. Young women who dismiss feminism as irrelevant or outdated are, I'm afraid, dead wrong. The struggle is never over.

Source: Caplan, 2017.

Victims of Sexual Assault

sexual assault assault of a sexual nature that violates the sexual integrity of the victim

In Canada, **sexual assault** is defined as an assault of a sexual nature that violates the sexual integrity of the victim. In 1987, the Supreme Court of Canada held in *R v Chase* that the act of sexual assault does not depend solely on contact with any specific part of the human anatomy, but rather defines sexual assault as any act of a sexual nature that violates the sexual integrity of the victim.

BOX 10.1 LEVELS OF SEXUAL ASSAULT

Sexual assault (level 1): An assault committed in circumstances of a sexual nature that violates the sexual integrity of the victim. Level 1 sexual assault involves minor physical injuries or no injuries to the victim (*Criminal Code*, s. 271).

Sexual assault (level 2): Includes sexual assault with a weapon, threats to a third party, or that causes bodily harm (s. 272(1)).

Aggravated sexual assault (level 3): Sexual assault that results in wounding, maiming, disfiguring, or endangering the life of the victim (s. 273(1)).

The victim of a sexual assault can be of any gender and the offender can be the same sex as the victim. A spouse may also be charged with sexual assault. Prior to 1983, "rape" was considered an offence only outside of marriage, meaning a husband could not be charged with raping his wife, and a wife could only charge her spouse with indecent assault, common assault, or assault causing bodily harm.

Sexual assault is one of the most traumatic types of victimization. Most victims of violence find it difficult to discuss their victimization, and sexual assault victims find it especially painful. A possible reason for this is the difficulty that many individuals have in discussing sexual topics. Another more problematic reason, however, is that many victims of sexual assault are traumatized not only by the humiliation of the physical violation, but by the fear of not being believed and the stress inherent in participating in the criminal justice system.

Many challenges arise when interacting with a sexual assault victim, and first responders and other helping professionals should keep the following in mind:

- Be prepared for any type of emotional reaction by the victim.
- Be supportive and permit the victim to express his or her emotions, which may include crying and screaming, and perhaps some less expected behaviour such as smiling and laughter, or no emotion at all.
- Avoid interpreting the victim's calmness or composure as evidence that a sexual assault did or did not occur. The victim could be in shock.
- Approach the victim calmly. Displaying your own reaction to the assault may cause the victim even more trauma.
- Ask the victim whether he or she would like a family member or friend contacted.
- Offer to contact a sexual assault crisis counsellor. Ask the victim whether he or she would prefer a male or female counsellor. In addition, ask whether the victim would prefer talking with you or someone of the opposite sex.
- Be careful not to appear overprotective or patronizing.
- Remember that it is normal for victims to want to forget, or to actually forget, details of the crime that are difficult for them to confront.
- Encourage the victim to get medical attention, especially to check for possible injuries. A medical examination may also provide evidence for the identification and prosecution of the offender.
- Be mindful of the personal, interpersonal, and privacy concerns of the victim. He or she may have a number of concerns, including the possibility of having contracted a sexually transmitted disease, the reactions of his or her family or friends, and potential media attention.
- Be aware that if the assault is reported to the police, a criminal investigation will be initiated. An officer will conduct a formal interview with the victim. Be mindful that every person the victim discloses the crime to could become a witness at a court proceeding.
- Offer to answer any further questions the victim may have and provide any further assistance required.
- Encourage the victim to seek follow-up counselling. Identify resources and support services available to the victim in his or her community.

Child Victims

child maltreatment includes all forms of physical, sexual, and emotional abuse, neglect, and exploitation that result in actual or potential harm to a child's health, development, or dignity

child physical abuse deliberate injury to a child that causes bruises, broken bones, burns, or cuts

child sexual abuse occurs when an adult or older adolescent uses a child for sexual stimulation

Child maltreatment is an unfortunate reality for many children in our society. The five primary forms of maltreatment are **physical abuse, sexual abuse**, neglect, emotional maltreatment, and exposure to domestic violence. In most cases of abuse the offender is known to the child, making these crimes difficult to identify because of the element of secrecy—the abuse is hidden behind the walls of the family home. Research has indicated that the immediate environment of children and youth can influence their risk of victimization (United Nations, 2006). Police-reported data support this assertion, as violent crime against children and youth most often involves someone known to the child (Sinha & Milligan, 2012, p. 57).

If a child does not disclose being victimized, it may be challenging to recognize the signs of abuse and neglect. The following is a guide for first responders and other helping professionals who work directly or have occasional contact with children.

Child Physical Abuse

Child physical abuse is the deliberate hurting of a child that causes injuries such as bruises, broken bones, burns, or cuts. In Canada, section 265(1)(a)

FIGURE 10.3 Number of Child Maltreatment Investigations and Risk of Future Maltreatment Investigations in Canada in 1998, 2003, and 2008

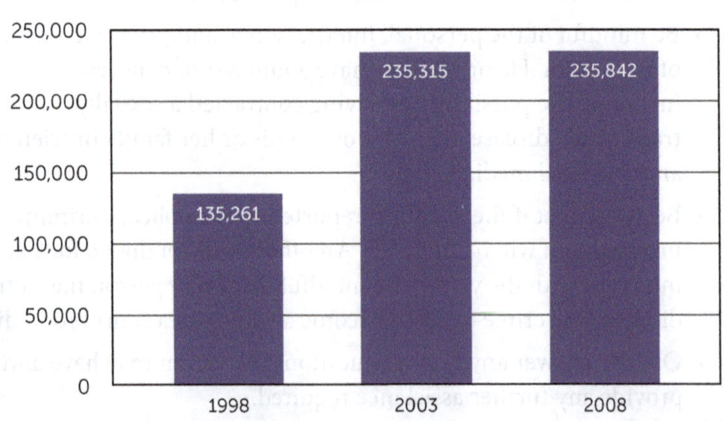

Canadian Incidence Study of Reported Child Abuse and Neglect–2008

* Based on a sample of 7,633 investigations in 1998, 14,200 in 2003, and 15,980 in 2008.

Source: Public Health Agency of Canada , 2010, p. 2.

of the *Criminal Code* states that a person commits an assault when "without the consent of another person, he applies force intentionally to that other person, directly or indirectly." The *Criminal Code*, however, still allows for a parent, caregiver, or teacher to use force on a child for disciplinary reasons. Section 43 reads:

> Every schoolteacher, parent or person standing in the place of a parent is justified in using force by way of correction toward a pupil or child, as the case may be, who is under his care, if the force does not exceed what is reasonable under the circumstances.

This controversial section of the *Criminal Code* is commonly referred to as the "spanking law" and was reviewed by the Supreme Court in 2004 and upheld.

BOX 10.2 HISTORIC DECISION ON ASSAULT

Several years ago, the Supreme Court of Canada made a decision about section 43 that helps to understand the law on assault today.

The Supreme Court said that the use of force on a child is only allowed to help the child learn. The parent, caregiver, or teacher who uses force must be correcting behaviour when it is happening, and the person must not use force on a child in anger.

The Supreme Court found that it was not appropriate to use force on a very young child or a teenager. The use of force will only be allowed under the exception in section 43 if the child is between two years old and twelve years old. Using force to punish a child under two is not appropriate because a child that young cannot learn from the situation. Using force on a teenager is not appropriate because there are better and more effective ways to respond to a teenager's behaviour.

Section 43 says that the force used on a two- to twelve-year-old child must be "reasonable under the circumstances." The Supreme Court defined "reasonable" as force that would have a "transitory and trifling" impact on the child. For example, spanking or slapping a child so hard that it leaves a mark that lasts for several hours would not be considered "transitory and trifling."

The Supreme Court also said that the force used must not be degrading, inhumane, or harmful. The person using force must not use an object, such as a ruler or belt, and must not hit or slap the child's head.

Finally, the Supreme Court said that the seriousness of the child's misbehaviour is not relevant. The force used must be minor, no matter what the child did.

The Use of Force When Managing a Child's Behaviour

There are times when parents, caregivers, and teachers may have to use force to control a child and keep the child, or other children, safe. Grabbing a child to keep that child from running across the street, carrying a screaming three-year-old out of a store, or separating two young students who are fighting may require a parent, caregiver, or teacher to touch or restrain the child.

Without [the protection of] section 43, parents, caregivers, and teachers could face criminal charges and might have to go to court to defend their actions when they use force to respond to a child's behaviour.

Summary

- The use of force to correct a child is only allowed in order to help the child learn and must never be used in anger.
- The child must be between two years old and twelve years old.
- The force used must be reasonable and its impact only "transitory and trifling."
- The person must not use an object, such as a ruler or belt, when applying force.
- The person must not hit or slap the child's head.
- The seriousness of what happened or what the child did is not relevant.

Using reasonable force to restrain a child may be acceptable in some circumstances.

Hitting a child in anger or in retaliation for something a child did is not considered reasonable and is against the law.

Source: Department of Justice, Canada, 2016.

Discussion Questions

1. Why is this a controversial topic?
2. Should section 43 be removed from the *Criminal Code*? Why or why not?
3. What impact would the removal of this section specifically have on teachers?

Any allegation of excessive force must be investigated by a child protection service agency, such as a children's aid society, jointly with the police service of the same jurisdiction. These agencies will determine whether an offence has been committed and will remove the child from his or her environment if it is deemed unsafe. It is very important for first responders and other helping professionals to understand the legal requirement to report any suspected abuse or neglect. The "duty to report" will be outlined below.

First responders and other helping professionals need to be aware of potential indicators of child physical abuse. Children who have been physically abused often demonstrate a variety of problematic behaviours that can include:

- aggression,
- anxiety,
- cognitive impairment,
- conduct disorder,
- depression,
- negative parent–child interactions,
- poor interpersonal relationship/social skills,
- self-injurious behaviour,
- substance-related disorders,
- suicidal thoughts and/or behaviours,
- trauma-related problems and/or post-traumatic stress disorder (PTSD), and
- violent and/or criminal behaviour (Lipovsky & Hanson, n.d., p. 4).

If any of the above behaviours are identified, consideration must be given to reporting the concerns and referring the child to the appropriate medical, mental health, or social service professional.

Child Sexual Assault

According to Statistics Canada, children and youth were five times more likely than adults to become sexual offence victims (212 versus 41 per 100,000 individuals), with level 1 sexual assaults accounting for three-quarters (75 percent) of these sex crimes. Another 22 percent of sexual offences committed against children and youth were child-specific, including sexual interference, invitation to sexual touching, luring a child via a computer, and corrupting children (Sinha, 2012, p. 57).

Child sexual abuse has been found to be associated with the development of a wide variety of mental and social problems in childhood and into adulthood (Lipovsky & Hanson, n.d., pp. 1–2). The following outlines some behavioural problems associated with child sexual abuse:

- anger/acting out,
- difficulty regulating emotional responses,
- anxiety,
- interpersonal problems,
- sleep problems and nightmares,
- post-traumatic stress disorder (PTSD),
- difficulties in school,
- sexualized behaviours,
- depression,
- suicidal thoughts and/or behaviours, and
- substance related disorders (Lipovsky & Hanson, n.d., p. 2).

Again, if any of the above behaviours are identified, consideration must be given to reporting the concerns and referring the child to the appropriate medical, mental health, or social service professional.

Child Neglect

child neglect includes acts of commission or omission by a parent or caregiver that result in harm, potential for harm, or threat of harm to a child

According to Statistics Canada, exposure to intimate partner violence (adult conflict) and **child neglect** were the most common forms of substantiated child maltreatment investigations, accounting for 34 percent each. Other categories of substantiated child maltreatment included physical abuse (20 percent), emotional maltreatment (9 percent), and sexual abuse (3 percent) (Sinha, 2012, p. 71).

According to the Canadian Child Welfare Research Portal (2011), child neglect is defined as "acts of commission or omission by a parent or other caregiver that result in harm, potential for harm, or threat of harm to a child." Examples include failing to provide medical and dental care, failing to properly feed a child, failing to supervise, permitting criminal behaviour, isolating and confining a child, and providing inadequate nurturing and affection. Neglect has been found to have a negative impact on a child's physical, intellectual, social, and emotional development. One life-threatening outcome of neglect is **failure to thrive**. Failure to thrive occurs when a child does not grow adequately over time. Children with untreated failure to thrive are at risk for having a short stature, behavioural and emotional problems, and developmental delays (Campbell & James, 2009). Some long-term problems that children experience due to ongoing neglect include:

failure to thrive
term used to describe a child who does not grow and/or develop over time

- poor intellectual and academic functioning,
- aggression,
- delinquency, and
- poor interpersonal relationships.

Treatment of neglect focuses on the importance of the relationships between the child, family, and community. As a result, treatment emphasizes the socio-economic needs, family dysfunction, and disconnection between the family and the community that are seen as important factors of neglect (Lipovsky & Hanson, n.d., p. 5).

If any of the above behaviours are identified, consideration must be given to reporting the concerns and referring the child to the appropriate medical, mental health, or social service professional.

Duty to Report Child Maltreatment

In civil society, there is a shared responsibility to protect children from harm. As mentioned, this includes situations where children are abused or neglected in their own homes. Ontario's *Child and Family Services Act* is legislation that provides protection for these children.

Section 72 of the Act states that the public, including professionals who work with children, must promptly report to a children's aid society (CAS) any suspicions that a child is or may be in need of protection. Section 37 of the Act defines "child in need of protection" and explains what must be reported to a CAS. It includes physical, sexual, and emotional abuse; neglect; and risk of harm. There is a high expectation that first responders and other helping professionals will report any suspected abuse or neglect. If it is unclear as to whether a concern should be reported, any member of the public can call a CAS for consultation (Ministry of Children and Youth Services, Ontario, 2016).

Each province has similar legislation outlining the legal responsibility to report suspected abuse and neglect. For example, Quebec's legislation is called the *Youth Protection Act*, British Columbia has the *Child, Family and*

Community Service Act, and Alberta has the *Child, Youth and Family Enhancement Act*. Please refer to the specific legislation pertinent to the province of interest.

Elder Abuse

elder abuse
intentional act, or failure to act, by a caregiver or an individual in a position of trust that causes or creates a risk of harm to an older adult

Like all Canadians, senior citizens deserve to be treated with dignity and respect. However various studies indicate that 4 to 8 percent of older adults are likely to experience abuse in this country. **Elder abuse** can occur in many forms and it can affect any senior regardless of socio-economic background, health status, or culture (Alberta Health, 2010). Elder abuse is a serious issue and can enter the realm of criminality. It undermines a senior's independence and dignity. Common forms of elder abuse include:

- **Physical abuse:** Use of physical force that may result in injury, physical pain, or impairment.
- **Emotional abuse:** Infliction of anguish, pain, or distress through verbal or non-verbal acts that diminish self-esteem or dignity.
- **Sexual abuse:** Non-consensual sexual contact of any kind with an elderly person.
- **Medication abuse:** The intentional or unintentional misuse of medications.
- **Financial/material exploitation:** Illegal or improper use of an elder's funds, property, or assets through fraud, theft, trickery, or force.
- **Neglect:** Refusal, or failure, to fulfill any part of a person's obligations or duties to an elderly person in relation to basic level of care.
- **Abandonment:** Desertion of an elderly person by an individual who has physical custody of the elder or by a person who has assumed responsibility for providing care.
- **Self-neglect:** Behaviours of an elderly person that threaten the elder's health or safety.

The two most frequently identified and reported types of elder abuse in Canada are financial and emotional. According to a government report, 40 to 70 percent of all reported cases involve financial and/or emotional abuse (Beaulieu, Gordon, & Spencer, 2003).

Similar to domestic violence and child abuse, elder abuse is often committed by someone known to the victim, such as a family member, caregiver, or friend. Victims may be reluctant to report the abuse or seek help. Shame or guilt may also limit reporting, while some elders may be fearful of repercussions, especially if the abuser is a family member who provides care and support. Specific concerns that elderly individuals might have with regard to reporting abuse may include loss of their home, loss of access to family members (for example, grandchildren), and fear of being relocated to unfamiliar surroundings or an institution. Similar to domestic violence, victims of elder abuse may regard the abuse as "normal" behaviour or may even blame themselves for the abuse. In some instances, victims may not even be aware that the treatment they are receiving is abusive. Victims may not have the capacity to report the abuse or know where to turn for help.

As with other types of family violence, elder abuse is complex. This type of abuse is often affected by the mental health and physical condition of both the victim and the abuser, and often there is a level of dependence between the individuals. Statistics from a government report indicate that approximately 25 percent of crimes against seniors are committed by family members, usually a spouse or an adult child (Sinha, 2012).

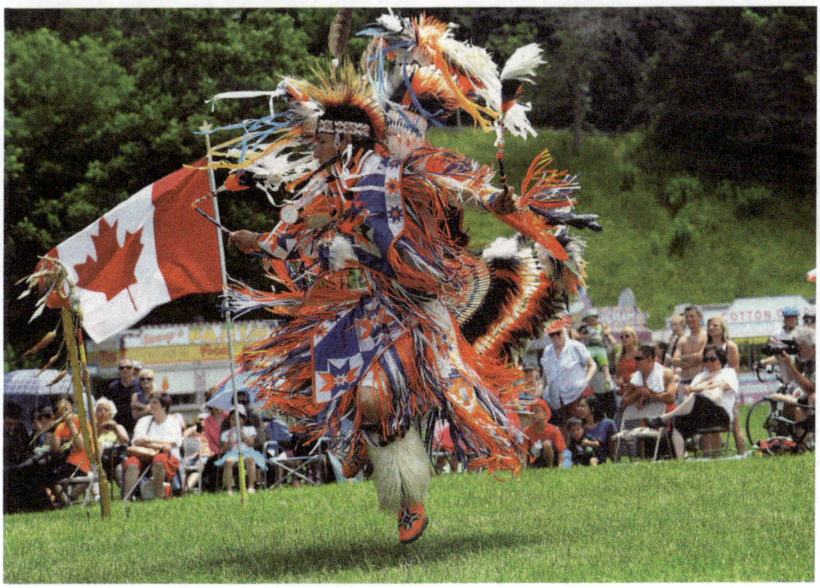

Indigenous traditional ceremonial dress.

Cultural differences also make this issue more complex. Senior members of immigrant communities may face additional challenges such as language barriers, limited social connections, and lack of familiarity with their surroundings, all of which can increase their dependence on an abuser. Seniors who are recent immigrants may also fear deportation if they report abuse.

Elder abuse is often hidden, and again, this is similar to domestic violence and child abuse. As such, similar approaches should be used when interacting with an older adult who is suspected of being a victim of abuse. The complex nature of elder abuse means that no single individual, social service, or law enforcement agency can address this challenge alone. Preventing and addressing elder abuse requires broad engagement and collective action by all sectors of society.

Issues Faced by Indigenous Communities

Mental health issues in Inuit and other Indigenous communities must be considered while keeping the unique historical experiences of these communities in mind. The collective cultural disruption experienced by Inuit and other Indigenous peoples as a result of colonization, in particular, has been profound. Past government policies, including the systematic dispossession of land, racial discrimination, and the weakening of social and political institutions, have had lasting effects on the collective sense of identity of Indigenous peoples. Because of their treatment at the hands of the government, substance abuse, addiction, depression, and suicide have greatly affected these communities.

BOX 10.3

Mental Health Challenges Among First Nations and Inuit

Suicide

The loss of human life through suicide is a tragic reality in First Nations and Inuit communities. These two communities experience a much higher suicide rate than the Canadian population as a whole.

Suicide rates among Inuit are shockingly high at 6 to 11 times the Canadian average. In Nunavut in particular, 27 percent of all deaths since 1999 have been suicides. This is one of the highest suicide rates in the world, and it continues to rise, especially among youth.

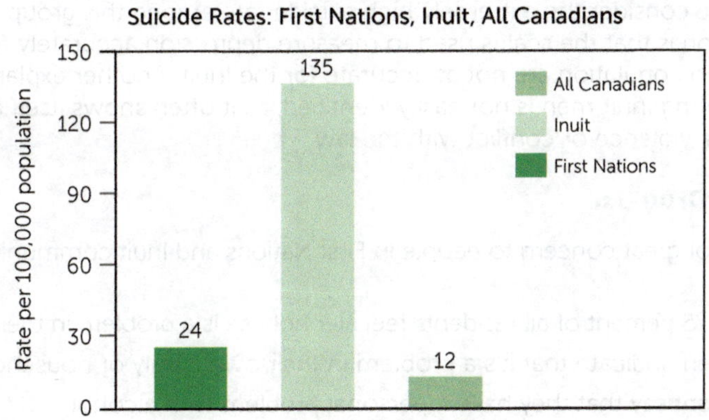

For the First Nations population, suicide rates are twice the national average and show no signs of decreasing. However, these rates differ from community to community. Some communities have had "epidemics" of suicide, while others have had few or no suicides for several years.

In both [Indigenous] groups, females attempt suicide more often than males. This trend is also seen in the general Canadian population, but the difference in rates is alarming. While the Canadian average is around 4 percent of females and 2 percent of males reporting they've attempted suicide, in the [Indigenous] survey, it was 19 percent of females and 13 percent of males.

Rates of completed suicides, however, are higher among males. And young adults aged 15 to 24 represent the age group with the highest rate of suicides. Completed suicides among First Nation young adults is five to seven times the Canadian average for the same age group.

Youth with a close family member who had committed suicide in the past 12 months, or who had a parent who attended a residential school, were more likely to have experienced suicidal thoughts.

Depression

Depression is a common and life-changing mental illness in the Canadian population. This is especially true for First Nations people, who experience major depression at twice the national average. A 1997 survey found that 16 percent of First Nations adults living on reserve experienced major depression, compared with 8 percent of the general Canadian population. Of the First Nations people in the study who experienced depression, 26 percent said that depression interfered with their lives, compared with 16 percent of the overall Canadian population.

Depression rates among the Inuit, however, are far below the Canadian average. In a Statistics Canada survey, only 3 percent of Inuit had suffered a major depressive episode. Only 6 percent were at high risk of depression. These findings don't make much sense when we consider the extremely high suicide rate among this group. One possible explanation is that the scales used to measure depression accurately for the rest of the Canadian population are not as accurate for the Inuit. Another explanation is that depression among Inuit men is not easily identified, as it often shows itself as alcohol or drug problems, violence or conflict with the law.

Alcohol and Drug Use

Alcohol use is of great concern to people in First Nations and Inuit communities. Surveys show that:

- Around 75 percent of all residents feel alcohol use is a problem in their community
- 33 percent indicate that it's a problem in their own family or household
- 25 percent say that they have a personal problem with alcohol

This is interesting in light of the fact that lower than average numbers of First Nations and Inuit people drink alcohol. Only 66 percent of First Nations adults living on reserve consumed alcohol compared with 76 percent of the general population. This suggests that those who do drink, drink heavily, consuming five or more drinks on one occasion on a weekly basis.

Figures drawn from hospital records in British Columbia and Alberta show that First Nations people, especially men, are admitted to hospital for problem substance use more often than other residents of these provinces. Cannabis use is also common among First Nations adults (27 percent) and youth (32 percent).

The good news is that about one-third of survey respondents reported that there was progress in reducing the amount of alcohol and drug use in their communities.

Source: Khan, 2008.

Discussion Questions:

1. **What barriers exist that impact the availability of social services to Indigenous and Inuit communities?**
2. **What steps could be taken to improve the availability of social services?**
3. **What factors contribute to the high suicide rate among Inuit and other Indigenous youth?**

The impact of the abuse that occurred in the residential school system transcends generations of Indigenous people.

VOICES FROM THE FIELD

Residential School Syndrome

by Charles Brasfield

Whether Indian residential schools are seen as an attempt at benevolence or a plan to annihilate a culture, many native people who attended the schools present with symptoms similar to those of post-traumatic stress disorder. This constellation of symptoms has come to be known as *residential school syndrome*.

• • •

For most people who attended Indian residential schools, there is no symptomology other than that similar to other people who have attended a boarding school for an extended period of time. However, for a significant minority of Indian residential school students, there is symptomology quite similar to post-traumatic stress disorder. More specifically, there are recurrent intrusive memories, nightmares, occasional flashbacks, and quite striking avoidance of anything that might be reminiscent of the Indian residential school experience.

At the same time, there is often a significant detachment from others, and relationship difficulties are common. There is often diminished interest and participation in aboriginal cultural activities and markedly deficient knowledge of traditional culture and skills. Often there is markedly increased arousal including sleep difficulties, anger management difficulties, and impaired concentration. As might be the case for anyone attending a boarding school with inadequate parenting, parenting skills are often deficient. Strikingly, there is a persistent tendency to abuse alcohol or sedative medication drugs, often starting at a very young age.

Some or all of the symptomology is referenced by the term *residential school syndrome*, but there is no formal agreement, even among health-care personnel dealing with the survivors of the Indian residential schools, on exactly what the diagnostic criteria should be. ... As all of the Indian residential schools are now closed, any person presenting with this constellation of symptoms presently has, by definition, a chronic disorder lasting months or years.

This definition of the term *residential school syndrome* is somewhat similar to that of *post-traumatic stress disorder* as defined in DSM-IV. Both residential school syndrome and post-traumatic stress disorder share criteria that the person has undergone or witnessed some degree of trauma and that his or her response was fearful or helpless. The two diagnoses share requirements of re-experiencing, avoidance, and increased arousal.

The residential school syndrome diagnosis is different from that of post-traumatic stress disorder in that there is a significant cultural impact and a persistent tendency to abuse alcohol or other drugs that is particularly associated with violent outbursts of anger. The residential school syndrome diagnosis also highlights possible deficient parenting skills.

• • •

Whether the residential school syndrome describes the children traumatized by the Indian residential school system or those in authority who created the possibility of such traumata, children were damaged. To deny the existence of the damage is to deny these now-adult survivors the possibility of redress and compensation.

Brasfield, 2001.

Discussion Questions

1. How is residential school syndrome similar to PTSD?
2. What is the specific cultural impact resulting from residential school syndrome?

Support Services for Victims

There are many different types of victim services in Canada. They are offered by governments, police services, courts, volunteers, non-governmental organizations, and others. At the government level, victim services in Canada are a shared responsibility between the federal and provincial governments. Federally, there are a number of departments and offices that offer specific types of information or assistance to all victims in Canada.

Crime victim assistance programs provide a range of services that include:

- information,
- crisis intervention,
- counselling,
- emergency shelter,
- advocacy,
- short- and long-term emotional support,
- court preparation,
- accompaniment through the justice system,
- information-sharing with victims of federally sentenced offenders (by the Correctional Service of Canada and the National Parole Board), and
- referrals that are suited to each individual's need.

Canada's Department of Justice has an online Victim Services Directory that is a thorough resource that can be used to search for victim services in every province and territory. Contact information is also available for specialized services for children, Indigenous people, survivors of domestic violence, and other victims of crime (Department of Justice, Canada, 2015).

POINTS TO REMEMBER

- ✓ As a first responder or other helping professional, it is important to be aware of the common concerns, behaviours, and symptoms that exist within and between various groups of victims. Although there are similarities, any professional working with a victim must provide individualized support that is unique to the individual and must provide care in an honest and transparent manner.
- ✓ It is also important for a first responder to remain aware of his or her own abilities and limitations as a professional, and to assess and refer victims to other levels of care when the support needed by the victim falls outside his or her role and/or abilities. Collaboration between helping professionals and various services is, in most cases, the most effective and comprehensive plan of care.

KEY TERMS

anxiety, 207
child maltreatment, 216
child neglect, 220
child physical abuse, 216
child sexual abuse, 216
crisis, 206
elder abuse, 222
failure to thrive, 221
panic attack, 207
sexual assault, 214
trauma, 206

REFERENCES

Alberta Health. (2010). Addressing elder abuse in Alberta: A strategy for collective action. Edmonton, AB: Government of Alberta. Retrieved from http://www.seniors-housing.alberta.ca/documents/ElderAbuse-Strategy.pdf

Beaulieu, M., Gordon, R.M., & Spencer, C. (2003, September). An environmental scan of abuse and neglect of older adults in Canada: What's working and why. [Report prepared for the Federal/Provincial/Territorial Committee of Officials (Seniors)]. Retrieved from https://www.seniorscouncil.net/uploads/files/For_Service_Providers/Senior%20Abuse%20Enviromental%20Scan.pdf

Brasfield, C. (2001). Residential school syndrome. *BC Medical Journal*, *43*(2), 78–81.

Campbell, D., & James, A. (2009). Pregnancy & babies: Failure to thrive. In *About kids health*. Toronto: The Hospital for Sick Children. Retrieved from http://www.aboutkidshealth.ca/En/ResourceCentres/PregnancyBabies/Babies/HealthIssuesinYourBaby/Pages/Failure-to-Thrive.aspx

Canadian Child Welfare Research Portal. (2011). Child abuse & neglect. Retrieved from http://cwrp.ca/child-abuse-neglect

Caplan, G. (2017, July 23). Honour killings in Canada: Even worse than we believe. *The Globe and Mail*. Retrieved from https://www.theglobeandmail.com/news/politics/second-reading/honour-killings-in-canada-even-worse-than-we-believe/article1314263/?service=print

Child and Family Services Act, RSO 1990, c C.11.

Child, Family and Community Service Act, RSBC 1996, c 46.

Child, Youth and Family Enhancement Act, RSA 2000, c C-12.

Criminal Code, RSC 1985, c C-46.

Department of Justice, Canada. (2015). Browse the victim services directory. Retrieved from http://www.justice.gc.ca/eng/cj-jp/victims-victimes/vsd-rsv/agencies-agences.aspx

Department of Justice, Canada. (2016). The criminal law and managing children's behaviour [Report]. Retrieved from http://www.justice.gc.ca/eng/rp-pr/cj-jp/fv-vf/mcb-cce/index.html

Khan, S. (2008). Aboriginal mental health: The statistical reality. Here to help: Mental health and substance use information you can trust. *Visions: BC's Mental Health and Addictions Journal*, *5*(1), 6-7. Retrieved from http://www.heretohelp.bc.ca/visions/aboriginal-people-vol5/aboriginal-mental-health-the-statistical-reality

Lipovsky, J., & Hanson, R. (n.d.). The treatment of child victims of abuse and neglect [Report to the Children's Law Center, University of South Carolina]. Retrieved from http://childlaw.sc.edu/frmPublications/TreatmentforChildVictimsofAbuseandNeglect.pdf

McBratney, L. (2007). Barriers to reporting crime. Here to help: Mental health and substance use information you can trust. *Visions: BC's Mental Health and Addictions Journal*, *3*(3), 8-9. Retrieved from http://www.heretohelp.bc.ca/visions/trauma-and-victimization-vol3/victimization-of-people-with-mental-illness

Ministry of Children and Youth Services, Ontario. (2016, July 19). Reporting child abuse and neglect: It's your duty. Retrieved from http://www.children.gov.on.ca/htdocs/English/childrensaid/reportingabuse/abuseandneglect.aspx

Public Health Agency of Canada. (2010). Canadian incidence study of reported child abuse and neglect—2008. Ottawa: Author. Retrieved from http://publications.gc.ca/collections/collection_2010/aspc-phac/HP5-1-2008-eng.pdf

R v Chase, [1987] 2 SCR 293.

Sinha, M., & Milligan, S. (2012, May 22). Family violence in Canada: A statistical profile, 2010. *Juristat*. Catalogue No. 85-0002-X. Ottawa: Statistics Canada. Retrieved from http://www.statcan.gc.ca/pub/85-002-x/2012001/article/11643-eng.pdf

Therapist Aid. (2016). Cycle of abuse [Diagram]. Retrieved from http://www.therapistaid.com/therapy-worksheet/cycle-of-abuse

Truth and Reconciliation Canada. (2015). *Honouring the truth, reconciling for the future: Summary of the final report of the Truth and Reconciliation Commission of Canada*. Winnipeg: Truth and Reconciliation Commission of Canada.

United Nations. (2006). *World report on violence against children*. Geneva, Switzerland: United Nations Publishing Services. Retrieved from http://www.crin.org/en/docs/UNVAC_World_Report_on_Violence_against_Children.pdf.

Women's UN Report Network. (2016, July 14). Canada—Violence against immigrant & refugee women with disabilities. Power & control [Diagram]. Retrieved from http://wunrn.com/2016/07/canada-violence-against-immigrant-refugee-women-with-disabilities/

Youth Protection Act, CQLR c P-34.1.

PART 4

EMERGING TRENDS

CASE STUDY 4

CURRENT PROBLEMS

Numerous studies have shown that the consequences of post-traumatic stress disorder (PTSD) and other mental health and life-affecting experiences are often felt by those working as correctional officers. A recent CBC article reported the results of some Canadian studies:

- One study estimated that a quarter of all prison guards live with PTSD.
- A 1992 study found that Canadian correctional officers will be exposed, on average, to 28 different critical incidents during their career.
- A 2003 Saskatchewan study showed that in a six-month period, correctional officers witnessed an average of five traumatic events (Purdon, 2015).

It turns out that the problem may be even worse than initially thought. The Department of Public Safety reported in 2016 that 36 percent of male correctional officers working in the federal system have reported living with PTSD (Galloway, 2016). A 2014 survey showed that 53 percent of the participating correctional officers displayed high psychological distress caused by factors such as time constraints, work environment, conflict on the job, and low recognition within their field of work (Union of Canadian Correctional Officers, 2016).

Further reviews of the literature regarding Canadian Correctional Officers showed "a psychologically inadequate environment, insufficient infrastructure, long workdays, lack of time for leisure, and inadequate work organization" among other issues such as "paradoxical missions," "dual tasks," and "conflict of roles" to be some of the "causes of suffering" for these officers (Bezerra, Assis, & Constantino, 2016). Canadian research also "noted that these professionals are more exposed to adverse psychosocial factors at work, and report more health problems (such as psychological distress, regular or poor health, and use of social or health services) than is found in a comparable sample of other workers" (Bezerra, Assis, & Constantino, 2016).

As detailed in this text and many others, these workplace issues and the psychological effects related to them can be found in varying degrees within numerous roles filled by first responders. This creates unique challenges for organizations recruiting personnel as first responders and for the helping professions.

DISCUSSION QUESTIONS

The following questions are to be answered from the perspective of a management team leader or policy maker working in the helping professions.

1. What are the key responses an organization such as a correctional institution can make to improve the mental and physical health outcomes associated with their employees based on the issues discussed above?
2. Are any of the changes recommended in your question 1 answer worth considering with regard to other first responder and helping professions such as policing, emergency medical technicians, firefighters, and front-line mental health professionals?
3. In general, what are the emerging trends in mental health and society that could connect potential recruits, help to improve their quality of life, and increase their satisfaction and mental safety at work?

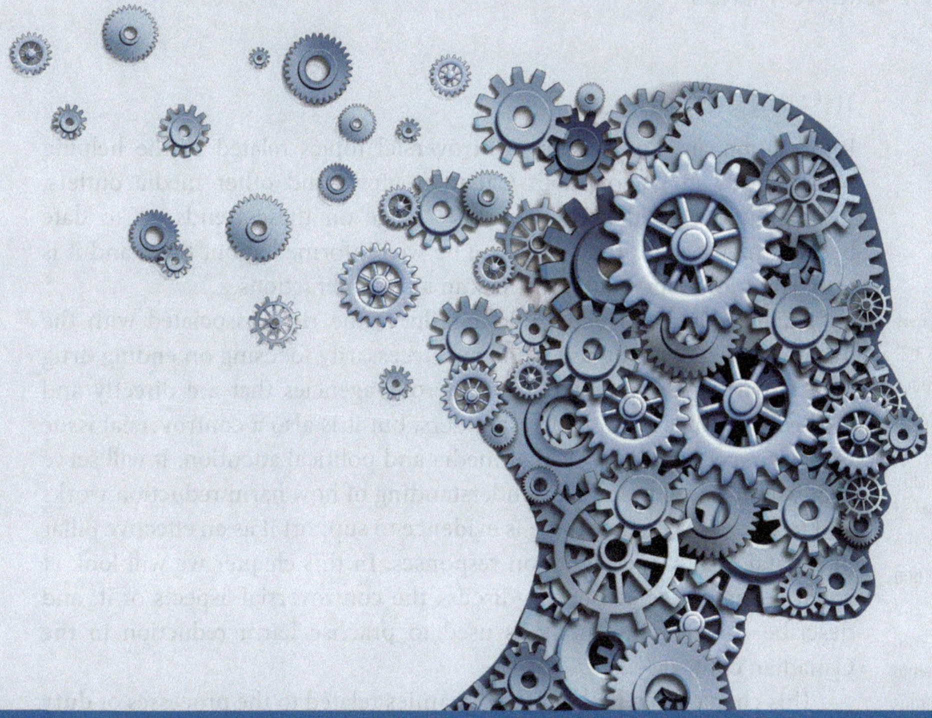

11 CONTROVERSIAL TOPICS IN THE HELPING PROFESSIONS

LEARNING OUTCOMES

After reading this chapter, you will be able to:

- Name a variety of harm-reduction programs and activities.
- Recognize challenging topics in the helping professions.
- Classify various legal and ethical duties related to reporting, case notes, confidentiality, and information-sharing in the helping professions.
- Critically assess positive and negative aspects of various oversight organizations in Canada that operate for the public good.
- Comprehend how systemic improvements and changes are motivated in the Canadian context.

Introduction

Information and updates on controversial topics related to the helping professions can be found in Canadian news and other media outlets. Professionals should keep their knowledge on these trends up to date because members of the public can be well informed about them and it is important to understand how this can affect interactions.

harm reduction
practices, policies, and programs designed to reduce the negative social, health, and economic consequences of drug use but not implicitly designed to reduce the rate of drug use—for example, the establishment of safe injection sites, which can reduce HIV infections, overdoses, and assaults related to sharing needles and doing drugs without supervision

duty to report
legal obligation to report certain types of abuse, neglect, or other crimes

consent
in mental health and related fields consent can occur where an individual gives a helping professional permission to share information with others; can also refer to informed consent, which is a legal term that means permission is given by an individual for a clinician to try a proposed therapeutic technique or for the individual to participate in research

confidentiality
individual's right to not have personal information disclosed without his or her prior consent

Harm reduction (activity that reduces the risks associated with the negative effects of drug use while not necessarily focusing on ending drug use) is part of the mandate of numerous agencies that are directly and indirectly connected to first responders, but it is also a controversial issue that has received a great deal of media and political attention. It will serve professionals well to have an understanding of how harm reduction works and to discover whether there is evidence to support it as an effective pillar of mental health and addiction responses. In this chapter we will look at harm reduction as a concept, discuss the controversial aspects of it, and describe some of the methods used to practise harm reduction in the Canadian context.

This chapter also looks at the dynamics related to the processes of **duty to report**, **consent**, and **confidentiality**, which are all used in the helping professions, and this includes first responders. It is vital to be aware of the rules that apply to these processes, because not following best practices can result in termination, poor service for individuals who are being helped, and unnecessary misunderstandings between organizations.

Watchdog groups and **ombudsman organizations** have made significant reports related to the helping professions, including justice and first responders. These reports make up a great deal of the discussion within the professions about how to improve and meet the needs of individuals and communities. What is the best approach in the long run for individuals and communities dealing with mental health–related crimes? What about standards in Canada and other jurisdictions? What suggestions are being made by industry experts with regard to the helping professions? How is the prevalence of mental health issues in the corrections system affecting service and how can this problem be addressed? This chapter will explore how watchdog groups and ombudsman organizations investigate these issues.

Harm Reduction

Harm reduction is a key piece in the public health approach to treating substance abuse. Access to harm-reduction services is generally a provincial or territorial responsibility that focuses on reducing the harm that persons who use substances may face as a result of their addiction (Hyshka et al., 2017). There are harms associated with substance abuse, including harms related to the acquisition of substances (risky and/or criminal behaviours), the use of substances (impairments, diseases, and other mental and physical health problems), and withdrawal from substances (symptoms and functioning issues) (Addy & Ritter, 2000).

watchdog groups
governmental and non-governmental groups that work to inform the public about the actions of organizations; these groups organize to help bring about change

ombudsman organization
arm's-length organization empowered to investigate complaints, resolve issues, and make recommendations for the betterment of the public and employees with regard to systemic issues in the ways that services are delivered; another word for "ombudsman" is "ombudsperson"

Harm-Reduction Programs and Policies

Harm-reduction programs and policies operate with an approach centred on the following principles.

- **Pragmatism:** Harm reduction recognizes that there will always be a percentage of the population who will engage in higher risk behaviour, for a range of social, economic, mental health, and personal reasons. Harm reduction recognizes that drug use is a complex and multifaceted phenomenon that encompasses a continuum of behaviour from abstinence to chronic dependence, and produces varying degrees of personal and social harm.
- **Focus on harm:** The priority for harm reduction is to decrease the negative consequences of drug use to the user and others, rather than to decrease or eliminate drug use itself. While harm reduction emphasizes a change to safer practices and patterns of drug use, it does not rule out the longer-term goal of abstinence. In this way, harm reduction is complementary to the abstinence model of addiction treatment.
- **Human rights:** Harm reduction respects the basic human dignity and rights of people who use drugs. It accepts one's decision to use drugs as fact; no judgment is made either to condemn or support the use of drugs. Harm reduction acknowledges the individual's right to self-determination and supports informed decision-making in the context of active drug use. Emphasis is placed on personal choice, responsibility, and self-management.
- **Maximizing intervention options:** Harm reduction recognizes that people with drug-use problems benefit from a variety of approaches. There is no one prevention or treatment approach that works reliably for everyone. It is choice and prompt access to a broad range of interventions that help to keep people alive and safe, and promote health.

- **Priority of immediate goals:** Harm reduction recognizes readiness to change as key to the process of individuals leading healthier lives. People may be anywhere along a continuum—from not thinking about change, to contemplating it, to taking action, to maintaining change—moving forward and back. Harm reduction starts with "where the person is" with his or her drug use, with the immediate focus on the most pressing needs. Harm reduction is based on the importance of incremental gains that can be achieved over time.
- **Involvement of people who use drugs:** The active participation of people who use drugs is at the heart of harm reduction. People who use drugs are seen as the best source of information about their own drug use, and are empowered to join with service providers to determine the best interventions to reduce harm from drug use. Harm reduction recognizes the competency of people who use drugs to make choices and change their lives (Canadian Liver Foundation, 2007; Thomas, 2005).

With these principles in play, harm reduction can help individuals who are living with addictions and their communities in many ways. Harm reduction can:

- keep persons with addictions alive until they are ready for successful treatment.
- expose persons with addictions to non-judgmental and non-coercive helping professionals at **supervised consumption services** so that they can learn to trust and reach out when they are ready for treatment.
- prevent overdoses through monitoring of substance users.
- prevent HIV, hepatitis C, and other blood-borne infections by providing clean needles and other substance-use paraphernalia that are not shared.
- prevent bystanders from exposure to drugs, drug paraphernalia, and persons who are under the influence of drugs by providing supervised consumption services that are accessible and private.
- provide persons living with addictions with more opportunities to participate in the activities of daily living.

supervised consumption services sites where illicit substance use is supervised in order to protect the users and the general public from issues related to drug abuse

- reduce the legal issues related to substance abuse to help reduce crime that is associated with drug use. This keeps individuals who are living with addictions out of jail and more likely and able to contribute to society.

Harm-Reduction Methods and Programs

Harm reduction can occur in a number of specific ways.

Methadone maintenance treatment is a harm-reduction technique that helps reduce cravings and the symptoms of withdrawal from opiate addiction—however, some argue that methadone simply replaces an opiate or heroin addiction with an addiction to methadone itself. While this may be true in certain cases, treatment with methadone can also allow addicted individuals to lead more productive and safer lives without having to engage in illicit or illegal activity to feed their addiction. If the message that addictions can be treated through medication becomes more mainstream it may create a shift in the number of persons willing to accept treatment. For example, persons who use insulin as a treatment for diabetes are not considered addicted to insulin. Instead they are encouraged to maintain a healthy treatment regimen to stave off the potentially dangerous effects of a disease. The same argument can be used to support helping individuals who are living with addiction to replace their use of illegal and dangerous substances with controlled medication.

methadone maintenance treatment type of treatment for those who are addicted to the use of opioids such as heroin; often carried out in clinics where methadone consumption is monitored by medical professionals to help users reduce or eliminate the use of opioids

Needle exchange programs have become more popular in cities across Canada and the United States (Golding, 2017). These harm-reduction programs focus on giving clean needles and syringes to persons living with substance abuse problems at no cost to the user. These programs also provide one or multiple locations where intravenous drug users can drop off used needles for safe disposal, which helps prevent public health risk. Health and other front-line workers are often made available at program locations so that they can establish a rapport with individuals and help connect them with other formal services (Canadian Liver Foundation, 2007).

needle exchange programs harm-reduction programs in which individuals can drop off used needles to be safely destroyed and pick up new needles and other drug-related equipment

Safe injection sites, also considered to be controversial, are another form of public health service harm reduction. They are also referred to as supervised consumption services. Safe injection sites provide a supervised, hygienic, and safe place for people to consume substances. As with needle exchange program sites, health and social service front-line workers are trained to supervise users and help them engage with other services when they are ready to take that step.

safe injection sites *see* supervised consumption services

There are many reasons why harm-reduction activities are considered to be controversial despite their success at maintaining life and quality of life as well as their cost-effectiveness. Reasons why some key stakeholders have expressed ambivalence toward supervised consumption services include:

1. lack of knowledge about the effectiveness of harm-reduction sites,
2. concerns that the goals of these programs are too narrow,
3. lack of certainty that the problem is large enough to warrant these programs,
4. feeling that there needs to be more known about proper locations for harm-reduction sites and programs so that they won't negatively affect community and business interests,
5. worries that problems that have not been seen since areas have become gentrified will reoccur,
6. concerns that resources that would go to prevention of drug use will be claimed to pay for these programs instead, and
7. worries about evaluation and community consultation relating to the fear that these programs will not be discontinued if any of the above problems arise (Strike, Watson, Kolla, Penn, & Bayoumi, 2015).

There are also concerns or fears that these programs will increase crime rates, which runs against the available evidence (Kerr, Mitra, Kennedy, & McNeil, 2017). Another way in which these and other justice or mental health–related programs sometimes become controversial is because of a popular phenomenon known as **NIMBYism**. NIMBYism has been a deterrent to finding locations for a variety of services related to the helping professions, including justice.

NIMBYism occurs when individuals or groups object to the development of programs within their own neighbourhoods; NIMBY is an acronym of the phrase "Not In My Back Yard"

The placement of harm-reduction facilities, correctional facilities, homeless shelters, and residential facilities in communities is often met with resistance from local residents who, although they may agree with the creation of these services, do not want to have to deal with the effects of having them in their neighbourhoods. Some harm-reduction programs in Canada have tried to accommodate this by creating mobile units that can travel through an area and do not require a fixed address (Kerr et al., 2017).

One of the problems that NIMBYism engenders with regard to harm-reduction services is a tension between the need for services to be accessible, central, and on public transit routes for users versus an established community's desire to not have to deal with something they find unappealing or are afraid of. This kind of opposition can further stigmatize individuals who are living with addiction and mental health issues.

In response to NIMBYism and the time-consuming bureaucracy that comes with getting approvals, organizations such as Overdose Prevention Ottawa and other similar groups in Vancouver and Toronto have been opening unsanctioned **overdose prevention sites.** These sites use a "pop-up" model, are opened in secret, and usually operate in a tent with chairs, tables, naloxone, and trained health professionals or peer-support persons available who can supervise persons living with addiction and help prevent overdose deaths (Kupfer, 2017).

overdose prevention sites sites where peer supporters, volunteers, and sometimes medical personnel observe individuals using drugs so that they can intervene to prevent overdoses and initiate intervention when overdoses occur

While harm-reduction efforts are sometimes controversial, an argument can be made that they really shouldn't be. Most people use harm-reduction practices regularly. When having sex, for example, many people use condoms to lower the risks involved (sexually transmitted diseases, unwanted pregnancies).

Many people engage in drinking behaviour that is not problematic because they take steps to reduce harm, such as using a designated driver, putting money aside for a cab, and making sure they eat plenty and drink lots of water on the day they are planning to drink. Individuals who are addicted to hard drugs may use cigarettes instead of heroin to help them quit.

Despite all this, there are those who feel that using harm-reduction methods to deal with illicit drugs, sex work, and other provocative issues will encourage illicit behaviour, and so—at least for the time being—these interventions generally remain controversial. However, they are becoming more accepted over time and through advocacy and education about their effectiveness.

VOICES FROM THE FIELD

B.C.'s Second Low-Barrier Supervised Injection Site, Safe Point, Opens This Week in Surrey

By Travis Lupick

June 6, 2017, *The Georgia Straight*—As of Thursday (June 8), Vancouver will officially no longer be the only city in British Columbia with a supervised injection site for drug users.

That morning, a new facility called Safe Point is scheduled to open on the Surrey Strip, at 10681 – 135A Street.

A second injection site in Surrey, attached to the Quibble Creek Sobering and Assessment Centre at 13670 – 94A Avenue, has also received Health Canada approval to offer supervised injection services, although users must be a member of the organization to use it.

Safe Point is low barrier, similar to Vancouver's Insite facility that has operated on the 100 block of East Hastings Street since 2003. Both Insite and Safe Point services are immediately accessible to anyone who walks in off the street. A user must give a name upon entry but it does not have to be one's real name. Intake staff also ask [individuals] for the name of the substance or substances that they are using.

Safe Point is funded by Fraser Health and will be operated in a partnership with Lookout Emergency Aid Society.

In a telephone interview, Dr. Victoria Lee, chief medical health officer for Fraser Health Authority, said that Safe Point will open with health care providers working there and offer connections to social services such as help with housing. There are also recovery services integrated into Safe Point where people who are ready to enter treatment can access methadone and Suboxone, both prescription drugs that suppress the mental and physical cravings that an addict feels for opioids.

Safe Point's location at 10681 – 135A Street is barely more than a few metres from a new RCMP community policing station. That attracted some criticism last December wherein concerns were raised about to what extent the presence of police officers might deter people carrying drugs from using the site.

Addressing those concerns, Lee noted that since January, an overdose prevention site has operated on the Surrey Strip very close to where the injection facility will open. According to Lee, that location came to see about 500 visits each week, and that should serve as evidence that drug users are okay with the presence of the RCMP.

"We've done surveys as well as focus groups prior to opening, and specifically asked about people's willingness to use services located at that site with RCMP services located nearby," Lee said. "We didn't see any concerns from people in the community or people that use substances on 135A Street."

The application that Fraser Health submitted to Health Canada for approval to open Surrey's two supervised injection sites requested that they also allow people to swallow and snort drugs.

Those sections of Fraser Health's applications remain under review. If approved, it would make Surrey's supervised injection sites—which would then be called consumption sites—the first government-sanctioned health care facilities in North America to offer that kind of service.

In Vancouver, an overdose prevention site at 62 East Hastings Street includes an outdoor area where people smoking drugs are observed for potential overdoses.

An overdose prevention site is different from a supervised injection facility in that the latter includes complementary health care services while the former does not.

Insite, for example, can connect users to drug counselling and has a detox centre, called Onsite, located on the building's second floor.

According to the latest B.C. Coroners Service report, the province is on track to see a record number of overdose deaths this year.

During the first four months of 2017, there were 488 fatal overdoses across the province. That suggests B.C. will see more than 1,460 overdose deaths by the end of this year, up from 935 in 2016, 518 in 2015, and 368 the year before that.

That report notes that Surrey is second only to the City of Vancouver for overdose deaths.

During the first four months of 2017, there were 51 fatal overdoses in Surrey, compared to 113 during all of 2016 and 76 in 2015.

In a June 6 media release, Surrey Mayor Linda Hepner said she hopes the city's new injection sites will help stem the tide of drug overdose deaths.

"Supervised consumption services in Surrey will play an important role in preventing fatal overdoses from occurring, while supporting people who are ready to begin their road to recovery with connections to treatment services," Hepner said.

On June 2, Mayor Gregor Robertson issued a media release where it's emphasized that Vancouver is all but certain to see an increase in its annual number of fatal overdoses for the fifth year in a row.

"The near-record number of drug overdose deaths in the fentanyl crisis is a bloodbath in all corners of Vancouver with no end in sight," Robertson said quoted there.

The coroner's report notes that no one has ever died at a supervised injection facility in B.C. or at any of the provinces more than 15 overdose prevention sites that opened last December.

DISCUSSION QUESTIONS

1. What kinds of harm-reduction activities have you or a loved one engaged in? Does this affect your own feelings about harm-reduction programs? Why or why not?
2. How would you rank the importance of the six principles found on pages 239–240 of this text? Explain the reasoning for your first and last picks.
3. What would be the positives and negatives to an overdose prevention site being created in your neighbourhood? Provide two or three examples for each side of the argument.

Duty to Report, Consent, and Making Decisions on Behalf of Others

In carrying out our duties as justice and helping professionals we sometimes have to make decisions on behalf of other people, investigate those making decisions on behalf of others, and work with other professionals who are making these kinds of decisions. The ethics, laws, and policies that are involved in these decisions can become, and can be perceived as, controversial by both the general public and those within the professions. It is therefore incredibly important to understand the concepts related to one's duty to report, substitute decision-making rights, and how one proceeds with gathering consent for treatment and information sharing.

There is no general duty to report a crime in Canada, with some exceptions around child abuse and abuse of persons with diminished capacity. The specifics about duty to report in terms of elder abuse vary from province to province. This text shared information with regard to the duty to report in child welfare cases in Chapter 10, Working with Victims. In this chapter, we will explore other aspects of the duty to report.

For example, in Ontario long-term care facilities and retirement homes it is mandatory for anyone (other than residents) who knows or has a reasonable suspicion that abuse, neglect, incompetence, or fraud are occurring to report it. Regulated health and helping professionals are released from their obligation of confidentiality to individuals and must report these issues if they become or are made aware of them.

Vulnerable adults such as those with developmental disabilities also fall under rules that allow helping professionals to report abuse. Helping professionals are allowed to breach confidentiality in these cases, too. Organizations that serve these groups are to immediately report abuse that is suspected, alleged, or witnessed. However, the abuse of adults who live in their own home or a private dwelling does not fall under a general legal duty to report. For example, a senior of sound mind who tells a helping professional that he or she was charged triple rent and verbally abused by his or her landlord but who does not want to report the problem is under no obligation to do so and neither is the helping professional.

Tension can arise between a helping professional's personal and professional sense of ethics. When working on these cases, there may be conflict with colleagues who don't understand the duty to report, principles of **self-determination**, and/or how to support an individual's wishes and confidentiality. However, the rights of the affected individual must be upheld. For example, an individual may have a number of good reasons to not want to report fraud and abuse to the police, but will still want to talk about it, vent about it, and strategize with a helping professional.

self-determination
a person's ability to determine and control his or her own life; the helping professions promote this concept

The duty of confidentiality is an important ethical and legal obligation. There are times when a helping professional may be *required* to disclose an individual's information, and other times a helping professional may be *permitted* by the individual to disclose information.

For example, a helping professional may be required to break confidentiality if the person he or she is aiding is a threat to themselves or someone else. This might occur in the following scenarios:

- The individual makes threats during an interaction with a helping professional about hurting or killing another person. In a case like this, some codes of ethics and laws in other countries have a **duty to warn** a person who is under threat from an individual as well.

- The individual makes comments that lead the helping professional to believe the person is at imminent risk of killing himself or herself.
- The individual discloses that he or she has medical issues that make it dangerous for him or her to drive.
- The individual is in the throes of a psychosis or a psychotic break and is acting in a way that could result in self-harm or harm to others.

duty to warn
responsibility that helping professionals have in some jurisdictions where they must break confidentiality with an individual in order to warn third parties that they are under threat by that individual

There are many ways that helping professionals can respond in order to maintain an individual's confidentiality. For example, some agencies, such as those who provide services to individuals who have been sexually assaulted, have gone so far as to not keep any clinical notes about those they are helping, other than attendance, in case they are subpoenaed. This might seem controversial, but there are valid reasons for this sort of response.

Imagine that a woman in her thirties is raped and accesses help from a sexual assault agency in the lead-up to a court appearance. While talking about her feelings regarding the sexual assault she discloses that in her early twenties she was emotionally, physically, and sexually abused by an ex-partner and forced into sex work by that ex-partner. The clinician writes this in a case note and this information is subpoenaed for the trial. Suddenly the focus of the woman's rape trial shifts to her previous abuse and her involvement in sex work.

Even when agencies do keep more detailed notes, it is very important for helping professionals to be thoughtful and selective about what they write down. This is different from training that is received in the justice system. Even events that seem relatively mundane can cause great harm in an individual's life.

For example, a person on long-term disability because of a workplace accident may become frustrated and want to speak with a helping professional. While consulting with the helping professional, the person mentions that he or she has looked at online job postings because he or she misses working, but none of the jobs would be possible because of the injury. The person was simply wistful on one occasion about not being able to work—that's all it was. In an effort to write a positive note about the individual, the helping professional includes a line in a case note about the individual "wanting to work and looking for work." The insurance company handling the claim sees this note as part of a review of the disability claim and uses it to threaten removal of or outright deny continuing coverage to the individual. The result of keeping such a case note is unneeded stress to the individual and his or her family, as well as a breakdown in trust in the therapeutic relationship between the individual and the helping professional.

These two examples show how important it is to keep thoughtful and carefully considered notes. In addition, it is increasingly important in this digital era to encrypt any case notes, use strong passwords, turn off screens when individuals enter a room, and implement any other measures that will help to maintain confidentiality.

Additionally, it is best practice to not talk outside of work about the individuals you work with as a helping professional. This goes beyond not mentioning names to include not mentioning anything that may identify individuals you work with, including nicknames, personal details, or unique identifiable situations. It is fine to say in broad terms to a loved one that you had a tough shift at work and you were working with someone who has suffered through many abuse issues. It becomes entirely possible, however, that you will accidently identify the person if you discuss things like the location or timing of the abuse, or provide any details that might be known in the community or have been reported in the media.

circle of care manifests when a number of helping professionals work together with an individual and are able to share information about their work and progress together through the implied consent of the individual

case conference formal meeting where a number of services and/or helping professionals meet to help with planning, goal setting, and coordination of services for an individual; whenever possible, the conference takes place with the individual present and at the centre of decisions

Freedom of Information and Protection of Privacy Act provincial legislation that provides the right of access to information that is under the control of institutions if criteria for disclosure are met

There is a concept called the **circle of care**, which is a term that is used to describe situations within the helping professions in which there is an implied consent that personal information about an individual is to be shared for the benefit of that person's care. If a helping professional is invited to a **case conference** where a decision will be made about where the individual will be placed in residential care, for example, it is reasonable to make the assumption that some information will be shared about the individual. In agencies where an individual might meet with numerous members of a multidisciplinary team, there is a sense of implied consent that those members will share opinions, relevant information, files, and case notes.

Many health and social agencies have formal processes for information sharing; consent requirements are explained to an individual and consent forms are signed. This is especially useful when another agency asks for information about an individual. Best practice dictates that it must be explained to those requesting the information that implicit consent is required and that information will not be released without it. Most agencies have detailed policies and standard forms that are used for consent purposes.

With regard to potentially dangerous individuals, opinions vary on disclosure and about how they should be treated in order to uphold public safety. There are those who believe professional judgment should be exercised. Others think clear and firm policies and laws, such as the ***Freedom of Information and Protection of Privacy Act***, are required and exceptions to confidentiality should be greatly expanded. Mandatory reporting in all cases might have an overall negative effect if it discourages people from getting the treatment they need and prevents them from making disclosures. Also, helping and health care professionals may make efforts to avoid working with difficult or potentially dangerous individuals because they do not want to be held legally responsible with regard to tricky issues that involve breaking confidentiality and the duty to warn.

Confidentiality issues can be avoided by having a frank and clear discussion with the individual you are working with about the limits of confidentiality and the consent requirements of your profession and your employer before providing service. This conversation normally takes place during an intake process so that all parties are clear about confidentiality issues from the outset. Even if a helping professional has to break confidentiality, it is possible to save or even enhance the therapeutic relationship afterward if everyone is clear about the process ahead of time.

DISCUSSION QUESTIONS

1. Do you think that duty to report provisions should be expanded to include more areas of crime and abuse? Why or why not?
2. List five types of information (not including names and specific addresses) about an individual that a helping professional could accidentally share in conversation that might identify the individual.
3. With a partner, role-play that one of you is an individual who is seeing the other as a helping professional. In two minutes or less, in those roles, discuss the limits of confidentiality. Take turns, and then try to do it again in one minute or less. Was this activity difficult to do? Why or why not?

Watchdogs, Ombudsmen, and Protestors

Oversight is an important aspect of the helping professions. Most of the industries related to these professions are regulated and involve some kind of professional membership or designation that has to be obtained. There are also a number of independent investigation units or other arm's-length groups that are able to analyze issues within the profession, make suggestions for the industries as a whole or even intervene in specific cases.

Sometimes called watchdog groups, these organizations are normally not-for-profit and they monitor the helping professions, including justice, and alert the public and media when they believe something is happening that is unethical or goes against the interests of the general public. There are differences from province to province in watchdog groups, regulatory bodies, and organizations, and this chapter provides province-specific examples. Professionals should research in-depth with regard to the dynamics of the province they live and work in.

Watchdog groups can be seen as hampering the abilities of front-line personnel, but they also work to help improve their lives, workloads, and policies as well. In 2016, the growing number of police officer suicides in Ontario resulted in the launch of a systemic review of how police handle mental illness within their services in an attempt to prevent further deaths and provide support for officers (Gillis, 2016).

LGBTQI2S+ stands for "lesbian, gay, bisexual, transgender, queer (or questioning), intersex, two-spirited, and other related ways" in which an individual may self-identify

Special Investigations Unit (SIU) civilian oversight agency in Ontario that investigates any incidents involving police and civilians that result in serious injuries, death, or allegations of sexual assault; organizations with similar mandates and powers exist in other parts of the country

Office of the Independent Police Review Director (OIPRD) Ontario organization that is responsible for collecting, managing, and overseeing public complaints about police; other provinces use different ministries, commissions, or committees to manage and oversee public complaints about police—British Columbia, for example, uses the Office of the Police Complaint Commissioner

Some watchdog groups are created by the government and have official powers granted to them to investigate and research, while others are non-governmental and usually run by interested parties who fundraise to help them organize, protest, and get their message out to the public. Both types of groups have been effective in bringing to light issues in the helping professions, including justice—even though at times these messages can be difficult to hear.

For example, Black Lives Matter (BLM) is a non-governmental grass-roots group that has had numerous successes in Canada in recent history, using a variety of tactics to challenge the relationship between police and the **LGBTQI2S+** community. This has created an atmosphere where many difficult discussions have occurred between Pride Festival organizers and police organizations about the role of police at Pride. More recently, BLM in Quebec has organized around a belief that "[p]olice should not be the first to intervene in mental health crises," and that an enhanced national mental health strategy should be developed, mental health data should be collected, and details of police interaction and the names of specific officers who are involved in shootings of mentally ill individuals should be released (Canadian Press, 2017).

There have been calls for the release of the names of police under investigation in Ontario as well. In 2017, journalist and activist Desmond Cole made public his critique of a government-commissioned review of the three oversight bodies that are involved with policing issues in Ontario. He is advocating that officers being investigated should have their names released in the same way that other adults under investigation for serious crimes do (CBC Radio, 2017).

Public demonstrations have an effect on policy-makers, although they can be controversial. The **Special Investigations Unit (SIU)**, the **Office of the Independent Police Review Director (OIPRD)**, and the **Ontario Civilian Police Commission (OCPC)** were all reviewed in the lead-up to a report aimed at making these government-approved watchdog groups more accountable and transparent. According to the report itself, the review took place because of "public demonstrations of dissatisfaction with policing and police oversight" (Tulloch, 2017, p. 3).

Among the 129 suggestions included in the report were the following:

- Police oversight bodies should collect demographic data that includes "gender, age, race, religion, ethnicity, mental health status, disability, and Indigenous status" (p. 18).
- It is recommended that "oversight bodies implement ongoing training and evaluation programs that address social and cultural competency issues, anti-racism, diversity, inclusion, accessibility, gender-based violence, and mental health" (p. 70).
- SIU staff should have "the skills and experience that allow them to address … trauma, counselling, crisis intervention, and mental health and addictions" (p. 78).
- The public complaints process should be made more accessible and persons who are vulnerable should be provided "assistance to navigate that process" (p. 147).

Ontario Civilian Police Commission (OCPC) independent oversight agency created to make sure adequate and effective policing occurs in Ontario within the parameters of the *Police Services Act*; hears appeals with regard to police disciplinary decisions and investigations about the conduct of officers, police chiefs, and police services board members as well as providing other services

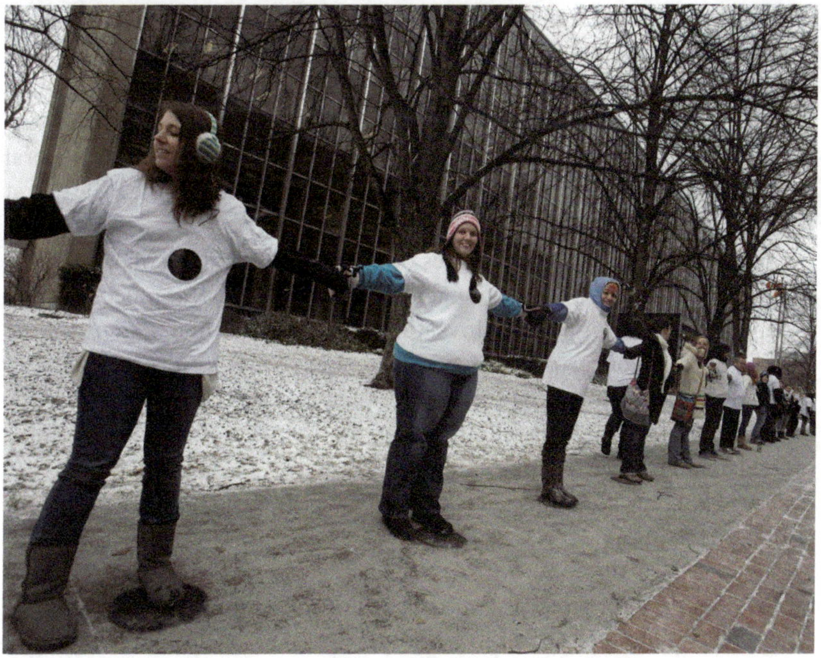

Concerned citizens at the "Connect the Dots" protest in Ottawa, Ontario hoping for improvement in mental health service delivery.

- "The SIU should create a public accountability office responsible for public communications and should be provided with adequate resources for this function" (p. 266).
- "At least 50 percent of the non-forensic investigators on an investigative team at the SIU should be investigators with no background in policing" (p. 267).
- "The OIPRD should actively recruit civilian investigators with relevant experience who were not former police officers. No more than 25 percent of the OIPRD's investigators should be former police officers" (p. 268).
- "The mandate of the SIU should include all incidents involving the discharge of a firearm by a police officer at a person" (p. 268).
- "The Ombudsman should have jurisdiction over all three police oversight bodies" (p. 94).

An ombudsman will take up, investigate, and resolve a variety of types of complaints. For the purposes of this chapter, the focus is on ombudspersons who are appointed to scrutinize public agencies related to the helping professions, including justice, and who may also intervene in and investigate issues related to mental health.

One of the most high-profile ombudsman offices in that context is the Government of Canada's Federal Ombudsman for Victims of Crime. This is an appointed position that addresses public complaints relating to crime victims, promotes federal programs for victims of crime, identifies systemic issues that hurt victims, and makes recommendations to federal policy makers in order to improve the victims' lives. More can be learned at www.victimsfirst.gc.ca.

Within the correctional services of Canada, the ombudsman's office is called the Office of the Correctional Investigator (OCI). This office provides independent oversight and investigation of individual and systemic complaints and concerns. Any federal offender or loved one of an offender can make a complaint about the Correctional Service of Canada. While the correctional service is not required to act on the recommendations of this ombudsman, they are required to respond.

The OCI has identified six key priorities that are the focus of ongoing concern:

1. access to physical and mental health care services;
2. prevention of deaths in custody;

3. conditions of confinement (e.g., segregation, lockdowns, use of force, population management);
4. Indigenous issues;
5. access to programs (e.g., case preparation, timely release); and
6. issues affecting federally sentenced women (Office of the Correctional Advisor, 2016).

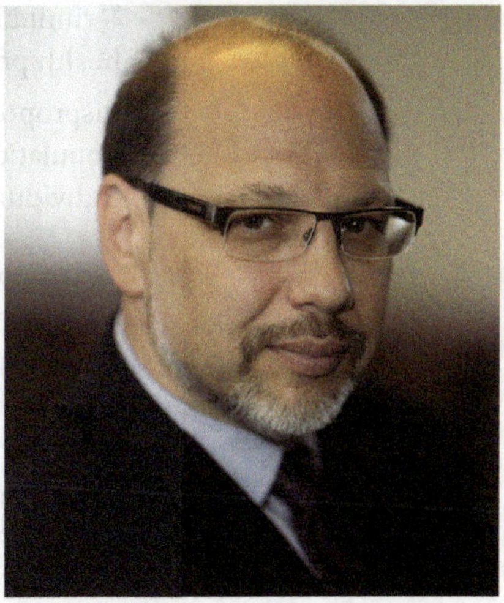

Former Correctional Investigator Howard Sapers.

The OCI has also released numerous reports of note on corrections and the treatment of persons living with mental health issues, as have many provincial ombudsman offices.

Former Correctional Investigator of Canada Howard Sapers made these observations in a groundbreaking 2011 report on mental health and corrections:

- Physical conditions of prison confinement (e.g., deprivation, isolation, and separation from family and loved ones) can be hard on mental health functioning.
- Prison environments are often crowded, austere, noisy, devoid of natural light, violent, stressful, volatile, restrictive, and unpredictable.
- These conditions are not conducive to therapy or rehabilitation.
- Some of the older penitentiaries lack the physical infrastructures, design, and capacity to adequately respond to rising needs and complexity of mental health problems.
- For staff, managing mentally disordered offenders in prison creates professional and operational dilemmas related to conflicting priorities and objectives—security versus treatment; inmate versus patient; assistance versus control; prison versus hospital (Sapers, 2011).

Sapers also made the case that prisons were becoming the new asylums and housing massive numbers of persons who were mentally ill as a result of the following cumulative problems:

- impact of the deinstitutionalization movement,
- inadequate and fragmented community services and supports,

- "criminalization" of behaviours associated with untreated mental health problems and "zero-tolerance" policies, and
- disproportionate incarceration of vulnerable and "at-risk" populations (Indigenous, homeless, impoverished, and addicted individuals) (Sapers, 2011).

In the OCI's 2014–15 annual report, Sapers weighed in on the Correctional Service of Canada's response to the Ashley Smith inquest regarding the use of segregation, calling it "frustrating and disappointing," and saying that "on many fronts, the response simply misses the mark" and is "backward-looking" (Sapers, 2015). This sort of blunt talk about important issues is a part of the advocacy process that is expected from ombudsmen for the good of the public interest. More resources, information, and special reports from this office can be found at www.oci-bec.gc.ca/index-eng.aspx.

Since the time of the 2014–15 report, Sapers has been appointed as the Independent Advisor on Corrections Reform to the Ontario provincial government where he has been heading a review of provincial solitary confinement measures and trying to find other ways to improve the provincial correctional system (Rushowy, 2016; White, 2016).

Lastly, the Veterans Ombudsman provides complaint resolution, system navigation, and other redress options for members of the Canadian Armed Forces, the Royal Canadian Mounted Police, veterans, and family members. The office of the Veterans Ombudsman can be a helpful source for RCMP or other front-line personnel who have served within the military and are living with stressors, including those brought on by mental health problems. Information on the Veterans Ombudsman can be found at www.ombudsman-veterans.gc.ca/eng.

When working with front-line personnel or with members of the community whose lives intersect with the helping professions, whether the individuals are victims of crime, service users, inmates, or others, there are a variety of watchdog groups, social/protest movements, and ombudsman offices they can be directed to. These referrals may help individuals with their cases or even help them create systemic changes in the way services are delivered, helping to make those services more effective and individual centred.

POINTS TO REMEMBER

- ✓ Controversies involving the helping professions will continue to arise. The topics will change and evolve over time as the discussion moves from one subject to another and new issues take precedence.
- ✓ Harm reduction is a great example of this—it has become less controversial over time as more and more programs and spaces dedicated to practising harm reduction have been created across Canada. However, there is still opposition despite evidence of program effectiveness and the use of harm-reduction methods in everyday life.
- ✓ NIMBYism is a mindset that is common when new services and programs related to the helping professions are proposed or created within communities. Fears regarding illicit behaviour and change can be navigated through a variety of methods that include consultation, education, and finding creative solutions to address local residents' concerns.
- ✓ The duty to report is an important aspect of work within the helping professions, and while law and policy are very clear with regard to child abuse and neglect issues, many people are unfamiliar with the intricacies that surround the reporting of other types of crime and abuse. For example, the duty to report can be unclear with regard to vulnerable adults or when working with those who threaten to hurt themselves or others. There are other related concepts that have yet to take a legal hold in Canada, such as the duty to warn. It will be worth keeping an eye on that for the future.
- ✓ Protecting an individual's confidentiality can be difficult in a growing digital world where so many different agencies are potentially involved in any given case as part of a circle of care. Helping professionals must be incredibly thoughtful about what they record (for example, in case notes) in order to avoid misunderstandings that can result in those they are trying to help suffering undue hardships. Two best practices that are worth adopting are discussing the limitations of confidentiality as well as the duty to report with an individual before beginning to work with that person and getting written consent before sharing a person's information with others.
- ✓ Social movements that protest controversial issues, governmental and non-governmental watchdog groups, and ombudsman offices all play roles in investigating and advocating in the best interests of the public. Sometimes their methods or choice of words can create tension within a given profession and in the general public. However, this tension can be a good thing when it helps to spur needed investigations and create positive changes for either workers or the public. Awareness of these groups and referrals to these groups can be part of good practice within the helping professions.

KEY TERMS

case conference, 248
circle of care, 248
confidentiality, 238
consent, 238
duty to report, 238
duty to warn, 247
Freedom of Information and Protection of Privacy Act, 248
harm reduction, 238
LGBTQI2S+, 250
methadone maintenance treatment, 241
needle exchange programs, 241
NIMBYism, 242
Office of the Independent Police Review Director (OIPRD), 250
ombudsman organization, 239
Ontario Civilian Police Commission (OCPC), 251
overdose prevention sites, 243
safe injection sites, 241
self-determination, 246
Special Investigations Unit (SIU), 250
supervised consumption services, 240
watchdog groups, 239

REFERENCES

Addy, D., & Ritter, A. (2000). *Clinical treatment guidelines for alcohol and drug clinicians: No 4: Reducing harm for clients who continue to use drugs*. Fitzroy, Victoria, Australia: Turning Point Alcohol and Drug Centre.

Bezerra, C.D.M., Assis, S.G.D., & Constantino, P. (2016). Psychological distress and work stress in correctional officers: A literature review. *Ciencia & Saude Coletiva, 21*(7), 2135–2146.

Canadian Liver Foundation. (2007). *Working with people who use drugs: A harm reduction approach*. Non Prescription Needle Use Initiative. Edmonton, AB: Author.

Canadian Press. (2017, July 2). "He was in crisis. They killed him": Black Lives Matter protest police response to mental health crises. *National Post*. Retrieved from http://nationalpost.com/news/canada/black-activists-hold-protest-in-response-to-fatal-police-shooting-in-montreal

CBC Radio. (2017, April 7). Police watchdog review doesn't go far enough, critic says. *CBC Radio's Ottawa Morning*. Retrieved from http://www.cbc.ca/news/canada/ottawa/ottawa-reaction-police-oversight-review-report-1.4058280

Freedom of Information and Protection of Privacy Act, RSO 1990, c F31.

Galloway, G. (2017, July 27). PTSD affects 36 per cent of male prison officers, federal data reveal. *The Globe and Mail*. Retrieved from https://beta.theglobeandmail.com/news/politics/ptsd-prevalent-among-male-prison-officers-federal-data-reveal/article31145169

Gillis, W. (2016, February 13). Ontario police watchdog to check on mental-illness help for cops. *Toronto Star*. Retrieved from https://www.thestar.com/news/crime/2016/02/13/ontario-police-watchdog-to-check-on-mental-illness-help-for-cops.html

Golding, N.J. (2017). The needle and the damage done: Indiana's response to the 2015 HIV epidemic and the need to change state and federal policies regarding needle exchanges and intravenous drug users. *Indiana Health Law Review*, *14*, 173–220.

Hyshka, E., Anderson-Baron, J., Karekezi, K., Belle-Isle, L., Elliott, R., Pauly, B., … & Wild, T.C. (2017). Harm reduction in name, but not substance: A comparative analysis of current Canadian provincial and territorial policy frameworks. *Harm Reduction Journal*, *14*(1), 50.

Kerr, T., Mitra, S., Kennedy, M.C., & McNeil, R. (2017). Supervised injection facilities in Canada: Past, present, and future. *Harm Reduction Journal*, *14*(1), 28.

Kupfer, M. (2017, August 24). Unsanctioned "overdose prevention site" to pop up in Ottawa, group says. *CBC News*. Retrieved from http://www.cbc.ca/news/canada/ottawa/overdose-prevention-site-supervised-injections-ottawa-1.4259634

Lupick, T. (2017, June 6). B.C.'s second low-barrier supervised-injection site, Safe Point, opens this week in Surrey. *The Georgia Straight*. Retrieved from https://www.straight.com/news/920736/bcs-second-low-barrier-supervised-injection-site-safe-point-opens-week-surrey

Office of the Correctional Advisor. (2016, January 11). *Making a complaint to the Office of the Correctional Investigator*. Retrieved from http://www.oci-bec.gc.ca/cnt/complaint-plainte-eng.aspx

Police Services Act, RSO 1990, c P.15.

Purdon, N. (2015, July 29). PTSD taking its toll on Canada's prison guards. *CBC News*. Retrieved from http://www.cbc.ca/news/canada/ptsd-taking-its-toll-on-canada-s-prison-guards-1.3166791

Rushowy, K. (2016, November 8). Howard Sapers to head segregation review. *The Toronto Star*. Retrieved from https://www.thestar.com/news/queenspark/2016/11/08/howard-sapers-to-head-segregation-review.html

Sapers, H. (2011). *Mental health and corrections: Scope of the problem* [Report]. Saint Francis Xavier University Department of Psychology Colloquium Series. Ottawa: Office of the Correctional Investigator of Canada. Retrieved from http://www.oci-bec.gc.ca/cnt/comm/presentations/presentations20120318-eng.aspx

Sapers, H. (2015). *Annual report of the Office of the Correctional Investigator 2014-2015*. Ottawa: Office of the Correctional Investigator of Canada. Retrieved from http://www.oci-bec.gc.ca/cnt/rpt/annrpt/annrpt20142015-eng.aspx#s5

Strike, C., Watson, T.M., Kolla, G., Penn, R., & Bayoumi, A.M. (2015). Ambivalence about supervised injection facilities among community stakeholders. *Harm Reduction Journal*, *12*(1), 26.

Thomas, G. (2005). *Harm reduction for special populations: Harm reduction policies and programs for persons involved in the criminal justice system*. Ottawa, ON: Canadian Centre on Substance Abuse. Retrieved from http://www.ccsa.ca/Resource Library/ccsa-003900-2005.pdf

Tulloch, Hon. M.H. (2017). *Report of the Independent Police Oversight Review*. Ottawa: Queen's Printer for Ontario. Retrieved from https://www.attorneygeneral.jus.gov.on.ca/english/about/pubs/police_oversight_review/.

Union of Canadian Correctional Officers. (2016). Operational stress injury and post-traumatic stress disorder among public safety officers and first responders presented to the Standing Committee on Public Safety and National Security [Brief]. Retrieved from https://www.ourcommons.ca/Content/Committee/421/SECU/Brief/BR8432474/br-external/UnionOfCanadianCorrectionalOfficers-CSN-Final-e.pdf

White, P. (2016, November 8). Ontario appoints Howard Sapers as corrections adviser. *The Globe and Mail*. Retrieved from https://www.theglobeandmail.com/news/national/howard-sapers-to-lead-ontario-segregation-review/article32724886/

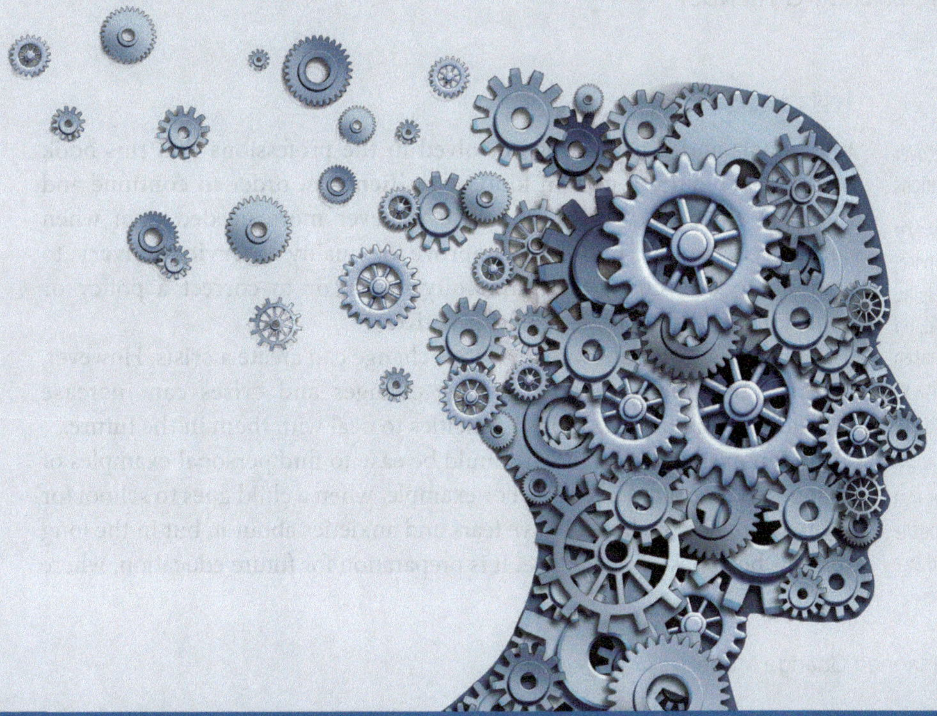

12 RESILIENCY AND ORGANIZATIONAL RESPONSES

LEARNING OUTCOMES

After reading this chapter, you will be able to:

- Distinguish examples of best practices for organizations that employ first responders.
- Discuss examples of positive organizational responses that have occurred because of difficult or tragic circumstances.
- Critically assess the services and gaps in service that are available for first responders living with PTSD and other work-related behavioural conditions.
- Reflect on factors that lead to resiliency and positive change in an organization's culture.

Introduction

resilience
the capacity to quickly recover from difficult situations

service delivery
the act of providing a service; in the justice and helping professions. This could, for example, be action taken by a policing, security, or mental health service

best practice
processes and procedures that are generally accepted to be the most effective based on evidence

Individuals and organizations involved in the professions that this book focuses on require a certain kind of **resilience** in order to continue and thrive in their work. That resilience is never more needed than when change is demanded in order to improve the quality of **service delivery**, to respond to ever-changing community needs, or to correct a policy or behaviour that is no longer a **best practice**.

Change is stressful. Even a positive change can create a crisis. However, learning to cope with and manage changes and crises can increase individuals' and organizations' capacities to deal with them in the future.

If you examine your life, it should be easy to find personal examples of changes that resulted in crises. For example, when a child goes to school for the first time he or she will have fears and anxieties about it, but in the long run this becomes an advantage. It is preparation for future education, where

FIGURE 12.1 Planned Change Model

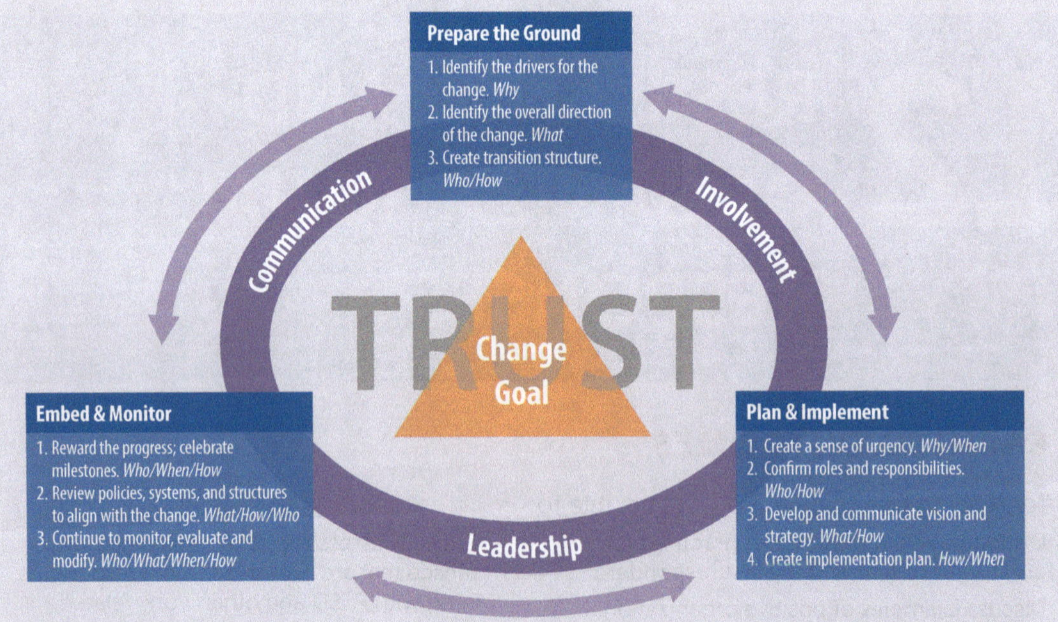
Prepare the Ground
1. Identify the drivers for the change. *Why*
2. Identify the overall direction of the change. *What*
3. Create transition structure. *Who/How*
Communication
Involvement
TRUST
Change Goal
Embed & Monitor
1. Reward the progress; celebrate milestones. *Who/When/How*
2. Review policies, systems, and structures to align with the change. *What/How/Who*
3. Continue to monitor, evaluate and modify. *Who/What/When/How*
Leadership
Plan & Implement
1. Create a sense of urgency. *Why/When*
2. Confirm roles and responsibilities. *Who/How*
3. Develop and communicate vision and strategy. *What/How*
4. Create implementation plan. *How/When*

There are many models for organizational change. Canada School of Public Service's Planned Change Model is a useful example of a method that can be used to reach the goal of specific change.

Source: Ace & Parker, 2010, p. 22.

those earlier experiences will inform behaviour and create a greater capacity to handle new and additional tasks and challenges more easily.

Individuals working in the justice and helping professions as well as the organizations they work for have, over time, greatly increased their capacities to deal with change. The level of training for police officers, correctional workers, military personnel, social workers, and other potential first responders has increased a great deal over the last several decades.

While many of the changes have been positive, they were often instigated by tragedy and unpleasant scenarios that unfolded over time. In this chapter we will look at some stories from front-line personnel and organizations and the responses to them that have resulted in improvements in service to the public and the health and well-being of working professionals, as well as some of the gaps that still exist.

Robert Dziekanski: Tragedy Results in Change

National headlines were made in October 2007 when Robert Dziekanski died after a **taser** was used on him during a physical altercation with four members of the RCMP. Dziekanski was a Polish immigrant who spoke no English. He became agitated after spending nine hours wandering through the Vancouver airport (Canadian Press, 2013).

The incident created quite a lot of controversy because the confrontation—including Dziekanski's death—was caught on video by an eyewitness. An additional unsavoury element to this story is that of two of the officers were convicted of perjury when the case went to trial (Theodore, 2016).

Dziekanski's tragic death was ruled a homicide by the coroner, and the pressure from public anger resulted in the B.C. provincial government conducting a **public inquiry** led by former judge Thomas Braidwood. The inquiry found that the RCMP officers were too quick to act and the repeated use of a taser resulted in excessive force (Canadian Press, 2013).

Braidwood also began a separate inquiry into police use of taser weapons. Before this inquiry took place, **conducted energy devices (CEDs)** such as tasers were placed in the category of "intermediate weapons" on most use-of-force continuums alongside items such as pepper spray, rubber bullet firearms, batons, and beanbag guns (Hall & Weaver, 2008).

These are Braidwood's recommendations that have been acted on:

- Tasers are to be used in "cases involving bodily harm or the threat of bodily harm";

taser
a device that uses electricity to temporarily incapacitate an individual; used in place of a more lethal weapon; also known as a conducted energy device (CED)

public inquiry
process where hearings are conducted and evidence is heard in a public forum about a specific issue of public interest; afterward, a report on the findings is submitted to government and made available to the public

conducted energy devices (CEDs)
devices that are used in place of more lethal weapons in order to temporarily incapacitate an individual; also known as tasers

- "Standardized training for police officers" who use tasers;
- Requirements to "file detailed reports whenever a Taser is deployed";
- "Independent testing" of devices;
- An increase in officers being equipped with "automatic defibrillators";
- Formation of an "independent body to investigate serious criminal allegations involving police." In British Columbia this office is called the Independent Investigations Office (Keller, 2012).

These changes were not simple and took years of investigation, study, and argument in public discourse and by experts in the field. Even so, some argue that tasers should not be used by police. The inquiry led by Braidwood also acknowledged that tasers have improved society and are valuable as an alternative to more lethal weapons. With an 87 percent decrease in the use of CEDs between 2007 and 2012, Braidwood suggested that "government and police officers [had heeded] his warning that stun guns are dangerous" (Canadian Press, 2012).

The report sought to balance and inform police decision-making processes on when to deploy CEDs. The report also helped to educate the public on the benefits and risks of CEDs, as exemplified in this portion:

> Experience suggests that, by deploying conducted energy weapons, officers can frequently avoid (or at least minimize) physical altercations with subjects.
>
> What is not so clear is whether injuries to subjects are reduced and, if so, to what extent. In many cases, a conducted energy weapon causes less injury than would a baton or a police dog, but that benefit must be balanced against the risk (however small) of death or serious injury from everything from a fall to ventricular fibrillation (Braidwood, 2009, pp. 283–284).

As discussed in Chapter 11, public outrage can help to foster needed change in the justice and other helping professions. Public concern raised by the death of Robert Dziekanski led to public inquiry, massive changes in policing and public safety training, and helped to create an independent oversight board for the investigation of police. These changes have helped to save lives, prevent injuries, and improve services for the community at large, and they show that government and police services take the need for change seriously.

Majencio Camaso: Tragedy Results in Constructive Recommendations

On July 11, 2004, British Columbia's 911 service received a call from Theresa Camaso about her husband Majencio. That morning Majencio had told Theresa that he believed a red balloon hanging on the wall in their apartment was a high-tech surveillance device. A while later he had taken a rolling pin and destroyed several items in the couple's apartment.

When called, police were told that Majencio was off his antipsychotic medication. The officers also saw that there had been a fire in the apartment and they could smell gasoline. When Majencio fled the scene, the police pursued him. They arrived at an elementary school playground where it is reported that Camaso ran at an officer while holding two metal objects—a crowbar and a pipe.

"Without calling for backup or firing a warning shot, the much larger police officer shot [Camaso] three times, ending his life," according to a report from CTV News (Lindsay, 2011). In 2011, the Supreme Court of British Columbia ruled that the shooting was unjustified and "grossly negligent" and ordered \$354,000 in damages to be paid to the Camaso family (CBC News, 2011). The B.C. Court of Appeal later overturned that ruling in 2013 (Petrescu, 2014).

Despite the legal back-and-forth, the Saanich Police still created a number of changes on their force after this incident. They became the first police service in British Columbia to adopt Crisis Intervention De-escalation (CID) training. This training "is mandatory training on the communication skills that promote effective, non-violent interventions in a crisis situation. The training emphasizes respectful and compassionate interactions and techniques suitable for use in mental health crisis situations" (British Columbia Ministry of Justice, 2013, p. 18, n. 11).

The Saanich Police also adopted 10 recommendations (known as the Camaso Recommendations) made by a former police complaint commissioner in response to this case. The recommendations included provisions that any investigation of a death suspected to involve police should be turned over to an external investigation department, that the scene of the death be secured for these **external investigators** and that police not make public statements about these cases before the deceased's family is notified (North, 2012).

external investigators investigators from outside an organization that is being investigated; use of external investigators helps to limit biased results

With the increasing numbers of mental health calls and new understandings about the way justice and mental health systems intersect, the need for change is ever-evolving. The Voices from the Field feature that

bobbies
nickname for a British police officer; similar to the word "cop" in North America

follows explores a variety of suggestions for improvements that police services have been encouraged to implement based on the types of front-line incidents in which officers are tasked to both serve and protect. A clear contrast can be seen in the feature article when Canadian, American, and British police services are compared. It is worth exploring differences in organizational responses to see how we can train, weaponize, and best support officers who are struggling with issues of mental health and justice.

VOICES FROM THE FIELD

More police officers carry guns in B.C. than in England and Wales combined

By Lori Culbert

Traditionally, since the 19th century, the vast majority of British ***bobbies*** *have been armed with just batons and tear gas to police the 57 million residents of England and Wales.*

March 30, 2015, *The Vancouver Sun*—Time slowed, the blaring police sirens became eerily silent, and some things—like the suspect's shotgun—looked much bigger than before.

As police sergeant Rick Parent pointed his service revolver at an armed suspect's head, his perception of time, sound, and sight blurred. "I ran up to the car even though the guy had a shotgun and smashed the window. What I didn't plan for was critical incident stress," the Delta officer, now retired, recalled. "Things went into slow motion and I could hear the glass slowly crackling and falling down."

The standoff ended without Parent firing his gun, but he still vividly remembers the exchange nearly 25 years later.

"I could have literally died and I could have killed somebody, those are things that went through my mind for days and weeks afterwards," said Parent, who is now an associate criminology professor at Simon Fraser University and a use-of-force expert.

Police shootings often happen very quickly and officers can be haunted emotionally and have flashbacks, Parent's academic research shows.

"We are quick to criticize police," Parent said, "but, in fairness, as long as we have human beings responding to these critical incidents, we are never going to have perfection."

There were six fatal shootings by police in B.C. in 2014, up from just one in 2013; all the deceased had a mental illness or were having a mental health crisis. Relatives and advocates have criticized how police handled some of these, such as the shooting of a 51-year-old schizophrenic man armed with a piece of wood on a Vancouver street last year.

But Parent argues police in Canada reach for their guns relatively rarely, especially compared to their colleagues in the U.S. On average, he said, there are a dozen fatal shootings by police in Canada each year compared to 400 south of the border.

In response to the 2007 death of Robert Dziekanski, who was Tasered at the Vancouver airport, B.C. introduced mandatory crisis intervention and de-escalation training to improve police interactions with mentally distraught people. It is a three-hour online and eight-hour in-class course, followed by an online refresher every three years.

Parent, though, said an 11-hour course does not turn an officer into a psychologist. He believes governments are taking the "cheap route" by sending police to mental health crisis calls that often devolve into the "worst of the worst cases" by the time 911 is dialed.

One answer, which he admits would be expensive, is to have a team of doctors and nurses respond to mental health calls, with police as backup.

"Police are not doing their best when they are killing people, but they are not the best people to send to these calls. ... It's unfair and unrealistic to expect we can train a police officer with the complexities required for drug treatment and counselling," Parent said. "We have it backwards. We think that a policeman with a gun will solve everything. But we know we don't need a gun in a hospital."

A Sun analysis of fatal B.C. police shootings shows at least 60 percent involved mentally unstable people in the past decade.

In an email, Justice Minister Suzanne Anton didn't talk about doctors or nurses responding to 911 calls, but said police and health authorities "have formed partnerships in various communities, where they share information and work together to better respond to people with mental health and addictions." One such example, she said, was Car 87 in Vancouver, in which a Vancouver Coastal Health nurse responds to psychiatric calls with a police officer.

While Car 87 is a valuable service, advocates argue many more are needed to respond to the increasing number of police calls involving mentally unstable people.

In his high-profile report into the 2013 police shooting death of a teenager on a Toronto street car, retired Supreme Court Justice Frank Iacobucci singled out one successful program used by Vancouver police: a "dashboard" system, which integrates police and mental health information into a database accessible on the road.

RCMP Supt. Norm Gaumont, who oversees the B.C. Mounties' mental health strategies, is working on a new province-wide review of how officers interact with those in a mental health crisis. "It's looking at what do we do now and what can we do," he said.

Some detachments, he said, already work with health boards through liaison officers, outreach programs, and teaming up nurses with officers for some calls.

The B.C. Coroner's Service holds an inquest into every police-involved death and many recommendations have been made about how to prevent the numbers from climbing.

Too many of the recommendations are left to collect dust, say justice advocates like Pivot Legal Society lawyer Doug King.

"There's a ton of public money and effort to get to these recommendations and conclusions, and there's absolutely no enforcement mechanisms to put them in place," King said.

A sample of mental health-related recommendations from police shooting inquests:

- Paul Boyd (Vancouver, 2007): A 24-hour drop in-centre so mentally distraught people have a place to go other than a hospital emergency room, and a joint Vancouver Police–Vancouver Coastal Health databank on people with mental illness.
- Gregory Matters (Prince George, 2012): A mental health professional at all police emergency response team calls.

- Matthew Wilcox (North Vancouver, 2010): Special teams including an officer and mental health professional at calls involving mentally ill people. Teams to have "intermediate weapons" (including Tasers).
- Jeffery Hughes (Nanaimo, 2009): A 24-hour link between the Health Ministry and police to share mental health information.
- Angus Mitchell (Maple Ridge, 2012): Doctors send assessments of people arrested under the Mental Health Act for a firearm-related offence to the Chief Firearms Officer and the police agency involved.
- Joseph Pagnotta (Langford, 2004) and Majencio Camaso (Saanich, 2004): Integration of plainclothes police into emergency mental health services.

The Justice Ministry did not give an update on these recommendations, but instead provided a general statement.

"We act on those recommendations that are practical and within our jurisdiction or control. In some cases, we commit significant resources to new initiatives that directly address coroner recommendations," said Clayton Pecknold, assistant deputy minister and director of police services.

In England and Wales, where fewer than five percent of police officers are authorized to carry guns, there were no fatal police shootings in 2013 or 2014.

In a tradition since the 19th century, the vast majority of British bobbies are armed with just batons and tear gas to police the 57 million residents of England and Wales.

Slightly more than 6,000 of the 130,000 officers are authorized to use firearms for dangerous situations, and since 2004 have fatally wounded 23 people.

In B.C., population 4.6 million, all 9,000 officers are armed and 42 people have been killed in police shootings since 2004, including six in 2014.

[A] recent debate about whether British police should be armed came in 2012, after two female officers were killed in a gun attack in Manchester.

But the U.K.'s Association of Chief Police Officers, including Manchester chief Peter Fahy, supported the status quo.

"We are passionate that the British style of policing is routinely unarmed policing," Fahy told reporters shortly after his officers were killed.

"We know from the experience in America and other countries that having armed officers certainly does not mean, sadly, that police officers do not end up getting shot."

Newfoundland was the only Canadian province with unarmed police, but that ended in 1998 when government permitted officers there to start carrying guns.

[In 2005,] B.C. became the first jurisdiction in Canada to arm transit police.

Simon Fraser University criminology professor Rick Parent said Newfoundland changed its policy because of the influx of guns from the United States.

According to United Nations figures, England and Wales have fewer guns per capita than Canada, which has far fewer than the U.S.

Parent doesn't think B.C., or the rest of Canada, will ever follow the lead of England and Wales.

"I think our model is not going to change, but we can see that reluctance (of Canadian police) to use firearms," Parent said. "And I think police need more alternatives than deadly force."

That could include access to more less-than-lethal weapons and more training on how to de-escalate tense situations.

Source: Culbert, 2015.

Discussion Questions

1. Reflecting on the high level of weapon usage of police services in the United States, the low number in British jurisdictions, and the moderate level found in Canada, what are your feelings on these difference? Which best suits your personal preferences?
2. Review the sample of mental health related recommendations from police shooting inquests and rank them based on which ones you believe to be most important. Which was your top-ranked choice and why?
3. From the list you made in answer to question 2, which was your lowest ranked choice and why?

Specific Treatment for First Responders

In 2017, Global News reported on the story of New Brunswick's Brad Calhoun, who served his community for nearly two decades as a firefighter and paramedic. When Calhoun began administering PTSD testing to other first responders he realized that he too might have acquired PTSD through his years on the job.

"As I'm looking at this checklist, I started to realize a lot of this stuff had related to me," he explained. "Misdirected anger, **hypervigilance**, I still suffer greatly with **night terrors**" (Keefe, 2017).

Not long after this realization, he was diagnosed officially with PTSD but found the treatment difficult and it sometimes even exacerbated his symptoms. Eventually he was able to receive a month of care in a facility in the United States that is run by the International Association of Fire Fighters (IAFF) and is specifically geared toward first responders and not the general public. Since having this treatment, Calhoun has been promoting the positive effects of treatment specific to first responders that is combined with "**aftercare**, continued counselling, and continued support" to help himself and others (Keefe, 2017).

It seems that this kind of first-responder specific treatment will likely become an organizational response to the rising number of PTSD-diagnosed first responders. The IAFF is on the cutting edge of a possible trend. Their 15-acre facility located just outside Washington, D.C. was designed from its inception to be specifically for firefighters. Treatment is based on a program that was created in the aftermath of 9/11 to treat first-responders who were at ground zero. The program focuses on PTSD,

hypervigilance
occurs when an individual shows abnormal levels of awareness and response to stimuli when it is not vital or required; for example, even though at home and not on duty, a soldier may be constantly screening his or her environment for threats

night terrors
episodes of intense fear that occur during a non-REM part of the sleep cycle; may manifest as screaming, flailing, sweating, heavy breathing, or racing pulse while still asleep; night terrors are distinctly different from nightmares

aftercare
continued care after intense treatment

addiction, and other behavioural health issues related to exposure to trauma, and it connects those living with these conditions to clinicians who "understand the fire service culture and the unique pressures of [that] job" (IAFF, 2017).

The Canadian Armed Forces (CAF) have also developed a number of resources specifically to help prepare their members for the mental toll that military service can take. The CAF currently have seven trauma and stress support centres across their jurisdictions that were created to treat operational stress injuries such as PTSD (Bogart, 2017).

With the goal of prevention, the CAF use programs designed to avoid the development of operational stress injuries. One such program is called Road to Mental Readiness (R2MR), which seeks to reduce mental health stigma for those who serve, encourages members to seek care, removes barriers to care, and helps those who serve to assist other members of the armed forces who might be living with mental health issues. It is a form of "resilience and mental health training that is embedded throughout [a] Canadian Armed Forces member's career, including the deployment cycle" (Government of Canada, 2015).

The foundation of the program is based around resilience, which is defined in relation to the military as "the capacity of a soldier to recover quickly, resist, and possibly even thrive in the face of direct/indirect traumatic events and adverse situations in garrison, training and operational environments" (Government of Canada, 2015). Versions of this training are provided during deployment, throughout a member's career, and even to the families of those serving. The Canadian Armed Forces also offer military-specific peer support programs, **bereavement groups**, telephone referral and information programs, recreation and fitness programs, and other support services for members and their families.

bereavement groups groups of peers (sometimes with a professional helper leading) that focus on recovering and healing from loss

This work has become especially important because in recent Canadian history information about the personal mental health of a number armed forces personnel has been breached. One example is the case of Gulf War veteran Captain Sean Bruyea. While Veterans Affairs Canada has a long history of providing specific programs and care to veterans and serving members of the armed forces, these individuals have sometimes had their mental health histories used against them. Bruyea had his confidential files viewed more than 4,000 times by as many as 850 people and shared widely in documents without his consent after he criticized the functioning of Veterans Affairs (Hébert & Sibbald, 2010). Furthermore, other critics, such as now-retired Veterans Ombudsman and army colonel Pat Stogran, had their mental health documents shared in an attempt to silence their critiques of the department and the government.

Bruyea and others having had their confidence betrayed shows that while, generally speaking, specific treatment for first responders is a positive organizational response to mental health and PTSD issues, it must not be accompanied by "inferior privacy standards for health information" and an "adversarial ... disability benefits process" (Hebert & Sibbald, 2010).

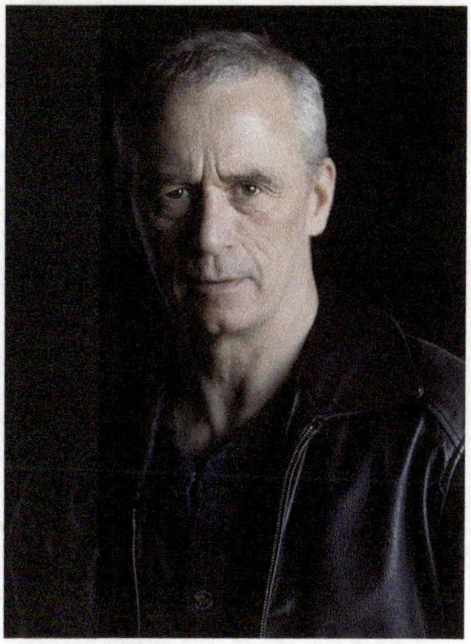

Pat Stogran

Further, Stogran's advocacy on this issue has continued and he recently put a spotlight on the need for Veterans Affairs Canada to institute routine formal reviews of suicides. He feels that this will help the organization respond more effectively to the mental health issues of veterans and serving members, and help prevent future suicides. As Stogran puts it, "there has to be a feedback loop to say where we are going wrong. They should be taking substantial and very visible steps to fight the problem. It's life and death" (D'Aliesio, 2017).

Another group that has decided to create specific treatment programs for first responders and uniformed personnel in Canada is Homewood Health. In late 2016, the organization opened an outpatient clinic in Mississauga, Ontario specifically for police, fire, EMTs, and other first responders. The program uses multidisciplinary teams that include psychiatrists, psychologists, trauma and addiction specialists, occupational therapists, social workers, treatment managers, and return-to-work specialists, and first-responders can access the program without having to get a referral from another agency (Clairmont, 2016; Homewood Health, 2016).

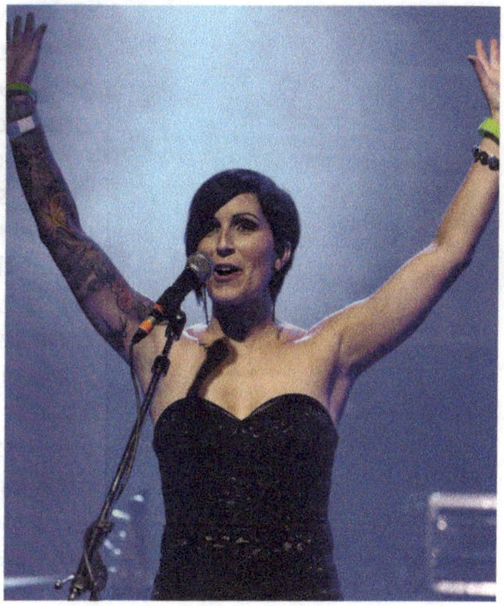

Natalie Harris

Natalie Harris credits the Homewood program with saving her life. Natalie, a paramedic, is one of Ontario's 73,000 first responders. Her story of how Homewood's first-responder-specific program helped her can be seen in the following Voices from the Field feature. Since her time in the program she has gone on to be a prolific speaker on mental health issues, founded a peer support program called Wings of Change, is a #BellLetsTalk Ambassador, and an author and blogger. Natalie can be followed on twitter @ ParamedicNat1 and her website is at paramedicnatsmentalhealthjourney.com.

VOICES FROM THE FIELD

New Outpatient Program Puts Trauma Help for First Responders Front and Centre

By Natalie Nanowski

October 24, 2016, CBC News—Natalie Harris is used to helping people, but it took responding to a grisly double-murder scene four years ago [for] the paramedic [to realize that] she needed help herself.

Harris was among the first responders called to a Barrie hotel in May 2012 where two women were found brutally killed. The murderer, she says, was her patient.

For years, Harris had been using alcohol along with prescription and over-the-counter drugs to self-medicate. But after that night, she says things got worse.

"Things really sort of came crashing down in 2012," she told CBC News. After the incident, she says she ended up in the hospital for an overdose and even tried to commit suicide.

She didn't know it then but says she later learned she'd been suffering from post-traumatic stress disorder.

Increase in First Responders Seeking Help

Two years after visiting the murder scene, Harris says she got help at the Homewood Health Centre for mental illness and addiction in Guelph.

That was before the Ontario government passed legislation that recognized PTSD as a work-related illness for police, firefighters, and paramedics. Since it passed this past April, specialists at Homewood Health Centre say they've seen an increase in first responders seeking help.

They say it's partially due to the fact that first responders don't have to prove that their PTSD is related to their job. In the past, an injured first responder needed to prove their diagnosis stemmed from a workplace injury in order to access benefits from the **Workplace Safety and Insurance Board (WSIB)**.

Workplace Safety and Insurance Board (WSIB) Ontario provincial agency that pays benefits to injured workers from a province-wide mandatory insurance fund

The higher demand for treatment has prompted the organization to open a new outpatient program in Mississauga that primarily caters to first responders.

The program offers access to specialists from psychologists to occupational therapists, is group based, and treatment is multiple hours per day.

"I Wasn't Taught About What PTSD Is"

Psychologist Ann Malain, the company's executive vice-president, says the approach is a good option for those who don't want or need to stay in a facility for long periods of time.

"PSTD really disrupts a person's sense of self and ability to trust anything around them," says Malain.

"People kind of say in general society, 'Oh, I'm depressed' and people kind of understand what that means. There's not the kind of language in general society [to say] 'I'm experiencing PTSD.'"

But even in the healthcare field itself, Harris says, that **literacy** is lacking.

"I do know that a lot of my colleagues, we use alcohol to help us cope just basically with the stresses of our career," said Harris. "I wasn't taught about what PTSD is. We didn't talk about it."

Malain says **waitlists** for PTSD programs at the health centre can be as long as four to five months. Through the new outpatient program, though, she says first responders can be assessed and start receiving treatment the next day.

The new program isn't covered by OHIP.

Source: Nanowski, 2016.

literacy
one's knowledge about mental health disorders, trends, dynamics, and how to manage or even prevent mental health issues

waitlists
ordered list of individuals who are waiting for something that is not readily available, such as mental health services or housing

DISCUSSION QUESTIONS

1. In your opinion, what are some of the characteristics found in the culture of first responders that would make their treatment alongside members of the general population difficult? Why is it better for first responders to be treated in facilities that are specific to them?
2. In what ways do you feel mental health literacy can be improved for persons who work as justice and helping professionals?
3. How would you react if your personal health and/or mental health records were shared widely without your consent?

Changes in Management, Change Fatigue, and Resilience

Whatever the reason for change, it can be difficult to implement. Even positive changes must be well managed and effectively communicated throughout organizations. Being able to work with change is a sign of resilience, but too many changes can create confusion, miscommunication, and **change fatigue**.

change fatigue occurs when an individual is exposed to too much change; can create frustration, cynicism, distrust, and confusion, among other negative results

Similar in dynamics to compassion fatigue, change fatigue occurs when people are asked to change too much and/or too often. People in a workplace suffering from change fatigue may exhibit "a sense of malaise, frustration, distrust, and cynicism that any change effort [would be] destined to fail" (Ace & Parker, 2010). David Garvin of Harvard Business School believes that change efforts fail for two primary reasons: poor design and poor communication (Morgan, 2001).

Elements of poor change design that are relevant to the justice and helping professions include a failure to address concerns about the allocation of resources and "not explicitly tackling the necessary behavioural changes" that are required to create change. Poor communication elements include a team leader's inability to clearly express the intent of proposed changes, no thorough explanation about how a particular change was decided upon, and failure to recognize and address employees' fears and apprehensions about change (Morgan, 2001).

A 2016 study involving 535 hospital staff nurses found some interesting correlations among change fatigue, resilience, and job satisfaction rates. The study found that as education increases, change fatigue decreases. Furthermore, the study found that education was a predictor variable for job satisfaction and that there was a significant positive association between resilience and job satisfaction (Brown, 2016). Education could be considered one of the factors that decreases change fatigue and increases overall job satisfaction—even in high stress and high-risk occupations such as the roles filled by first responders and other helping professionals.

But what about resilience? Unlike the Canadian Armed Forces definition shared earlier in this chapter, Professor George A. Bonanno, looking through a psychological lens, offers a fuller definition of the word when he describes it as the "ability of adults in otherwise normal circumstances who are exposed to an isolated and potentially highly disruptive event, such as the death of a close relation or a violent or life-threatening situation, to maintain relatively stable, healthy levels of psychological and physical functioning" (Bonanno, 2004).

Research has shown that, generally, first responders are resilient people even in the face of critical incidents (Gunderson & Grill, 2014; Pietrantoni & Prati, 2008; Timmons & Vernon-Evans, 2013; Wyche et al., 2011). Some research has even referred to this as a "resilience phenomenon," which is described as

> [a]t least in part accounted for by the identification of enabling core beliefs about one's role, one's capacity, and about the meaning of negative and positive outcomes for self. It is clear that these factors, loosely described as a philosophy, provide the individual with protection against the development of adverse reactions to stress or from becoming unduly concerned about negative outcomes. This in turn enables them to operate optimally in the situations they are exposed to without experiencing the negative psychological consequences that might otherwise arise" (Davies et al., 2008).

One could argue that first responders have to be generally resilient in order to work in their professions in the first place. They are human and sometimes, as this book and others have shown, tragedy can strike no matter how much resiliency an individual may have. It is believed that first responders also have traits related to self-efficacy, collective efficacy, and a strong sense of community that "could be considered resilience factors that preserve first responders' work-related mental health" (Pietrantoni & Prati, 2008). Whatever one's natural aptitude for resilience is, it is also believed that resilience can be supported and enhanced through educational efforts (Gunderson & Grill, 2014).

In Vancouver, first responders are getting resiliency training to help them with the relatively new issue of fentanyl overdoses that are taking that city and others in Canada by storm and putting those responding to these scenes in crisis (Johnson, 2017). Vancouver Fire and Rescue has even hired a full-time, in-house health and wellness coordinator to deal with similar issues. One type of training that is spreading across British Columbia helps first responders learn strategies that will turn off their brain's **acute adrenaline surge mode** so that these individuals can recuperate when their shifts are over or when they are on their days off (Johnson, 2017).

acute adrenaline surge mode
sudden surge of adrenaline that can be helpful in acute situations that require fight-or-flight type responses, but that is not helpful if it occurs for prolonged periods when rest and recuperation are required

Whenever new trends, problems, and issues arise in the justice and helping professions, change will be required to meet the challenges that arise. Education and open minds are required to increase successful outcomes for the professionals involved and the communities they serve. First responders and the organizations that employ them have a long history of adaptation and resilience in the face of crisis, but individuals also have to be honest with themselves and others about their limitations, and all those involved need to advocate for appropriate mental health services. Suitable changes in management approaches and processes can help create a culture of positive change overall within the professions and the communities they serve.

BOX 12.1 WAYS TO BUILD RESILIENCE

The American Psychological Association has developed the following recommendations for individuals who want to build resilience.

Make connections. Good relationships with close family members, friends, and others are important. Accepting help and support from those who care about you and will listen to you can strengthen your resilience. Some people find that being active in civic groups, faith-based organizations, or other local groups provides social support and can help with reclaiming hope. Assisting others in their times of need also can benefit the helper.

Avoid seeing crises as insurmountable problems. You can't change the fact that highly stressful events happen, but you can change how you interpret and respond to these events. Try looking beyond the present to how future circumstances may be a little better. Note any subtle ways in which you might already feel somewhat better as you deal with difficult situations.

Accept that change is a part of living. Certain goals may no longer be attainable as a result of adverse situations. Accepting circumstances that cannot be changed can help you focus on circumstances that you can alter.

Move toward your goals. Develop some realistic goals. Do something regularly—even if it seems like a small accomplishment—that enables you to move toward your goals. Instead of focusing on tasks that seem unachievable, ask yourself, "What's one thing I know I can accomplish today that helps me move in the direction I want to go?"

Take decisive actions. Act on adverse situations as much as you can. Take decisive actions, rather than detaching completely from problems and stresses and wishing they would just go away.

Look for opportunities for self-discovery. People often learn something about themselves and may find that they have grown in some respect as a result of their struggle with loss. Many people who have experienced tragedies and hardship have reported better relationships, a greater sense of strength even while feeling vulnerable, an increased sense of self-worth, a more developed spirituality, and a heightened appreciation for life.

Nurture a positive view of yourself. Developing confidence in your ability to solve problems and trusting your instincts helps build resilience.

Keep things in perspective. Even when facing very painful events, try to consider the stressful situation in a broader context and keep a long-term perspective. Avoid blowing the event out of proportion.

Maintain a hopeful outlook. An optimistic outlook enables you to expect that good things will happen in your life. Try visualizing what you want, rather than worrying about what you fear.

Take care of yourself. Pay attention to your own needs and feelings. Engage in activities that you enjoy and find relaxing. Exercise regularly. Taking care of yourself helps to keep your mind and body primed to deal with situations that require resilience.

Additional ways of strengthening resilience may be helpful. For example, some people write about their deepest thoughts and feelings related to trauma or other stressful events in their life. Meditation and spiritual practices help some people build connections and restore hope.

Source: American Psychological Association, 2017.

✓ POINTS TO REMEMBER

- ✓ Change is necessary but it can be stressful for individuals and organizations even when the change is positive or desired. The changes that have occurred in the justice and helping fields have created an increased capacity for the professions and have generally created improvements around how organizations respond to external and internal mental health concerns.
- ✓ Change is often spurred on by public pressure or instances of tragedy that have entered into the public consciousness. These changes can result in unintended consequences, so it is vital for justice and helping organizations to create systems that allow them to receive feedback.
- ✓ Mental health is beginning to be seen as intersecting with the health care, justice, and labour systems and, as a result of this, resources specific to first responders and other related personnel are being created. Treatment specifically geared toward the professional cultures of first responders and those in the justice professions is now available.
- ✓ First responders are resilient, but changes are needed to make sure there is less tragedy and more longevity. Numerous protective factors exist to help first responders and their families succeed in their lives and work. Educational opportunities such as courses, conferences, online materials, telephone services, apps, and traditional publications are available to help change the culture around mental health in the justice and helping professions. This has occurred in great part because of the resilience and the efficacy of first responders, their loved ones, persons with lived experience of mental health issues, and community advocates who have spoken out and demanded change.

KEY TERMS

acute adrenaline surge mode, 273
aftercare, 267
bereavement groups, 268
best practice, 260
bobbies, 264
change fatigue, 272
conducted energy devices (CEDs), 261
external investigators, 263
hypervigilance, 267
literacy, 271
night terrors, 267
public inquiry, 261
resilience, 260
service delivery, 260
taser, 261
waitlists, 271
Workplace Safety and Insurance Board (WSIB), 270

REFERENCES

Ace, W., & Parker, S. (2010). Overcoming change fatigue through focused employee engagement. *OD Practitioner*, *42*(1), 21–22. Retrieved from http://citeseerx.ist.psu.edu/viewdoc/download?doi=10.1.1.471.2400&rep=rep1&type=pdf

American Psychological Association. (2017). The road to resilience. Retrieved from http://www.apa.org/helpcenter/road-resilience.aspx

Bogart, N. (2017, January 8). PTSD: What happens when Canadian military members ask for help? *Global News*. Retrieved from https://globalnews.ca/news/3162225/ptsd-what-happens-when-canadian-military-members-ask-for-help/

Bonanno, G.A. (2004). Loss, trauma, and human resilience: Have we underestimated the human capacity to thrive after extremely aversive events? *American Psychologist*, *59*(1), 20.

Braidwood Commission on Conducted Energy Weapon Use (BC) & Braidwood, T.R. (2009). *Restoring public confidence: Restricting the use of conducted energy weapons in British Columbia*. Victoria, BC: Braidwood Commission.

British Columbia Ministry of Justice. (2013, December). *British Columbia policing and community safety plan*. Retrieved from http://www2.gov.bc.ca/assets/gov/law-crime-and-justice/criminal-justice/police/publications/community/bc-policing-plan.pdf

Brown, R.J. (2016). *Determining the relationship among change fatigue, resilience, and job satisfaction of hospital staff nurses* (Doctoral dissertation). Retrieved from South Dakota State University, Open Prairie: Public Research Access Institutional Repository and Information Exchange. http://openprairie.sdstate.edu/etd/964/

Canadian Press. (2012, October 16). Former inquiry chair "very impressed" with B.C.'s response to taser report. *CTV News*. Retrieved from http://www.ctvnews.ca/canada/former-inquiry-chair-very-impressed-with-b-c-s-response-to-taser-report-1.998117

Canadian Press. (2013, April 9). Death of Polish man tasered by RCMP was a homicide, BC coroners rule. *The National Post*. Retrieved from http://nationalpost.com/news/canada/death-of-polish-man-tasered-by-rcmp-was-a-homicide-bc-coroners-rule

CBC News. (2011, April 14). "Negligent" police shooting nets family $354K award. *CBC News*. Retrieved from http://www.cbc.ca/news/canada/british-columbia/negligent-police-shooting-nets-family-354k-award-1.1094207

Clairmont, S. (2016, October 24). First responders get PTSD treatment program. *The Waterloo Record*. Retrieved from https://www.therecord.com/news-story/6926567-first-responders-get-ptsd-treatment-program/

Culbert, C. (2015, March 30). More police officers carry guns in B.C. than in England and Wales combined. *The Vancouver Sun*. Retrieved from http://www.vancouversun.com/health/More+police+officers+carry+guns+than+England+Wales+combined/10930364/story.html

D'Aliesio, R. (2017, January 12). Ottawa ignored calls to probe veteran suicides despite troubling 2014 audit. *The Globe and Mail*. Retrieved from https://beta.theglobeandmail.com/news/national/ottawa-ignored-calls-to-probe-veteran-suicides/article33593650/?ref=http://www.theglobeandmail.com&

Davies, E., Maybury, B., Colquhoun, M., Whitfield, R., Rossetti, T., & Vetter, N. (2008). Public access defibrillation: Psychological consequences in responders. *Resuscitation, 77*(2), 201–206.

Government of Canada. (2015, August 13). Road to mental readiness (R2MR). Retrieved from http://www.forces.gc.ca/en/caf-community-health-services-r2mr/index.page

Gunderson, J., & Grill, M. (2014, March 3). An evidence-based program for improving and sustaining first responder behavioral health. *JEMS: Journal of Emergency Medical Services, 39*(3). Retrieved from http://www.jems.com/articles/print/volume-39/issue-3/features/an-evidence-based-program-for-improving-and-sustaining-first-responder-behavioral-health.html

Hall, N., & Weaver, C. (2008, May 10). Submission to the Braidwood Inquiry into the use of tasers: A perspective from the Canadian Mental Health Association BC Division. Retrieved from http://www.cmha.bc.ca/wp-content/uploads/2016/07/Braidwood_Inquiry_Submission5.pdf

Hébert, P.C., & Sibbald, B. (2010). Protecting privacy of health information for those who serve and protect us. *Canadian Medical Association Journal, 182*(17). Retrieved from http://www.cmaj.ca/content/182/17/E755.short

Homewood Health. (2016). Helping first responders and uniformed personnel. Retrieved from http://www.homewoodhealth.com/employers/responders

International Association of Fire Fighters [IAFF]. (2017). IAFF center of excellence for behavioral health treatment and recovery: Our center. Retrieved from http://www.iaffrecoverycenter.com/

Johnson, L. (2017, May 16). "We're starving for it": Paramedics get new resiliency training due to overdose crisis. *CBC News*. Retrieved from http://www.cbc.ca/news/canada/british-columbia/first-responders-overdose-trauma-stress-1.4115497

Keefe, J. (2017, September 15). New Brunswick firefighter calls for first responder specific treatment in Canada. *Global News*. Retrieved from https://globalnews.ca/news/3748003/new-brunswick-firefighter-calls-for-first-responder-specific-treatment-in-canada/

Keller, J. (2012, December 16). Thomas Braidwood, taser inquiry chair, "very impressed" with BC's response. Retrieved from http://www.huffingtonpost.ca/2012/10/16/taser-inquiry-chair-impressed-bc-response_n_1971105.html

Lindsay, B. (2011, April 14). B.C. cop negligent in shooting death of disturbed man. *CTV News*. Retrieved from http://bc.ctvnews.ca/b-c-cop-negligent-in-shooting-death-of-disturbed-man-1.631826

Morgan, N. (2001, September 10). Do you have change fatigue? Harvard Business School. *Working Knowledge*. Retrieved from http://hbswk.hbs.edu/item/do-you-have-change-fatigue

Nanowski, N. (2016, October 24). New outpatient program puts trauma help for first responders front and centre. *CBC News*. Retrieved from http://www.cbc.ca/news/canada/toronto/new-outpatient-program-puts-trauma-help-for-first-responders-front-and-centre-1.3817648.

North, N. (2012, January 23). Police board adopts Camaso recommendations. *Victoria News*. Retrieved from http://www.vicnews.com/news/police-board-adopts-camaso-recommendations/

Petrescu, S. (2014, November 2). Investigators seek witnesses to fatal police shooting in James Bay. *The Times Colonist*. Retrieved from http://www.timescolonist.com/news/local/investigators-seek-witnesses-to-fatal-police-shooting-in-james-bay-1.1492300

Pietrantoni, L., & Prati, G. (2008). Resilience among first responders. *African Health Sciences*, *8*(Suppl. 1), S14–S20.

Theodore, T. (2016, July 14). RCMP officer convicted of perjury in Robert Dziekanski taser case loses appeal. *The Toronto Star*. Retrieved from https://www.thestar.com/news/canada/2016/07/14/rcmp-officer-convicted-of-perjury-in-bc-taser-death-loses-appeal.html

Timmons, S., & Vernon-Evans, A. (2013). Why do people volunteer for community first responder groups? *Emergency Medicine Journal*, *30*(3), e13.

Wyche, K.F., Pfefferbaum, R.L., Pfefferbaum, B., Norris, F.H., Wisnieski, D., & Younger, H. (2011). Exploring community resilience in workforce communities of first responders serving Katrina survivors. *American Journal of Orthopsychiatry*, *81*(1), 18–30.

GLOSSARY

12-step recovery program group programs whose goal is to help others in recovery avoid negative lifestyle choices related to addiction

absenteeism missing work, school, or other responsibilities

absolute discharge the lowest-level adult sentence that an offender can get; if an offender gets an absolute discharge, a finding of guilt is made but no conviction is registered, and the person is not given any conditions to follow (for example, not even a probation order)

active listening form of communication that is helpful in a variety of therapeutic situations; it involves listening to another individual with full concentration and encouraging that person with verbal and non-verbal cues to demonstrate that the listener is paying close attention to what is being said; also sometimes called intentional listening

acute adrenaline surge mode sudden surge of adrenaline that can be helpful in acute situations that require fight-or-flight type responses, but that is not helpful if it occurs for prolonged periods when rest and recuperation are required

adaptive behaviours positive skills that people learn in order to adapt to and function in the activities of daily life

addiction habitual or compulsive use of a mood-altering substance or engagement in activities such as gambling

affect how a person expresses emotions or feelings physically; for example, through a change in facial expression, body language, and/or tone of voice

aftercare continued care after intense treatment

Alcoholics Anonymous (AA) 12-step program the primary purpose of which is to help alcoholics achieve a state of sobriety; Narcotics Anonymous provides a similar service for those trying to recover from drugs

antidepressants prescription drugs used to treat depression

anxiety disorder characterized by excessive, intrusive, and persistent fear, uneasiness, and apprehension; may also include elements of obsessive and/or compulsive behaviours and panic

avoidance behaviour in which an individual becomes insistent that he or she will avoid particular activities, environments, or situations because of a perception of negative consequences (such as becoming anxious or experiencing painful feelings) if they come into contact with the things they wish to avoid

bail hearing court session in which a judge or justice of the peace decides whether an accused will remain in custody prior to their court date; if the police decide not to release an accused on his or her own, the person must receive a bail hearing with 24 hours of arrest

bereavement groups groups of peers (sometimes with a professional helper leading) that focus on recovering and healing from loss

best practice processes and procedures that are generally accepted to be the most effective based on evidence

black market trafficking and trade of legal or illegal goods and services in a way that is against the law in order to avoid inspection, quality standards, and/or taxes

bobbies nickname for a British police officer; similar to the word "cop" in North America

brain reward system several parts of the brain that are activated by pleasurable stimuli such as food, sex, water, drugs, and alcohol

brief psychotic disorder shares at least one of the symptoms of schizophrenia but for less than one month; can occur as a response to an extreme life stress

case conference formal meeting where a number of services and/or helping professionals meet to help with planning, goal setting, and coordination of services for an individual; whenever possible, the conference takes place with the individual present and at the centre of decisions

change fatigue occurs when an individual is exposed to too much change; can create frustration, cynicism, distrust, and confusion, among other negative results

child maltreatment includes all forms of physical, sexual, and emotional abuse, neglect, and exploitation that result in actual or potential harm to a child's health, development, or dignity

child neglect includes acts of commission or omission by a parent or caregiver that result in harm, potential for harm, or threat of harm to a child

child physical abuse deliberate injury to a child that causes bruises, broken bones, burns, or cuts

child sexual abuse occurs when an adult or older adolescent uses a child for sexual stimulation

circle of care manifests when a number of helping professionals work together with an individual and are able to share information about their work and progress together through the implied consent of the individual

closed questions questions that can usually be answered very briefly or by a yes or no response; for example "when is your birthday?" and "did you bring your lunch to school?" are closed questions

cognitive behavioural therapy (CBT) structured form of talk therapy with a limited number of sessions that helps individuals build an awareness of distorted, negative, or inaccurate thought patterns; the focus of this style of therapy is to change behaviours and thinking to help solve problems

community capacity relates to the resources (physical and intellectual) that exist within a community to solve a community problem

community engagement process with the specific purpose of working with identified groups of people, whether they are connected by geographic location or special interest, to address issues that affect their well-being

community mobilization process whereby a group of professionals meet on equal terms in order to facilitate a participatory decision-making process

community outreach program program designed to provide flexible and individualized mental health services for people living with mental illness in their home or community

community treatment order (CTO) a legal order that sets out the terms under which a person must accept medication and therapy, counselling, management, rehabilitation, and other services while living in the community

concurrent disorders a state wherein a client lives with co-occurring mental health and addiction issues that affect and interact with one another

conducted energy devices (CEDs) devices that are used in place of more lethal weapons in order to temporarily incapacitate an individual; also known as tasers

confidentiality individual's right to not have personal information disclosed without his or her prior consent

consent in mental health and related fields consent can occur where an individual gives a helping professional permission to share information with others; can also refer to informed consent, which is a legal term that means permission is given by an individual for a clinician to try a proposed therapeutic technique or for the individual to participate in research

coping use of skills to help tolerate stresses and conflicts and make it easier to live with them

core values foundation upon which an organization makes decisions, plans strategies, and interacts with its own members and external groups, organizations, and stakeholders

crisis acute emotional reaction to a powerful stimulus

Crisis Outreach and Support Team (COAST) one of several mobile crisis teams made up of mental health workers and police officers that assist in mental health-related crisis situations

cycle of addiction a circular and often repetitive process in which a person living with addiction uses, tries to stop, relapses, experiences guilt, and is triggered into using again

deinstitutionalization societal push to move away from confining people living with mental health issues in institutions and instead offering treatment in community settings

delusional disorder a mental health issue in which delusions exist for at least one month without the other symptoms of schizophrenia or mood disorders

depersonalize make something impersonal; for example, helping an individual who is troubled by the actions of another understand that it is not because of or directed at him or her

depression or depressive disorder feelings of sadness, hopelessness, low self-worth, and/or reduced ability to enjoy previously enjoyable daily activities that persists for a period of longer than two weeks

***Diagnostic and Statistical Manual of Mental Disorders* (DSM)** the standard North American text for classifying and diagnosing mental disorders

distress centre crisis lines confidential helplines that are available 24 hours a day, 365 days a year to any person experiencing emotional distress

distress tolerance skills developed in dialectical behavioural therapy when a situation that causes distress cannot be changed by the person experiencing distress

duty to report legal obligation to report certain types of abuse, neglect, or other crimes

duty to warn responsibility that helping professionals have in some jurisdictions where they must break confidentiality with an individual in order to warn third parties that they are under threat by that individual

elder abuse intentional act, or failure to act, by a caregiver or an individual in a position of trust that causes or creates a risk of harm to an older adult

electroconvulsive therapy medical treatment that has been shown to be effective for treating clients with severe depressive disorders: brief electrical stimulation is focused on the brain while the person is under anaesthesia

emotional regulation a person's ability to manage his or her emotions when responding to experiences that are emotional

etiology the cause of a condition

exposure therapy used in the treatment of anxiety disorders: an individual is gradually exposed to a feared object or situation while in a safe environment; exposure is increased in the hope of normalizing the object or situation to the individual, thereby, in time, extinguishing the phobia or anxiety

external investigators investigators from outside an organization that is being investigated; use of external investigators helps to limit biased results

failure to thrive term used to describe a child who does not grow and/or develop over time

fentanyl a synthetic opiate originally used as a prescription medication for cancer patients dealing with intense pain; 2 mg of fentanyl (about the same size as 2 grains of salt) can be deadly

fight-or-flight response acute response to stress during which a physiological reaction occurs in response to an event that is perceived as harmful or threatening; may include increased cortisol in the body and increased heart rate, blood pressure, and blood glucose levels

first responders all law enforcement officers, firefighters, paramedics, correctional staff, search and rescue personnel, dispatchers, and nurses

a fix common slang term that describes an addict getting and using his or her drug or substance of choice

Freedom of Information and Protection of Privacy Act provincial legislation that provides the right of access to information that is under the control of institutions if criteria for disclosure are met

grieving process normal process through which an individual deals with the loss of something or someone from their life

group therapy psychotherapy practised in a group setting with a trained therapist guiding the sessions

harm reduction practices, policies, and programs designed to reduce the negative social, health, and economic consequences of drug use but not implicitly designed to reduce the rate of drug use—for example, the establishment of safe injection sites, which can reduce HIV infections, overdoses, and assaults related to sharing needles and doing drugs without supervision

harm-reduction strategy strategy meant to reduce the negative consequences of substance use for an individual who is unwilling or unable to completely end his or her use of drugs or alcohol; for example, a counsellor may work with a person who drinks 30 beers a week to try to get them to drink only 15 beers a week

helping professions all helping professionals (other than first responders) who work in the justice, health care, mental health, or social service sectors; for example, social workers, social service workers, counsellors, clergy members, human services workers, child and youth workers, employment counsellors, and others

a high feelings of elation, excitement, and euphoria brought on by intoxication

human rights approach a framework in which respecting a person's rights and his or her value as an individual is the driving principle of care

hypervigilance occurs when an individual shows abnormal levels of awareness and response to stimuli when it is not vital or required; for example, even though at home and not on duty, a soldier may be constantly screening his or her environment for threats

Indian residential schools (IRS) system of federally run boarding schools that was forced upon Indigenous children and operated in Canada into the late 1990s; more than 150,000

children were removed from their families and communities; spiritual, emotional, physical, cultural, and sexual abuse was widely reported to have occurred

individual therapy psychotherapy practised in a one-on-one process between a trained therapist and an individual

institutionalization the practice of confining individuals or groups of people in residential institutions such as asylums, prisons, and mental health hospitals

intoxication state wherein mental and physical control is diminished by the use of alcohol or drugs

justice system all professions related to the administration of the law and the criminal justice system, including police, attorneys, paralegals, court workers, probation officers, and so on

Kids Help Phone Canadian organization established in 1989 initially for children to report abuse and access telephone counselling 24-hours a day; now also provides web counselling and referrals for children and youth

LGBTQI2S+ stands for "lesbian, gay, bisexual, transgender, queer (or questioning), intersex, two-spirited, and other related ways" in which an individual may self-identify

light therapy method of treating seasonal affective disorder (SAD) that uses exposure to artificial light that approximates sunlight; sometimes referred to as phototherapy

literacy one's knowledge about mental health disorders, trends, dynamics, and how to manage or even prevent mental health issues

long-term treatment program (residential) type of program that provides 24-hour care in a non-hospital setting and lasts from 6 to 12 months—the focus is on "re-socialization" of an individual living with addiction and substance abuse issues

maladaptive behaviour behaviour that hinders a person's capacity to adjust to situations in a healthy manner

mania symptom of bipolar disorder that is characterized as a state of persistent and abnormally elevated arousal or mood that can have characteristics of both euphoria and irritability

medication/pharmacological treatments treatment using legal drugs recommended or prescribed by a medical professional

***Mental Health Act* (MHA)** law that regulates the administration of mental health care in Ontario; the main purpose of this law is to regulate the involuntary admission of people into a psychiatric hospital

mental health court specialized court for those who have exhibited criminal behaviour due to mental illness; focuses on treatment and rehabilitation of the individual, rather than punishment

methadone maintenance treatment type of treatment for those who are addicted to the use of opioids such as heroin; often carried out in clinics where methadone consumption is monitored by medical professionals to help users reduce or eliminate the use of opioids

mindfulness-based cognitive therapy (MBCT) form of psychotherapy that combines principles of CBT with education about a major depressive disorder as well as mindfulness training and meditation techniques

minimal encouragers subtle verbal ("uh huh") and non-verbal actions (nods, open and attentive posture) that make speakers feel comfortable and listened to

mission statement brief summary of the goals and values of an organization

mood disorder psychological disorder that is marked by an elevation and/or lowering of a person's mood that interferes with daily functioning

multi-sectoral approach approach to solving systemic problems where collaboration between governments, not-for-profits, non-governmental organizations, communities, and individuals occurs

multidisciplinary team an approach in which professionals from a variety of professions work together with an individual on a topic or a specific set of problems

naloxone a medication that can reverse the effects of opioid overdose

needle exchange programs harm-reduction programs in which individuals can drop off used needles to be safely destroyed and pick up new needles and other drug-related equipment

night terrors episodes of intense fear that occur during a non-REM part of the sleep cycle; may manifest as screaming, flailing, sweating, heavy breathing, or racing pulse while still asleep; night terrors are distinctly different from nightmares

NIMBYism occurs when individuals or groups object to the development of programs within their own neighbourhoods; NIMBY is an acronym of the phrase "Not In My Back Yard"

not criminally responsible (NCR) when the court finds that a person, because of a mental illness, could not appreciate the nature or consequences of his or her actions, or did not know that the actions were wrong at the time of the act, that person is NCR

Office of the Independent Police Review Director (OIPRD) Ontario organization that is responsible for collecting, managing, and overseeing public complaints about police; other provinces use different ministries, commissions, or committees to manage and oversee public complaints about police—British Columbia, for example, uses the Office of the Police Complaint Commissioner

ombudsman organization arms-length organization empowered to investigate complaints, resolve issues, and make recommendations for the betterment of the public and employees with regard to systemic issues in the ways that services are delivered; another word for "ombudsman" is "ombudsperson"

Ontario Civilian Police Commission (OCPC) independent oversight agency created to make sure adequate and effective policing occurs in Ontario within the parameters of the Police Services Act; hears appeals with regard to police disciplinary decisions and investigations about the conduct of officers, police chiefs, and police services board members as well as providing other services

Ontario Court of Justice judges and justices of the peace deliver independent, impartial, and timely justice to thousands of people who come before this court in more than 200 locations across the province; the court deals with approximately 500,000 adult and youth criminal charges, hears millions of provincial offence matters such as traffic tickets, and serves more than 20,000 families

open-ended questions questions that cannot be answered with a yes or no response; fuller and more meaningful answers are encouraged: "how did that make you feel?" is an example

overdose/overdosing accidental or intentional consumption of a substance in excess of safe parameters

overdose prevention sites sites where peer supporters, volunteers, and sometimes medical personnel observe individuals using drugs so that they can intervene to prevent overdoses and initiate intervention when overdoses occur

panic attack sudden onset of disabling anxiety

paraphrasing restating an individual's words in a new way to demonstrate that he or she has been understood

perinatal depression severe depression during or after giving birth that involves extreme sadness, exhaustion, and anxiety; also known as postpartum depression

pre-charge diversion option for police to enter an individual into the mental health system instead of the criminal justice system when certain criteria are met

pre-trial diversion option for the Crown attorney to enter an individual into the mental health system when certain criteria are met instead of proceeding through the court system

predictor piece of data that is used to foretell some aspect of future well-being; for example, if individuals with more education tended to have greater economic opportunities, education would be said to be a good predictor of economic opportunity—this does not mean everyone with an education is well off or that everyone without one is poor, but that trends exist that show one is a good predictor of the other

presenteeism attending work, school, or other responsibilities but with reduced productivity because of mental or physical illness

procedural justice refers to due process, equity, and fairness in policing

protective factors variety of factors that may decrease the risk of someone completing suicide

psychotherapy talk-therapy method used to treat mental disorders

public inquiry process where hearings are conducted and evidence is heard in a public forum about a specific issue of public interest; afterward, a report on the findings is submitted to government and made available to the public

relapse a recurrence of use after a period of abstaining from use

resilience the capacity to quickly recover from difficult situations

rigidity resistance to adaptation and change

risk factors variety of factors that may increase the risk of someone completing suicide

safe injection sites see supervised consumption services

schizoaffective disorder shares the symptoms of schizophrenia as well as mood disorder symptoms such as those seen in depressive disorders

schizophreniform disorder shares the symptoms of schizophrenia for more than one month but less than six months

self-determination a person's ability to determine and control his or her own life; the helping professions promote this concept

self-harming behaviour deliberate harm or risky behaviour that can lead to physical harm of oneself; sometimes called self-injury

self-help a variety of processes that are self-directed to improve health or well-being; methods may include using books, online resources, and peer-run support groups with some basis in psychology

self-medication behaviour in which drugs and/or alcohol are used without the consent or recommendation of a doctor or other professional in order to treat physical or psychological pain; an example of this is when someone drinks alcohol to deal with depression or post-traumatic stress disorder (PTSD) symptoms

self-stigma socialization of individuals with mental illness that leads them to the belief that they are devalued members of society

service delivery the act of providing a service; in the justice and helping professions. This could, for example, be action taken by a policing, security, or mental health service

sexual assault assault of a sexual nature that violates the sexual integrity of the victim

short-term treatment program type of program that provides intense yet brief treatment based on a 12-step approach

silo service providers who work in isolation from one another are said to be working in a silo; working in a silo contributes to a lack of teamwork, collaboration, and information sharing

soft/behavioural/process addictions compulsive behaviours not related to substance use but that are similar in many respects, including dependency and tolerance; for example, gambling

Special Investigations Unit (SIU) civilian oversight agency in Ontario that investigates any incidents involving police and civilians that result in serious injuries, death, or allegations of sexual assault; organizations with similar mandates and powers exist in other parts of the country

stay (a charge) stop or suspend court proceedings either indefinitely or until the occurrence of a condition imposed by the court

substance abuse harmful and excessive use of substances such as alcohol and drugs

substance dependence a tolerance to repeated exposure to or ingestion of a substance; stopping regular usage causes symptoms of withdrawal

substance-induced disorders medical or mental health disorders that are caused directly by the use of substances; an example is substance-induced psychosis

substance-use disorder pattern of substance or alcohol use that is problematic, impairs daily living, and causes distress

suicidal behaviour any action that could reasonably cause one's own intentional death

suicidal ideation suicidal thoughts, be they momentary and transitory, or longer-lasting and detailed

suicidal intent conscious aim or desire to end one's own life

suicide voluntary and intentional act causing the death of oneself

suicide by cop (SBC) suicide method in which an individual deliberately behaves in a threatening manner with intent to provoke a lethal response from a law enforcement officer

suicide plan specific plan a person may have to end his or her life

summarization condensing and clarifying an individual's statements; this is helpful in expressing what has been said as a theme or in helping to draw a conversation or session to a close

Superior Court of Justice this court has jurisdiction over criminal, civil, and family cases, and is the largest superior trial court in Canada; the Divisional Court, Small Claims Court, and Family Court are all branches of the Superior Court of Justice

supervised consumption services sites where illicit substance use is supervised in order to protect the users and the general public from issues related to drug abuse

supported housing an individual lives in the community and has supports such as homecare and counselling when required

supportive housing an individual receives 24-hour assistance within a housing unit

taser a device that uses electricity to temporarily incapacitate an individual; used in place of a more lethal weapon; also known as a conducted energy device (CED)

therapeutic relationship relationship between an individual and a helping professional that aims to create beneficial changes in the life of the client; also sometimes called a therapeutic alliance or a helping alliance

trauma injury to the body or mind

waitlists ordered list of individuals who are waiting for something that is not readily available, such as mental health services or housing

watchdog groups governmental and non-governmental groups that work to inform the public about the actions of organizations; these groups organize to help bring about change

withdrawal often painful set of symptoms that occur when a person stops using a substance that he or she has been using on a regular basis

Workplace Safety and Insurance Board (WSIB) Ontario provincial agency that pays benefits to injured workers from a province-wide mandatory insurance fund

INDEX

CREDITS

Chapter 1

Page 9 (photo): asiseeit/iStock
Page 12 (photo): CP photo
Page 13 (photo): CP photo
Page 18 (text): Dorothy Cotton, Ph.D., C. Psych., Psychologist. *Canadian Police Chief Magazine*, Winter 2014. Reprinted with the permission of the Canadian Association of Chiefs of Police.
Page 19 (photo): juefraphoto/iStock

Chapter 2

Page 33 (text): Forced-treatment orders a growing controversy for mental health advocates, by Sue Bailey, the Canadian Press, February 26, 2016. Reprinted with the permission of The Canadian Press.
Page 44 (text): Man who beheaded Greyhound passenger wins right to live on his own-with daily monitoring, by Steve Lambert, the Canadian Press, February 25, 2016. Reprinted with the permission of The Canadian Press.
Page 48 (Figure 2.2): Reprinted with the permission of the Centre for Addiction and Mental Health.

Chapter 3

Page 55 (photo): CP photo/Tibor Kolley
Page 57 (photo): CP photo/Jeff McIntosh
Page 57 (text): Suicide by Cop: A growing phenomenon, *CBC News*, February 27, 2013. Reprinted with permission.
Page 62 (text): Royal Canadian Mounted Police. (2014, April 3). De-escalation training for police. *Gazette magazine, 76*(1). Reproduced with the permission of the RCMP Gazette.
Page 64 (photo): KatarzynaBialasiewicz/iStock

Chapter 4

Page 77 (photo): Todd Wright/Thinkstock
Page 79 (photo): Creatas/Thinkstock
Page 82 (photo): Marjan_Apostolovic/Thinkstock
Page 85 (photo): ClarkandCompany/Thinkstock
Page 88 (photo): Jupiterimages/Thinkstock
Page 89 (text): © All rights reserved. *A Report on Mental Illnesses in Canada.* Public Health Agency of Canada, 2002. Adapted and reproduced with permission from the Minister of Health, 2017.
Page 91 (photo): Jupiterimages/Thinkstock
Page 92 (photo): KatarzynaBialasiewicz/iStock

Chapter 5

Page 108 (text): Fentanyl Can Kill, by Sean Allen, *Brant News*, March 22, 2017. Reprinted with the permission of Sean Allen.
Page 108 (photo): Reprinted with the permission of Lucas Duguid, Octopus Red.

Page 115 (text): Adapted with permission from The Centre for Addiction and Mental Health (CAMH).

Page 118 (text). Reprinted with permission from The Centre for Addiction and Mental Health (CAMH).

Chapter 6

Page 126 (photo): Peter Badge/Wikipedia

Page 129 (Table 6.1): © All rights reserved. *A Report on Mental Illnesses in Canada.* Public Health Agency of Canada, 2002. Adapted and reproduced with permission from the Minister of Health, 2017.

Page 132 (text): Ashley Smith's sister disappointed by federal solitary confinement bill, by Patrick White, *The Globe and Mail*, June 22, 2017. Reprinted with permission.

Page 138 (text): Sean Clifton's search of forgiveness: Follow-up film tracks notorious Cornwall "NCR" case, by Blair Crawford, November 20, 2016, *Ottawa Citizen*. Reprinted with the permission of Postmedia.

Page 138 (photo): CP photo/Lars Hagberg

Chapter 7

Page 145 (photo): © All rights reserved. *Suicide in Canada.* Public Health Agency of Canada, 2016. Adapted and reproduced with permission from the Minister of Health, 2017.

Page 147 (photo): DGLimages/Thinkstock

Page 148 (text): © All rights reserved. *Working Together to Prevent Suicide in Canada. The Federal Framework for Suicide Prevention.* Public Health Agency of Canada, 2016. Adapted and reproduced with permission from the Minister of Health, 2017.

Page 150: (Table 7.1): Wilson, M.G., & Gauvin, F.P. (2012). Evidence brief: preventing suicide in Canada. Reprinted with the permission of McMaster Health Forum.

Page 152 (Table 7.2): © All rights reserved. *Working Together to Prevent Suicide in Canada. The Federal Framework for Suicide Prevention.* Public Health Agency of Canada, 2016. Adapted and reproduced with permission from the Minister of Health, 2017.

Page 154 (text): Canada's lack of first-responder suicide stats is a national disgrace, by Mack Lamoureaux and Alex McPherson, *Vice News*. Reprinted with the permission of Mack Lamoureaux and Alex McPherson.

Page 158 (text): Juhnke, G. A., Granello, P. F., & Lebrón-Striker, M. A. (2007). IS PATH WARM? A suicide assessment mnemonic for counselors (ACAPCD-03). *Alexandria, VA: American Counseling Association*. Reprinted with permission.

Page 160 (text): Preventing Suicide: a resource for police, firefighters and other first line responders. © WHO 1999. Reprinted with permission.

Chapter 8

Page 172 (photo): bowdenimages/ Thinkstock

Page 177 (photo): MivPiv/iStock

Chapter 9

Page 183 (Table 9.1): Coleman, T., & Cotton, D. (2014). Tempo: Police interactions: A report towards improving interactions between police and people living with mental health problems. Ottawa and Calgary: Mental Health Commission of Canada. Reprinted with permission.

Page 186 (text): Study Shows Mentally Ill More Likely to Be Victims, Not Perpetrators, of Violence, by Matt Shipman, *NC State News*. Reprinted with the permission of NC State University.

Page 188 (photo): Stéphane Groleau / Alamy Stock photo

Page 189 (text): Ministry of the Attorney General. @ Queen's Printer for Ontario. Reprinted with permission.

Page 191 (photo): DigitalVision/Thinkstock

Chapter 10

Page 204 (photo): Alamy Stock photo

Page 209 (Figure 10.1): Power and Control, Women's UN Report Network, 2016.

Page 210 (Figure 10.2): Reprinted with the permission of Therapist Aid LLC.

Page 212 (text): Honour killings in Canada: even worse than we believe, by Gerald Caplan, *The Globe and Mail*, July 23, 2010. Reprinted with the permission Gerald Caplan.

Page 216 (Figure 10.3): © All rights reserved. *Canadian Incidence Study of Reported Child Abuse and Neglect*. Public Health Agency of Canada, 2010. Adapted and reproduced with permission from the Minister of Health, 2017.

Page 217 (text): Department of Justice Canada. (2016). The Criminal Law and Managing Children's Behaviour. Reprinted with permission.

Page 223 (photo): Jonny White / Alamy Stock photo

Page 227 (text): Residential school syndrome, by Charles Bradfield, *BC Medical Journal, 43*(2), March 2001. Reprinted with permission.

Chapter 11

Page 239 (text): Adapted with permission from The Canadian Centre on Substance Abuse by the Canadian Liver Foundation's Non-Prescription Needle Use Initiative.

Page 243 (text): B.C.'s second low-barrier supervised-injection site, Safe Point, opens this week in Surrey, by Travis Lupick, *The Georgia Straight*, June 6, 2017. Reprinted with permission.

Page 251 (photo): CP photo/David Smith

Page 253 (photo): Reprinted with the permission of Howard Sapers.

Chapter 12

Page 260 (Figure 12.1): Ace, W., & Parker, S. (2010). Overcoming Change Fatigue Through Focused Employee Engagement. *Od Practitioner*, *42*(1), 22. Reprinted with permission.

Page 264 (text): More police officers carry guns in BC than in England and Wales combined, by Lori Culbert, March 30, 2015, *The Vancouver Sun*. Reprinted with the permission of Postmedia.

Page 265 (photo): Photo by Stephen Thorne. Reprinted with the permission of Pat Stogran.

Page 265 (photo): Reprinted with the permission of Natalie Harris.

Page 270 (text): New outpatient program puts trauma help for first responders front and centre, by Natalie Nanowski, October 24, 2016, *CBC News*. Reprinted with permission.

Page 274 (text): American Psychological Association. (2017). The road to resilience. Reprinted with permission.